MW01077797

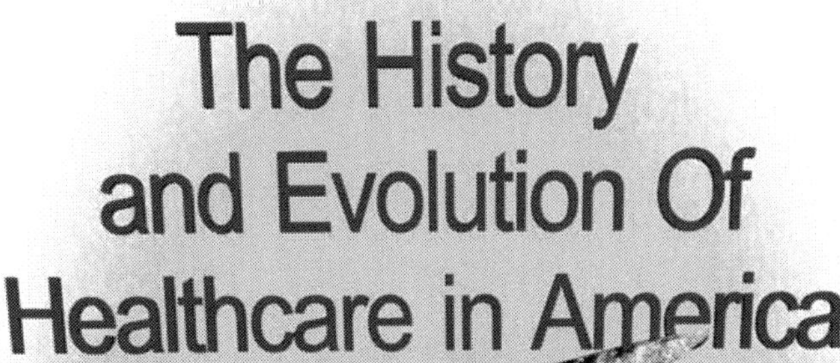

The History and Evolution Of Healthcare in America

The Untold Backstory of Where We've Been, Where We Are And Why Healthcare Needs More Reform

Thomas W. Loker

iUniverse, Inc.
Bloomington

The History and Evolution of Healthcare in America
The Untold Backstory of Where We've Been, Where We Are, and Why Healthcare Needs Reform

iUniverse books may be ordered through booksellers or by contacting:

iUniverse
1663 Liberty Drive
Bloomington, IN 47403
www.iuniverse.com
1-800-Authors (1-800-288-4677)

ISBN: 978-1-4759-0073-6 (sc)
ISBN: 978-1-4759-0075-0 (e)
ISBN: 978-1-4759-0074-3 (dj)

Library of Congress Control Number: 2012906094

Printed in the United States of America

iUniverse rev. date: 4/11/2012

Advance Praise for the History and Evolution of Healthcare in America

In Tom Loker's latest book, "The History and Evolution of Healthcare in America," his many years as Chief Operating Officer for Ramsell Holding Corporation, a company comprised of four healthcare business entities that coordinate the management and care of healthcare benefits and related services for the underserved, helps him both understand and explain how we have arrived at the ineffective and unsustainable system we have today.

As a champion for those most in need of healthcare and related services, Loker has traveled to Washington, D.C. extensively meeting with legislators helping them understand private-sector solutions to the daunting task at hand, fixing a system that is great in delivering services, but financially unsustainable.

Mr. Loker explains with wit, in his introductory remarks in, "From the Mayflower to Medical Mayhem" that democrats, in their hastiness, may have over-reached in order to deliver Obamacare. Tom Loker's understanding and guidance should certainly be requested as a more effective system accomplishing the same goals but at far less expense replaces the current law. This book is, a must read, for anyone interested in healthcare, frustrated with the current system, or who would like to learn more about America. Heck, it should be a required read for anyone in Congress or in our state legislatures!

–Jim Campbell, Staff Writer, The National Examiner

Tom Loker's keen insight and skill applying the history and evolution of American healthcare today is an apt and readable primer for Obamacare and beyond.

–Don Perata, President Pro Tempore, California Senate Emeritus

In The History and Evolution of Healthcare in America, Thomas Loker provides a comprehensive overview of Obamacare, putting it in lively historical perspective, and shedding light on its inadequacies and false hopes. From his considerable real-life experience in business and healthcare, he explores ideas for more coordinated, workable approaches.

–Ellen Brown J.D., Author

Loker puts healthcare and healthcare reform in historical context, while challenging the orthodoxies of both left and right. This out-of-the-box analysis provides unique insights and a new way of thinking about healthcare that should inform future public policy debates."

-Daniel M. Crane is a Washington and Sacramento-based government relations consultant and former Legislative Director to the late Senator Daniel Patrick Moynihan (D-NY).

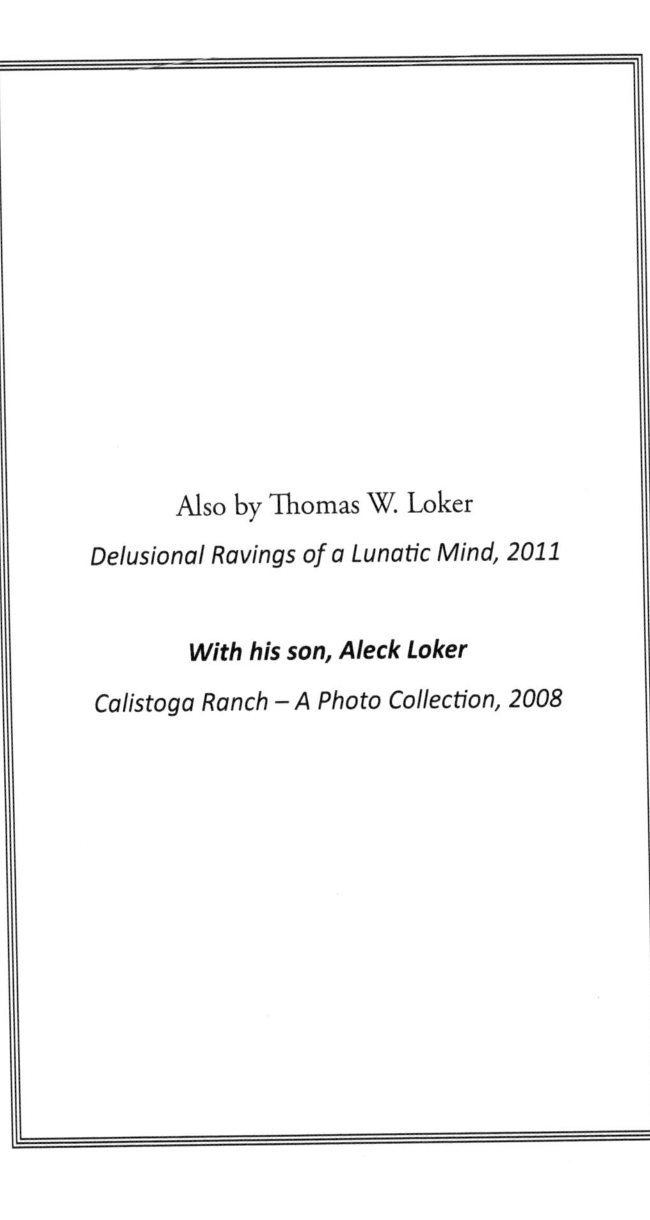

Also by Thomas W. Loker

Delusional Ravings of a Lunatic Mind, 2011

With his son, Aleck Loker

Calistoga Ranch – A Photo Collection, 2008

THE HISTORY AND EVOLUTION OF HEALTHCARE IN AMERICA

The Untold Backstory of Where We've Been,

Where We Are, and Why Healthcare Needs More Reform

Thomas W. Loker

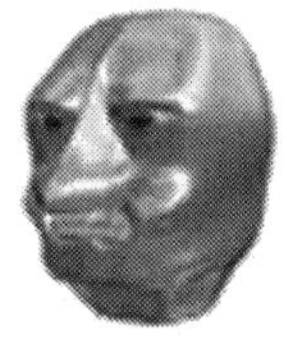

SYDK Press

California

2012

This book is dedicated to my wife, Teresa, who always graciously allows me the time to focus, think, and create. To my son Aleck who tolerantly gives me extended periods of peace and quiet even though he would prefer to be playing with his dad. To my son Tom who showed tremendous character when his brother Justin was born and throughout his life. And, to my son Justin who has experienced first-hand the benefits and detriments of our current healthcare system, my passion for these issues comes from you all.

I also dedicate this book to those that have encouraged me to take action and get involved in Washington, DC: Michael Shiffman, Don Perata, Jerry Crank, Dan Crane, Lucie Gikovich, Steven Churchwell, Tim Howell, Jordanna Burgo, and Sophia Byndloss. Additional thanks go to my editor, who took my words and made them speak much clearer. I heartedly express my many thanks to those of you who read all my rough drafts and were kind enough to give me your comments. Your guidance and suggestions unquestionably helped me improve the book. To all the people I met on Capitol Hill who anonymously struggle every day trying to make a real difference. You may not be many in number— but you are large in spirit! Specifically, To Britt Weinstock *(senior health policy advisor in the Office of Congresswoman Donna M. Christensen)* and Connie Garner, *(Policy Director for Disability and Special Populations for Massachusetts Senator Edward M. Kennedy)* who shared your frustrations and aspirations and helped lead me to understand my own convictions. A special thanks to Governor Jerry Brown who helped me make my first solid contacts in Washington, D.C. and always has been a strong advocate for the underserved.

Finally, to my family, who throughout these years continue to communicate the stories and lessons from our past, and build a strong interest in understanding who, and what, went before, and how not only the times were different, but people and their expectations were different, as well. All important to understanding why we have the healthcare system we do today.

Contents

It is thus compromise on the basis of tolerance for others' opinions that lead us to good solutions . . .

—Benjamin Franklin

Introduction: From the *Mayflower* to Medical Mayhem

It is March 23, 2010, and the East Room of the White House is swarming with people. Members of the congressional leadership, White House aides, and Democratic supporters all chat nervously as they await the arrival of the President. The enormous media contingent, with its omnipresent TV cameras and crews, nearly outnumber the participants awaiting this historic moment. The mood is electric, charged by the sheer symbolism, ceremony, and sweeping importance of the event they are about to witness.

Into this tumult, walks, rather almost glides, the 44th President of the United States, Barack Obama. His effect on the crowd is like oil cast on water; the waves of movement subside; the crowd grows silent. Into the deafening stillness, thirty-three words from the President ring out:

> *"Today, after almost a century of trying; today, after over a year of debate; today, after all the votes have been tallied—health insurance reform becomes law in the United States of America—Today."*

With the strokes of twenty-two separate pens (presented as gifts to invited guests), President Obama signs into law the Patient Protection and Affordable Care Act, otherwise known as healthcare reform, or Obamacare. The ceremony, repeatedly interrupted by cheers, applause, and standing ovations, marks one of the singular achievements of the Obama presidency.

Despite the visible excitement, in the East Room on this day few of the people responsible for crafting the new healthcare reform law actually like the end-result. Too many deals were struck, and too many compromises were made in order to reach this day. No one can say for sure how many people will be helped by the law, whether the law will actually save the government money, or how high some health insurance premiums will rise in order to cover mandated lowered rates for others.

Conservative Republicans think the bill goes too far, and they doubt its constitutional legitimacy. Liberal Democrats think the bill does not go far enough and that too many concessions were made to insurance and pharmaceutical companies. Following the passage of one of the most divisive, costly, and contentious pieces of healthcare legislation in the entire history of the U.S., even the many groups that supported the legislation have misgivings about its efficacy. The East Room ceremony had barely ended when almost immediately everyone with a stake in healthcare reform began to try and fix what they saw as the flaws in the new law. These debates continue today, as many of the final rules required by the law are now in the hands of numerous governmental committees, commissions, and departments, while other provisions of the law are being contested in the courts.

The purpose of this book is to take you, the reader, on a journey through the history of American healthcare, so you can see where we have been, understand how we arrived where we are today, and determine where we might need to go tomorrow. The book will show how various evolutionary changes in the practice of medicine have led to the high costs and inefficiencies that continue to defy resolution in the new healthcare reform law. The history also illustrates how parts of the problem have been solved in the past and helps us understand what might be necessary to solve our remaining problems in the future.

The chief problem with the current healthcare delivery system in America is that it is neither integrated, nor practical, nor functional. It has mutated in its form over decades with hit-and-miss solutions that tend to put the interests of industry players ahead of the interests of their patients. Having grown weed-like in an unbounded field the system is a tangled mess that defies comprehension. The result is such wasteful consumption of resources that, in the U.S., we think that we pay more for our healthcare system than any other advanced nation. We think we get poorer results despite our massive expenditures. But, do we?

My personal journeys to understand this system and its problems began a number of years ago when I became Chief Operating Officer of a company that contracted, with state governments, to deliver medical treatment to under-served populations. In my role, I observed just how difficult it is to decide who is really underserved, how difficult it can be to address the needs of this vulnerable population, the kinds of challenges the existing system creates for its participants, and how easy it is for many to game the system. I have observed first-hand how the current system fosters the waste of almost two-thirds of the moneys spent on healthcare in duplicated procedures, defensive/unnecessary services, and purposeful fraud and abuse. Along the way, I learned a few things about what we can do, simply, to vastly improve how we define healthcare, how we deliver quality care, and how we can spread the burden of serving the needs of the underserved across the widest base to make it affordable, efficient, and effective. At the end point of this process, we should be able to reduce by at least one-half the waste of funds lost in the current system, improve by two-thirds the access to quality care, and redefine the healthcare supply chain and better allocate the provision of care services to the most appropriate providers in the chain.

Over the years, it became increasingly clear to me that providing an effective healthcare safety net depends on much more than any government can or will provide. I learned that we asking the government for too much while taking on too little of the responsibility amongst ourselves. We underestimate the ability of our society to do good, and then supplant this fear with clumsy government regulations and mandates. Finally, we avoid remedying the real issues in healthcare by deferring to the expertise of its major interest groups, allowing them to descend into "us vs. them" infighting that serves no one. All of these problems have persisted so long that I've come to believe we are running out of time and money. If we don't agree soon to identify and address these difficult issues systemically, with a thoughtful retooling of the system (and not a series of legislative patches), our country could collapse under a mountain of debt and divisiveness.

From my work in the healthcare field, I also came to the realization that in order to understand where we are, we must understand from where we have come. It may be difficult for some to believe, but the quality of routine care we expect today is a very recent development. From the settlement of the first colonies in the New World up until the early 1950s, nearly all of what we see today in healthcare simply did not exist. Life itself was tenuous for most citizens throughout our history, and in the early days of this country life expectancies were less than half of those today. Medicinal interventions, if they existed at all, were often more deadly than the disease they purported to treat. Surgeries, prior to 1846, were done without anesthesia in a quick and brutal fashion that ended in fatality more often than not. Nearly all the wonder drugs and antibiotics we rely on today are inventions of the past half-century.

At the beginning of each chapter of this book, I've included a fictional vignette to try to bring to life the particular medical concerns that were prevalent during that chapter's corresponding time period. The central characters in these stories are people who really existed, drawn from my own family history. Their stories to varying degrees represent amalgamations of accurate historical information, in some cases; I have augmented the stories and altered specific dates and events in order to more vividly represent certain historical periods. I hope these sections will help introduce you to the chapter's time period and provide you a relevant framework to understand what the people of the era felt and experienced. Writing these sections was very difficult but also very rewarding. My fondest wish is that they provide you with an enjoyable perspective on how different our ancestors' outlook on healthcare was from our own modern view.

The practice of healthcare, after all, is largely a war with other species (bacteria, viruses, and other complex pathogens), a war with our environment (accidents, violence, and pollution), and also a war with ourselves (diet, exercise, work habits, and sleep). From time to time, we can see gains for ourselves in these battles, but our mortality assures us that we will all eventually lose the war. Basic biology and the laws of nature have stacked the deck against us. Innovations in technology, science, and medication have helped many of us delay the day of our ultimate surrender, but these advances have also fostered the false belief that no price is too high to pay for an extra day or week of life.

This sort of thinking, I hope to show, has effectively put all of us at greater risk by encouraging the allocation of too many resources in medical areas where doctors can achieve only minimal incremental gains in health and quality of life. Every expensive, exciting new medical treatment has a way of distracting us from making sure that sound, and basic, healthcare is fully available to more people. As Pablo Picasso once said, "Every positive value has its price in negative terms. The genius of Einstein leads to Hiroshima."

Following the historical chapters that make up the bulk of this book, I conclude by offering a series of proposed changes to Obamacare that I believe are both significant and achievable. In the end, such changes will lend themselves to a series of simple steps that we can effectively implement both legislatively and in our own lives in different ways. I believe you will discover that there is an effective and appropriate role for government, an appropriate role for healthcare professionals, for non-profits, for corporations, for religious organizations, for us as potential recipients, and most importantly, for every American striving to achieve the closest thing to an ideal healthcare package we can attain.

Once you have finished reading, I hope you will have gained a fresh perspective on the issues that we face. Writing this book was my own journey of discovery; an attempt to help us all define the fundamental questions, find some answers and identify the right path and the right priorities. For that to happen, I believe we need to look beyond the rhetoric, reset our expectations, and accept that while we all want some ideal form of universal healthcare, what we can actually obtain cannot—and never will—be ideal. I believe instead that we should follow the words of Ben Franklin who said, ". . . it is thus compromise on the basis of tolerance for others' opinions that lead us to good solutions . . ."

I. (1492 – 1776)
Health and the New World

Imagine . . .

It is the early evening of November 1, 1633. A cool, dark, fog envelops you in a disquieting silent shroud as you make your way down the dark cobblestone streets of Gravesend in northwest Kent. The night airs settle around you as oil lamps and candles cast faint, flickering light through the salt glass windows. From a short distance, you can hear the soft roar of England's mighty river Thames. Sticking to the shadows, you search for a tavern called, "The Gravedigger's Refuge."

The soles of your hobnail boots click and clack as you creep down the dark streets. Your broadcloth shirt is damp, and the chill seeping into your bones is unbearable. You don't feel well. The shivers grip you, and they are not just from the cold. You pray this is not the first sign of consumption, dropsy, or the dreaded cholera that held your homeland in its grip when you fled.

As you made your way across Europe through Flanders to England, you left each and every town just as disease and pestilence took hold of them, devastating the populations. The plague or fever seemed to follow you. Each time you found a home in a town and commenced to develop some skill, disease began to rip the town apart, along with your hope to learn a trade and make a living. So you fled west—always farther west.

At last you see a tilted tombstone slung above a doorway, the sign of The Gravedigger's Refuge. A wave of weariness and hunger nearly overcomes you as you push open the door. You worry that your poor command of English and your Flemish accent will betray you. You feel close to salvation, and fulfillment of your simple wish for escape to the New World. But, at this very moment your most pressing need is for a warm hearth, a few morsels of food, and a place to rest.

"Eay Yo" calls the portly man behind the bar, "what's yer pleasure be?" His waistcoat is bursting at its seams, and the few remaining hairs on his head are askew. There is a dangerous air to this man, as well. On your guard, you respond, "A simple draught and some palaver 'el do." As you sit to make your drink, you inquire as to how a man can find some "bed for the night and fair and safe work for

the future." "S' yer trade mate?" asks the barman. You say but one word, "carpenter."

The barkeep fixes his gaze on you and slowly moves from behind the bar. The code word "carpenter" has worked. The man pulls up a stool and leans forward, which causes you to recoil. His breath emits a foul stench, for sure, but it also makes you nervous, for you have heard that vapors cause disease.

"So," he begins. "You's a papist?" You nod solemnly, though it is a lie. "I wouldn't have reckoned that from yer accent," he says, "but then again, I ain't been far."

He pauses to look over your shoulder before continuing. "I knows ya needs fast and complete passage, and yer lucks good, mate. There's two ships leaving tomorrow morning. You reports to the Master of the ones called The Dove. Tells him yer name is Thomas Loker. Tells him, you's good with maul, trunnel, and caulk and he will be sure to take you as carpenter's mate."

You ask about the cost, and the man replies, "Yer bed and yer drink is six pence apiece, but the palaver is eight shilling. And mind you, you'll need give me another eight for the Master if'n you expect to get the job." You are startled by the expense, but you dig in your purse and pay out sixteen shillings twelve pence.

"That's all there is," he says, grinning from the feel of coins in his hands. "Get there early, as I ain't the only bookie in Gravesend." You mount the stairs to your bed, only to find that your bed-mate is a frail man with a hacking cough. There is more comfort to be found on the floor, and you make your bed there for the night.

As you drift off to sleep, you wonder why the barkeep assumed you were a Catholic. You have been accused of many things as you made your way from your homeland over the past year. You've been called a bagger, bumbler, bounder, and stranger, but never a religious. Certainly you're no carpenter, either! But, if you need to be a Catholic to make this voyage, then a Catholic you'll be!

You wake at dawn the next morning and make your way down to the docks on the south bank of the river. Two ships stand ready for sailing. One is a giant vessel of 400 tonnes or more, while the other seems too tiny for oceangoing, no more than 50 tonnes. You find the Master, and, as instructed, you tell him your name is Thomas Loker and that you're good with maul and other carpenter's tools. He assigns you to the Dove, the smaller of the two ships, but first, he insists that you make the oath to Lord Baltimore and the Crown. You pledge to do your best to make passage and to stay true to the Catholic faith. You learn the terms of your passage. You promise 10 years carpenter's service in the new land, and you will be granted a parcel of land and earned status as a freeman. What luck! All you seek is simple passage out of Europe and its disease, famine, and pestilence. Now you will have both a trade and soil of your own in the new world of freedom called Mary's Land.

Within a few hours of leaving England on November 2, 1633, you find out that the papists are leaving to avoid arrest and persecution because of their Catholic faith. By the second day, the Dove is caught up in a pounding storm and, while the larger 400-tonne Ark is barely making way, your boat, the Dove, is foundering badly. The ship is taking water, and you are deathly sick, as is most of the motley crew. You have forgotten all about the luck of this venture, your oath to Lord Baltimore and the King. Now all you want is to be back on dry land. Taking on any of the diseases you are fleeing would seem a welcome relief to how you feel now. Even an English jail would serve a man better than this sickly, bouncing, and leaking coffin. Finding some shelter back at the Isle of Wight, your Captain anchors the ship in the sheltering bay, keeping all hands on the ship and away from shore. After a few days respite, you are back at the rolling sea.

After a few weeks, most have their sea legs; but other problems rear their ugly heads. Your bunk mate catches his thumb in the mizzen sheet and skin and nail are torn from the end. Having no ships surgeon, treatment of the injury is left to the captain. A plaster of roots and white powder is applied—yet the next day he complains of the pain. The Captain orders an additional draught of rum to help. The infection worsens. While your larger sister ship, the Ark, is nowhere in sight, you do come upon another ship, the Dragon, a large well-armed merchant vessel, and you sail in trail to her during the dangerous passage. In the next week, consumption shows itself in some of the crew. Again, the Captain provides his medicinal ministrations. The first unfortunate crew members pass within two weeks. The captain remarks at one of the buggers' good luck, "Aye, with a surgeon on board treating him instead of me, he would have only lasted a few days. You know I read this philosopher, Francis Bacon, who said, 'The remedy is worse'n the disease!'"

Always feeling ill, you pray to God that you don't get sick, because you know that the Captain is correct. More people are dying from the treatments than from the illnesses or injuries themselves. You are left to wonder—if they had just left some of these poor, sick people alone instead of giving them these awful tasting remedies, would they still be alive today?

Within a day of the discovery of the crewmen with the consumption, your bunk mate's thumb is still not healed and begins to smell bad. He is suffering from fever. With a healthy dose of rum for both the Captain and the patient, the Captain takes a meat knife in hand from the cook and quickly hacks off the man's thumb at the base. Once again, he provides a poultice to stem infection; he pours rum down the amputee's throat for the pain. Later, as you lay next to him in sleep you still hear the echo of his screams; yet there is something else about this difficult voyage you will never forget. The fever never breaks; your bunk mate dies within days. His corpse, with its skin mottled from infection, is cast over the side.

Over the next few weeks, others succumb to consumption, fever, and other mysterious diseases. Everyone is worried about the pox or plague, but none shows its lethal countenance. The ship's stores were packed well, not just in barrels, but in the new-fangled lead cans. While the meat packed this way has a bit of distaste, it is much better than the daily salted meat and fish. Even though the ship has no surgeon, the Captain has some patent remedies. They include cinchona bark (quinine), "Anderson's Scotts Pills," "Daffy's Elixir" and "Lockyear's Pills." He also has a book of recipes showing how to mix other curatives with the new drugs—quicksilver (mercury), strychnine, and arsenic.

If asked, the captain proudly tells all who will listen that, with these wonders, he can cure; "The Stone" in babes and children, Convulsion fits, Consumption and Bad Digestives, Agues, Piles, Surfeits, Fits of the Mother and Vapors from the Spleen, Green Sickness, Children's Distempers, whether the Worms, Rickets, Stones, Convulsions, Gripes, King's Evil, Joint Evil, or any other disorder proceeding from Wind or Crudities, Gout and Rheumatism, Stone or Gravel in the Kidneys, Colic and Griping of the Bowels, the Phthisic both as cure and preventative provided always that the patient be moderate in drinking, have a care to prevent taking cold, and keep a good diet, Dropsy, and Scurvy. It seems the captain believes no surgeon or physician is needed on board as he can fix anything with these cures. So far they ain't worked. Just like back home, people are still dying from injury and disease.

In January 1634, you make Barbados and find your larger sister ship, the Ark, getting ready to depart. After only a day or so to resupply, you are again off to the New World. Just like on the Dove, many on the Ark are also sick with fever and injury. While you didn't know "doodly squat" about carpentry when you left Gravesend, you have learnt to keep at it till it stops leaking . . . You learned that if 'n you just keep working hard somehow it'll all come together.

On March 3, 1634, you make your way from the Atlantic Ocean into a large, rough, but beautiful, bay called Chesapeake. On March 25th you make land at St. Clements Island. The papists, of whom you are now one, make a mass to thank the Almighty for his good graces and your safe arrival. Two days later, you catch your first glimpse of the land that is now to be your new home.

Pulling up the St. Mary's River early in the morning, you see two fingers of land that come to an opening on the bay. On deck, the air is cool and heavy. All sounds muted—the eerie quiet wraps you just like that evening in Gravesend when you found the barkeeper and began this journey. Large trees stand on either side of the river. You welcome them as good shelter from the storm. The land ahead gently slopes to a sandy beach in the north of the inlet, forming a marsh where the fingers join. The creaking in the rigging almost drowns out the moans of the sick below. Muskrat, mink, and otter are abundant on shore. Deer, duck, swan, goose, and many other fowl are everywhere. The days are warm and nights cool. This land looks perfect, except for the dampness of the air and the bugs that appear everywhere, and bite you.

You are thankful for your final arrival—and none too soon either. As for the godforsaken Dove, it is full of shipworms and leaking mightily. Despite all your effort, to you your repairs are all too obviously ill-fitting and improper. As you disembark from what has become your ship, now moored in the St. Mary's River right next to the Ark, and go ashore; the remoteness and isolation of this new place, like the damp morning air, begins to settle on you. You know that Indians are about because at night you have seen their torches and fires, but so far no contact has been made. You know that the Potomacs are fierce warriors and that the Susquehannocks and other nations are equally as fierce. Not ten years ago, the venerable Captain John Smith in the Virginia colony had much of his detachment murdered by the Powhattan Confederacy of the Algonquins.

Arriving at the shore of this small bay, at the joint of the fingers with a gradually slopping sandy beach in front of a stand of tall trees, you realize that everything you will need to survive will have to be made. And, that you, along with the only other carpenter, who sailed on the Ark, will need to hew by hand all the building boards and fashion stools, benches, tables, chairs, bowls; carve treenails, spoons, and all manner of implements. Farm tools like hoes and axes will need new handles. Carts will need new wheels. Homes will be built and then rebuilt due to rot, storm damage, and from fires started by the rendered fat oil lamps and fireplaces. Each house will need a kitchen—located away from the main structure to help protect the house from fire. And, here you have no idea how to do most of this. As you sit on the beach and watch others disembark, you see dozens come off with fever, scurvy, and mental prostrations. Some no longer seem right in the head. This adventure has been a trial from the beginning, and here you sit: no house, not much in supplies, few soldiers to protect you, and many people counting on you, and a few others, to form a new colony in order to survive.

You spent nineteen years fleeing disease and pestilence across Europe only to arrive in this land with even more sickness at your heels. Over one-third of your ship's company and that on the Ark as well, has perished on the trip. Over one-half of the settlers that have arrived are sick with one malady or another. The treatments, salves, patent medicines, and mixtures brought from England have shown no benefit during the voyage. The papists are buoyed that their prayer to God will bring Providence, but with your own faith not yet formed, you feel it will be the hands of Man that brings the cures. Still you feel at last you have a chance, a hope that you can finally build a life and make a family. Yet your stomach aches, your back spasms; still you don't feel well.

Little do you know that your small, ill-prepared, sick collection of Catholics fleeing the persecution of the Protestants in England will not only survive but found a new community that they will call Maryland. You have no idea that, in only a few hundred years, your descendants will thrive in this small town. That, the area in which you sit, will become, 300 years later, the campus of St. Mary's College of Maryland on the very land that was once part of your original grant. No, today you rightly focus on the tenuousness of your life and the fact that Indians, disease, fire, crop failure, or failure of resupply by subsequent trips from Lord Baltimore's company could spell the death of you and all with you. For you, and all the others, the daily struggle for survival is a simple fact of life and it will largely remain such until the birth of your great, great, great, grandson in 1872. Not many will feel well, most of the time.

Disease and Conquest

The history of the New World is a history shaped by violence, illness, and contagion. Within ten years of Columbus's first voyage in 1492, England, France, and Spain had all laid competing claims to what would someday become the United States. These were the disputes that could only be extinguished by colonial settlement of territories in question, which guaranteed that the price for acquiring these new lands would be paid, not just in treasure but in human lives.

Early settlers in America faced numerous disease and injury-related maladies from the day, they set sail from Europe. Those who went to sea were generally poor in health to begin with, and the fundamental lack of knowledge about basic sanitation, germ epidemiology, and control of infectious diseases caused many to die during the Atlantic crossings, and many more to perish once they reached the relative safety of land.

The French and Spanish feuded over Florida in the 1500s, with repeated attempts at colonization by the Spanish failing before the founding of St. Augustine in 1565. The first English attempt at a permanent North American settlement was made in 1587 on Roanoke Island in what is now North Carolina. By 1590, it had vanished without a trace.

In 1607, a new colony was established in Jamestown, Virginia, through the ambitious effort of the London Company (later renamed the Virginia Company). The settlers left England on three ships with a company and crew of 143 men and boys, only 103 of which made it to Virginia alive. No women were permitted on the first trip, due to the dangers of sea travel.

Not long after the founding of Jamestown, it became apparent why the local Native Americans did not occupy the site. Jamestown Island was in a low, marshy area, infested with mosquitoes, and other airborne pests. The brackish water of the tidal James River was not a good source of drinking water. The area was also isolated from the preferred foraging areas of big game like bears and deer.

A staggering 80 percent of the Jamestown's settlers perished during the first two years. Malaria spread by mosquitoes killed over 135 settlers in the first year alone. Drinking unfiltered seawater killed more. Outside supplies came infrequently due to an ongoing war with Spain, and all the small game in the area was hunted down and killed off, leaving the settlement with a severe food shortage.

Effective medical treatment within early settlements was non-existent. There was no way reliably to repair a broken limb. There was no effective medicine to salve an open wound, and no medicine to ward off other ailments, such as gout. They had no understanding of the cause of disease, nor did they understand the need for basic sanitation. Furthermore, either most available medicines were composed of completely ineffective agents or, even worse, they often included toxic chemicals, such as mercury, antimony, and other compounds. The death rate for indentured settlers was overwhelming for the Virginia Company. As many as 30 percent of the passengers would fall ill and perish due to disease and the stresses of travel. Additionally, 50 percent of those that arrived were doomed to an early demise within the first years of service.

It is no wonder that, faced with the potential devastating impact of disease and death that awaited them in a new world with few, or no, physicians, early settlers were noted for their determined self-reliance. Many surely focused their attention not just on sustenance and shelter but also on health and well-being for themselves and family. It is little wonder that the self-dosed magical elixirs—the "patent medicines" from their homeland—were a strong staple of the colonial medicine kit.

Like the Virginians, the Pilgrims made their way to the New World on a voyage marked by disease and death. Composed of 102 English separatists and sixty-six crewmen, the *Mayflower* expedition left England September 6, 1620 and landed sixty-six days later on November 11, 1620.

During the first winter in the New World, the *Mayflower* colonists suffered greatly from diseases like scurvy, exposure due to lack of shelter, and heinous conditions onboard ship—forty-five of the 102 immigrants died the first winter and were buried on Cole's Hill. Over one-half of the ship's crew died during the first winter, as well. Of the eighteen adult women, thirteen died the first winter. Additional deaths during that same year meant that only fifty-three settlers were alive in November 1621 to celebrate the harvest feast, the one that modern Americans know as "The First Thanksgiving." Only four adult women were left to celebrate Thanksgiving. Despite these problems, and through continued immigration of indentured settlers, by 1643, the European population of the area had miraculously grown to approximately 2,000.

Early settlers in Maryland experienced very similar problems. During the voyage from England, many suffered from saltwater poisoning which often led to infection, fevers, and dysentery. Upon arrival, and as a result of the harsh conditions, most of these early settlers died of disease and starvation.

Much of this early migration to America was driven by the yearning for freedom and a new life because life in the Old World was not much better. European cities had grown substantially since the Middle-Ages and had become squalid and crime-ridden. The average life expectancy was in the early thirties due to epidemics of small pox, chilblain, pneumonia, scarlet fever, rickets, cholera, diphtheria, dropsy, dysentery, influenza, and plague. Lives were also shortened by poor nutrition food poisoning, infection, and violence. Many who were lucky enough to survive these afflictions suffered from mental illnesses. The common diet was deficient in iodine and vitamins C and D. Rye bread was often contaminated with ergot fungi, which could bring on hallucinations, convulsions, and even death. Lead and mercury poisoning, both of which led to neurological disorders, was widespread because mercury was in many popular medicines while food cans and eating utensils often contained lead. Little importance was placed on keeping sewage and animal waste out of the drinking supply, and alcohol was not only a regular part of daily food consumption, it was also a main ingredient in most medicinal preparations.

Those of means and property in London, Paris, and other cities could afford some shelter from the afflictions of the day. Their diet was better, and they generally had better access to fresh air and clean water. For the poor, the risk of the journey to the New World far outweighed the risk of their current circumstance in Europe. As a result, most of the people who took the deal were riddled with addictions, disease, and years of dietary imbalances. These issues, even before the willing and eager departed for America, left many of them mentally unstable and often quite ill upon arrival. Having hailed from such unhealthy surroundings many of the first settlers in the New World were poor candidates for survival.

For several centuries after Columbus and well into the late 1700s, some 15 to 20 percent of those who chanced a voyage to the New World, either succumbed to illness during the crossing or perished within the first two years of arrival. The settlers continued to come, nonetheless. By 1776, the population of Philadelphia climbed beyond 40,000, most of them European working class immigrants and indentured servants. City fathers of the era regarded Philadelphia as "a melting pot for diseases, where Europeans, Africans, and Indians engaged in the free exchange of their respective infections."

II. (1777 – 1849)
Hospitals & Physicians
Never the Twain Shall Meet

Imagine . . .

Boston, June 21, 1816
Mistress Rebecca Loker Smoot
Bards Fields
St. Mary's, Maryland

My Dearest Mother,

It has now been 1 year since our loving father has passed to the great beyond, and the anniversary of his passing reminds me how fine a father he was. He instilled in all of us such a love of God and respect for man's better nature that all of us, Robert, Elizabeth, and myself, have continued to see the better of the world as time has passed.

I trust that your recent ordeal at the hands of the foul British during the war has not left you bereft of your soul. I am sure the same fiery spirit you possessed in protecting our land and livestock with your broom, the same that caused your arrest, was not quenched in the hold of that British frigate. Now that, General Andrew Jackson has once again driven the bounders from our shores, perhaps like General Washington he will soon take leadership of our country.

This city of Boston is so chocked full of the widest breadth of human immigrant. The air is difficult to breathe, and the water smells so foul. No matter where you look there are people. Rich man, poor man, beggar man, thief, and multiplied by the thousands, crowded along the Charles River. The simple pleasure of a clear drink from the stream behind our home has been replaced by a game of chance as to what color, taste, or smell I can expect from a simple draught, from any source. I feel as though I have not only left the peace and Catholic faith of our father's land, but that I have lost a part of my health and safety, as well.

I am finding Harvard College is a fine place for the study of modern medicine. It is truly an amazing collection of the most dedicated science and the most liberal philosophy. I am learning all the medical arts of bleeding and of balancing the 4 Humors with compounds of mercury, antimony, arsenic, strychnine, and others. The mysteries of disease are revealed to us, such as the source of the plague, which we now know arises from spontaneous generation within the body's various closed systems.

As Physicians, we are training this month at setting broken limbs, which takes great practice to perfect. As long as the bone is not too badly splintered, and the skin is not pierced by bone, we are able to achieve quite good results. However, proper setting requires us to squeeze and manipulate the injured limb in order to locate the fracture and determine the proper type of splint. These manipulations cause such great distress to our patients that even the strongest of tradesman with a fracture will scream out in pain during the setting. It is quite upsetting to cause such great distress in those who we as healers are seeking to help. The application of strong drink helps these patients little, so I endeavor to be gentle in this practice. But, my Master has repeatedly yelled at me—often louder than the patient can scream: "Squeeze right hard! Drive out the bad humors and find the bloody break!"

Some breaks, we know, will leave these limbs all but unusable. Other patients will get the fever whether the skin is broken or not. So we bleed them, and a goodly number die in our care from their broken arms, legs, and other afflictions. I find resolve in those I am able to help, though I wish sometimes that I had a magic candle, so I might peer inside and find the break without causing these poor souls so much suffering.

I am content, like others in my profession, to leave the cutting of surgery to barbers. I find the practice of these surgeons repulsive, as the act of surgery must be completed with much haste, and as such the process itself is as barbaric as any amputation, inelegantly done, by the gladiators in the coliseum of Rome. In witness of some surgical processes, in the auditorium, the patients screamed in such acute pain I prayed they fainted fast, as my ears simply could not stand the assault.

I sometimes wonder what father would make of the profession I have chosen. As with his own father, and his grandfather Tom, he abjured all medical practice, whether by a physician, surgeon, doctor or apothecary. I remember father telling us children how only the incantations, roots, barks and berries of the old Mattaponi medicine man made him feel well. Perhaps, there was something to it in that recently the science is discovering that tea from the bark of some willow trees contains an acid that may truly reduce dropsy and relieve a bit of pain.

In my discussion with the learned chemists and apothecaries, I find that most of their solutions, powders, and plasters are just as father described. They seem to be more drawn from superstition than science. Many of the most popular simply seem to do more harm than good, but woe unto the student that contradicts the teacher! We are expected to memorize all of these ministrations, including the old standbys like Anderson's Pills, Daffy's Elixir, and Lockyear's Pills, as well as, the growing crop of new ones: Dr. Batemen's Pectoral Drops, Dr. Hooper's Female Pills, and Robert Turlington's Balsam of Life. I am convinced that soon even Mr. Turlington will apply the affectation doctor as well so as not to be left behind—most of the purveyors of these concoctions are neither doctor, physician, nor have they had the least bit of scientific training. The ingredients in most of these remedies are the same that great-grandfather Tom likely had on his voyage aboard The Dove!

Less, and less, we write the old medicinal prescriptions to be compounded and prepared by the apothecary. Now druggists simply sell these packaged elixirs, nostrums, and powders to their patrons, who take whatever dose, and at whatever frequency they desire. Private physicians complain their business is suffering, as fewer seek their learned advice and now self-medicate. More and more I fear the result!

I heard the other day that Sir Humphrey Davy has discovered that the oxide of nitrogen will help reduce the sensation of pain during dentistry, but the effect is small and fleeting. There are rumors that many are trying other chemistries that yield a more sustainable result. In a few weeks, I am going to a demonstration by a student of Sir Davy, at my new place of work, which promises to help extend the daylight without an open flame. This invention they call the incandescent light, offers the promise of great results but like so much of the promises from this new science, I am waiting to see with my own eyes.

At first, I had wished these elixirs could have cured father, who for many years suffered from stomach problems, dropsy, and ague. Now, I am starting to listen again more attentively to the memory of father's exhortations against medicines, as too many of these new nostrums make the users lost in spirit, despondent, dependent, and often in much worse shape than when they started the treatment.

Recently, I have seen some small infants of our poor indentured, whose mothers have administered one of the new syrups for children. When I have seen them at hospital, they appear in such a state of stupor that I have had to wonder if they will ever regain their faculties. And, this is often after just one single teaspoon! I must see them at hospital, as we who work here are prohibited from seeing patients in their home as that is the realm of the private physician. Private physicians are allowed to recommend admittance to the hospital, and if they have a patient in the hospital, can minister to the patient here, but they are prohibited from charging for such services performed inside the hospital. Few do this, as almost none would refer a patient here in the first place. Further, if they do refer a "pay" patient to the ward, they become the responsible party for payment to the hospital. If the patient dies, the physicians are on the hook for the burial cost, as well. This often "puts that nail square in the coffin" as father used to say.

Now Mother, I have some news that I know, will distress you greatly. Since I started this correspondence a few weeks ago it is now clear to me that I am about to run out of funds, and therefor, my studies at Harvard, along with my hopes to become a physician, are suspended. I have instead found a job at the new Massachusetts General Hospital. I know that, like many others, your expectation of hospitals and their doctors is that they exist only as a secluded and quiet location to escort the deranged and infirm safely to the next life—and little else. I know you will not be impressed that, like many others, this institution has been founded to treat the sick-poor. There is a second facility within the same corporation that is established to treat the insane. As I have decided to apprentice for the role of doctor, I am not expected to spend much time in that horrible place. Instead, as an apprentice house doctor, I will be administering to the sick-poor—the indentured working class of Boston—who as "ordinary" patients can get their bed and care free of charge. Since few private physicians will set foot in such a squalid place, let alone refer their wealthy patients to such an institution, I do fear the methods that I will learn, may be more on how to usher these unfortunates to their next life than ways to help extend their journey in this one. Just the same, as I have little money left, and few prospects, I am happy for what physician education I received from Harvard, and the opportunity to work anywhere as a doctor. Despite the well-deserved squalid reputation of most hospitals, there are some good things about this institution.

Only open these past 4 years, the new hospital is rapidly growing in size as wealthy town leaders bequeath homes, land, and monies to support the endeavor. While their public voice cries out for the acts of Christian conscience and kindness for the poor, our father's skepticism keeps me grounded in the healthy understanding that the true reason for this and other such institutions now founding in New York, Baltimore, Philadelphia, and others is much more pragmatic. As more and more indentured souls arrive with all the maladies common in Europe, many simply are unfit for duty upon arrival. The poor businessman or landowner that has spent his good money, and not a paltry sum either, to retain the required servants and pay for their board and transport, often finds himself very economically disadvantaged when these vital workers arrive unfit. At the time of its founding, the hospital was partnered with another venture, The Massachusetts Hospital Life Insurance Company. Both institutions work, in tandem, to help solve the problem for the wealthy businessman or landowner. Upon the signing of the contract with the immigrant laborer, and even before they leave their distant shore, an agreement is struck with this "Life Insurance" company whereby the holder of the policy receives payment if the covered servant dies, becomes unfit for service by illness or injury, or is deemed insane upon arrival—thereby insuring the investment in this servant and their production is not simply a sorry loss. How many times did father and grandfather face ruin of just such a result in their early days?

This policy is a great boon for the economic interests of Boston, as no longer are businesses and wealthy merchants failing due to the economic hardship caused by loss of production.

The hospital benefits mightily, due to the support of the payments from the Insurance Company as grants for operations. The Life Insurance Company also benefits, as for every one of the poor souls we can recover, the Insurance Company is saved the casualty payout to the policy holder. The wealthy citizens of Boston benefit, because the sick-poor no longer simply waste away on the streets, neither in the alleyways, nor in the sick rooms of their masters' estates, exposing them, or the general population, to all manner of contagion. The general citizens benefit, because they now have a place they can find a bed. And although the wealthy say they would not be caught dead in this house, some beds are placed for those that can "pay." And, since most come here to die as it is, the few gentry that do pay often find their conceit fulfilled.

As for the insane, both rich and poor are treated equally in this institution as "ordinary" non-paying patrons. We all know that insanity may come in the night to anyone, and the vapors know no difference from the fineness of the linen on which one lays or the roughness of the cloth in which one huddles—rich or poor alike, the insane are treated for free. The city fathers and the wealthy gentry know that to do otherwise would destroy all their fortunes equally. In this affliction, the hospital has a ready vehicle to seek endowment; as they tell their patrons, for a donation of one-hundred dollars, a "pay" patron will get a bed free for a year; for $1,000 a free bed for life. As the threat of insanity is so high and increasingly commonplace, regardless of social standing, many are willing to "donate" to assure a place outside the home. I wonder how long this offer will truly stand, as the insane may be mentally unfit, but few die from the malady. Truly, it seems that the afflictions suffered by the rest of us are afraid to inhabit these lunatics. It is as if the one disease is so bad, the Almighty refuses to grant them another. Often, they linger in restraint and filth for years. How many beds can this institution afford to create, if this curse continues to grow?

I continue to base my hope for medicine in certain breakthroughs we are now learning, such as, Bernard Courois' discovery of Iodine as a necessity in the diet. Its lack is now believed to be the cause of goiter and perhaps lunacy, as well. More of us are now using the "inoculation" technique of Edward Jenner, to forestall small pox. We pass a small thread through the blister of a sickened person, and then pass the same string through an open incision made upon the skin of an uninfected. This procedure provides a strong prophylactic benefit to the uninfected subjects. They often get very mild cases of the small pox but quickly recover and thereafter remain immune from its terrible predations. Please promise me that you will seek out this procedure, as it may well save your life!

At Harvard, I have grown most curious about a new class of afflictions defined collectively as "cancers," which are increasingly appearing among the citizenry. With their slow, wasting effect on their victims, I am now wondering if these "cancers" might be what afflicted father with so many frailties and illnesses in his declining years and finally took his life. While I have chosen Allopathic practice, in some ways I often find myself subscribed to the teaching of the Eclectic Physicians, which suggest that it was just the travails of father's early life that set the stage he occupied for the remainder of it. I know that as a doctor at this Massachusetts General Hospital I will see and learn much more than I will elsewhere and perhaps discover some of my own truths in this area.

Now that, Meverell has passed on, and Elizabeth has wed Joseph Clarke, I count the days when I can complete my apprenticeship and return to you and to Bard's Fields with all the medical knowledge that I have gained. I look forward to being reunited with you and with the place of my birth, to share what I've learned as a healer, and to make my living by helping our neighbors rid themselves of the prostrations and afflictions to which so many have already succumbed.

As I recall father's life on this anniversary of his passing, I remember him, like his father before him, as master of Bard's Fields, kind to his children, kind to his servants, kind to his neighbors, and the epitome of what Maryland breeds. With his grace, I hope to live up to his ideals.

With the humblest of God's grace, I remain your devoted son;

William Loker

Humorous Bleedings and Cathartics

On December 14, 1799, former President George Washington was suffering from a severe sore throat. His throat had swollen so badly that swallowing became almost impossible. Doctors arrived that morning and followed the customary treatment for swelling by cutting open a vein and bleeding him of twelve ounces of blood. Typically, doctors restricted bleeding to an every-other-day regimen, but the President's doctors were so eager to ease the great man's suffering that they bled him that same afternoon of another twenty-four ounces. Later that evening another physician arrived to consult on Washington's condition. He ordered the bleeding of another thirty-two ounces. At that point, those present noticed that the President's blood was no longer running freely. No wonder. He had been drained of one-third of all the blood in his body. That night, George Washington died at the age of sixty-seven. Had he been killed by his sore throat? Not likely. Today we are all but certain that Washington's physicians bled him to death in the course of treating an ailment he likely would have survived if they had merely left him alone.

In the early years of the American republic, physicians were aware of only a small bit of the medical science we know today. Much of the medical education of the day was driven by the dictates of mysticism and classical dogma. Belief in the power of evil spirits and the presence of the devil continued to influence medical practice and the choice of treatments.

The principles of education and training for physicians during this time were based largely on the theories of Herman Boerhaave (1668 – 1783). Boerhaave combined the best parts of the medical theories he had studied, including those of the ancient Greeks: Aristotle and Galen. He did so in a manner that was based on the new science and discoveries, while maintaining harmony with fervent religious tradition and historical myth.

It was Galen, in 300 BC, who described the four factors thought to cause all illness and disease. He theorized that the body had four elements called Humors: blood, phlegm, melancholy (yellow bile), and choler (black bile). When these elements were in good balance, the body was healthy. If the body had too little or too much of any one of these elements, then disease was either clearly present or would soon follow.

Boerhaave refined Galen's theory and taught that blood was formed by the liver; melancholy by the spleen; choler by the gall bladder; and phlegm by the stomach. The role of the physician was to identify which of the humors was out of balance and to use appropriate methods to bring the fluids back into check. This process of diagnosis was also done on the basis of a person's evident temperament. An individual could be diagnosed as sanguine, melancholy, choleric, or phlegmatic—all terms that remain in use today to describe broad personality and character traits.

This "philosophy" of medicine gave rise to some fanciful notions of treatments. For instance, people with scarlet fever, measles, small pox, or any disease with a red eruption on the skin were kept in beds surrounded by scarlet bed-curtains. Jaundice and other diseases casting a yellow hue were treated with powdered turmeric, a yellow spice. Asthma and shortness of breath were treated with the lung of the long-winded fox. Memory loss was treated with heart of nightingale.

Boerhaave's system also described three physical states that could lead to disease: salty, putrid, and oily. The physician-prescribed remedies from the apothecary aimed to sweeten the acid, purify the stomach, and rid the body of impurities by catharsis. The alternative to the catharsis remedy was bleeding. Since fever was an affliction of the blood, bleeding was the preferred form of treatment. The typical bleeding called for the removal of ten ounces, which didn't seem like much at the time because the circulatory system was thought to hold nearly 400 ounces of blood—about twenty-four pints. In fact, there are only ten pints, or 160 ounces, of blood in the human body. With no practical limitation on the number of bleedings that physicians ordered to rid the body of impurities, this simple miscalculation often produced fatal results.

Bleeding was only the most outrageous example of the ignorance rampant in medical practice at the time. With no knowledge of bacteria, germs, viruses, or the benefits of sanitation, physicians had no notion as to the cause of most deadly diseases or how they spread. They did not practice any form of sterilization on their tools, nor did they even see the need to wash their hands. Physicians were often the very cause for the spread of contagion and infection that was killing their patients. Even their rudimentary understanding of anatomy was flawed by historical, religious, and cultural biases, all of which were firmly entrenched in the mores of the day.

Religious doctrine drove science and medicine up until the time of the Protestant reformation—a revolution of sorts that ignited the age of free-inquiry. We recall today William Harvey as the discoverer of the circulatory system upon his publication of *"De Motu Cordis"* (On the Motion of the Blood and Heart), published in 1628. The Spanish theologian, Miguel Serveto, known also as Michael Servetus, published a remarkably sound and accurate description of the circulatory system in a religious tract, in 1553, almost one-hundred years earlier. The Protestant reformer John Calvin, who was an intellectual correspondent with Serveto, took offense at Serveto's religious beliefs, however, and had both Serveto and his publications burned for heresy in Geneva.

The continuing power of this form of religious authority and mystical beliefs into the nineteenth century should not be underestimated. Bad ideas had a way of taking root and hanging around. Van Helmont's *"Oriantrike: Physick Refined,"* published in 1662, asserted that since nauseating medicine impaired mental vigor (as anyone with a hangover can attest), then the stomach is the seat of human intelligence. This misconceived notion took almost a century to refute.

You may ask how people in that "scientific age" could come to such preposterous conclusions. A better question might be, why do mystical and nonsensical beliefs continue to hold sway over some of our medical decision-making to this day. Why do so many people still believe in copper bracelets and magnet therapies for arthritis and other ailments? Why do many major league baseball players wear titanium-threaded necklaces in the belief that they draw energy and healing powers from them? And, why did Steve Jobs, the supremely rational founder of Apple computers, put off surgery on his cancerous pancreas for months so that he could first try various unproven herbal remedies? Even after decades of scientific study, the root causes of cancer remain a source of superstition. An Australian study recently showed 1 percent of cancer sufferers attributed the cause of their illness to "stress" even though no scientific study has ever suggested such a link.

Throughout the first half of the nineteenth century, expectations from the medicinal arts were quite low. Physicians were judged on their few successes, rather than their many failures. Most illnesses and diseases either passed in due time, persisted as chronic conditions, or proved fatal. The root-cause was often attributed to diabolic acts, God's wish or, from the scientific theory of spontaneous generation. As a result, the physician and his various concoctions were usually forgiven any role in the patient's demise.

However, it was also during this era that some of the most profound advances in medicine and technology first began to change the fundamental practice of healthcare in America. The invention of the stethoscope and microscope, the theory of germs, the practices of inoculation, anesthesia, and antiseptic principles all originated during this time period though most would not reach widespread use until much later.

Table 1 shows the wide assortment of medicines from the apothecary that would have been available to William. What is most ironic is that most of us likely have many of these "remedies" in our kitchen cabinets today. Like many medicines in our history, when their effectiveness was disproven they found new lives as soft

Table 1: The Nineteenth Century Medicine Cabinet

Basil	Birch	Catnip
Chickweed	Dandelion	Dill
Dogwood	Evening Primrose	Holly
Lavender	Lemon Balm	Magnolia
Mallow	Mandrake	Marigold
Mountain Ash	Oak	Oregano
Parsley	Peach Tree	Peppermint
Jewel Weed	Poplar	Queen Anne's Lace
Rosemary	Sage	Sassafras
Spearmint	Sweet Gum	Sycamore
Thyme	Tulip Tree	White Pine

drinks, condiments or candies, such as Coca-Cola, catsup, and horehound candy drops.

In addition to the natural remedies described in the table, there were a number of mixtures available—concoctions of mercury, antimony, arsenic, and strychnine—that were used as cholerics, phlegmatics, and purgatives. These, like bleedings, were often used with no positive results, and sometimes fatal ones.

It was also during this era that physicians had to contend with the emergence of two decidedly less "heroic" and less painful forms of treatment—the Eclectic and Homeopathic schools of medicine. Eclectic medicine, founded around 1813, placed an emphasis on plant remedies, bed rest, and steam baths, while Homeopathic medicine, founded around 1825, prescribed a different set of medicines in much smaller doses, as well as allowing the body to heal itself. Improved diet and hygiene played a huge role in Homeopathic medicine, as did methods for stress reduction.

The name for traditional medicine, Allopathic medicine, was coined as a pejorative term by Homeopaths. The Allopathic emphasis, on bloodletting, purging, high-dose injections, and enemas, containing mercury and antimony, were heroic methods of fighting illness (*allo* meaning "other"), while homeopathy stressed the use of more gentle remedies.

As we have seen, Allopathic medicine usually consisted of painful treatments that yielded results that often proved worse than nothing. By contrast, Eclectic and Homeopathic treatments were rarely painful. They sometimes created a mild, beneficial placebo effect or, on the downside, an allergic reaction. The most common effect they provided was no discernible effect at all. The practice of Eclectic and Homeopathic medicine rose quickly as most of the medicines they required became more readily available and significantly less expensive. As a result, private Allopathic physicians and apothecaries both grew concerned about an ominous drop in demand for their services.

Hospitals and the Birth of Health Insurance

In 1751, Benjamin Franklin and Dr. Thomas Bond founded the first American hospital in Philadelphia to "treat the sick-poor and the insane." Disease, addiction, and mental illness continued as a blight to all in the colonies. Philadelphia, the largest city in the thirteen colonies, was suffering from an onslaught of immigrants who were diseased, disabled, or insane. The city simply needed a place to put them.

Similar hospitals were rapidly established in New York City and Baltimore. The Massachusetts General Insane Asylum and Hospital was chartered in Boston, in 1811, the result of a $5,000 bequest by William Phillips on his death, in 1797, to build a place "for the reception of lunatics and other sick persons."

The word hospital comes from the Latin term for immigrant home or visitor home. In America, the name referred to warehouses that isolated the sick-poor and insane from society. The wealthy either endowed these institutions or had them supported through taxes so that the "ordinary" person suffering from illness could be kept there and off the streets at no cost.

"Extraordinary" was a term in those days to refer to those above the common or "ordinary" class. The "extraordinary" people, who had means to pay private physicians for treatment in their homes, viewed hospitals as filthy and deadly places where "ordinary" people went to die. Private physicians also avoided hospitals, but for economic reasons. Hospitals forbade physicians for charging for their services on their premises. And, should a patient expire under the care of a physician in a hospital, the physician was on the hook for the cost of burial.

While hospitals were typically established, as a place, to isolate the sick-poor and insane from the lives of the upper class, they did provide for "pay" patients as an additional means to help secure endowments. In its early days, and keeping with the original promises, people who were insane, regardless of their class, were provided a bed.

There were many environmental factors in nineteenth century life that could create symptoms of mental illness, no matter one's station in life. The prospect of insanity provided hospitals with a ready vehicle to seek endowment. At Massachusetts General Hospital, patrons would be promised, for a donation of one-hundred dollars, a free bed for a year. For one-thousand dollars, patrons would be allowed a free bed for life. The threat of insanity was so high and commonplace that many were willing to "donate" to assure, themselves a place of care outside the home.

These endowments constituted an early form of catastrophic health insurance. But, Massachusetts General was instrumental in the development of the first practical medical insurance product. At the time of its founding, the hospital was cofounded with another venture, The Massachusetts Hospital Life Insurance Company. Both institutions worked, in tandem, to help solve one specific and serious problem for wealthy businessmen and landowners.

More and more immigrants were coming to America as indentured servants at the time of the founding of Massachusetts General. They gained a free passage to America, in exchange for years of service to their sponsors, after which they could become "titled" landowners and free men. But, after a lengthy voyage, packed in with others who had different diseases and mental problems, indentured servants who arrived on these shores were often ill-prepared to fulfill their indenture. Those in the colonies who put up the money for their passage, in exchange for their commitment to many years of servitude, often lost their risky investment. Instead, they were responsible for their newly arrived diseased and insane charges.

The hospital gave society a central location to house these people, which addressed one half of the problem. The formation of hospital life insurance companies, starting with the Massachusetts example, addressed the other half of the problem, by protecting the sponsor's investment. Upon the signing of the contract with the immigrant laborer, an agreement was struck with the life insurance company whereby the holder of the policy would receive payment if the covered servant either; dies, becomes unfit for service by illness or injury, or is deemed insane upon arrival. The investment in an indentured servant was thus assured by granting compensation to the unlucky sponsor whose asset is dead, dying, or insane in the hospital. This basic concept would go on to shape the coverage if other healthcare losses. It was, you might say, way ahead of its time.

Physicians, Apothecaries, and the Patent Medicine Manufacturers

"Patent" medicines came about in the early seventeenth century in Europe. They evolved over the following one-hundred years and made their way to America. While the initial medicines in the eighteenth century were indeed patented, near the end of that century the expense and disclosure of ingredients required in patents were being rethought. Manufacturers suddenly began to regard their formulas as being closely held secrets, and they used registered trademarks as protection instead. Nevertheless, until the early nineteenth century, these nostrums were hard to come by. They were expensive and often less trusted than traditional home remedies.

Initially, patent medicines like, Daffy's Elixir and Bateman's Pectoral Drops were shipped to the colonies from England. The first American-made patent medicines, like everything else in those days, were poor counterfeits of their British cousins' products. By the end of the War of Independence, Americans were importing empty vials and filling them with their own versions of the name-brand elixirs, sometimes even importing actual printed wrappers to perfect the counterfeit. As was the custom of the day, most of these patent medicines were purported to cure just about anything and everything. The principal ingredient in all these medicines was alcohol. The colonial customers had no idea that the products they were purchasing were not the originals. Since they actually had little to no medicinal value, it didn't matter.

The domestic manufacture of medicinal nostrums and patent medicines in America did not begin in earnest until, after the War of Independence was over. Soon the patent medicine industry was one of the largest and most profitable in the colonies. A combination of poor health in the population, the sorry record of physicians and their apothecary formulations, lack of education and superstition all helped fuel the large and rapid growth of the industry.

As medicine manufacturers prospered, they looked for increasing means to gain more customers. The growing almanac and newspaper industry provided the answer. In 1796, Samuel Lee Jr. of Windham, Connecticut, secured the first American patent for "Lee's Bilious Pills," which were purported to fend off biliousness, yellow fever, jaundice, dysentery, dropsy, worms, and female complaints. When confronted with a counterfeit version from another Samuel H. P. Lee, also from Connecticut, the original Mr. Lee Jr. not only sued, but he waged his war against the charlatan by using a rising star of the day: newspapers! Mr. Lee Jr. noticed that the articles they posted against one another created a demand so great that, by 1810, Bilious Pills could be found in all territories, even south to Georgia and in the newly acquired territories to the west of the Mississippi.

In the nineteenth century, the adage oft quoted, that the "cure was often much worse than the malady," rang particularly true, for the American public, regarding the Allopathic practices of bleeding and purging. Many sick men and women did not want to be subject to such painful measures, and there was no shortage of charlatans and unethical practitioners willing to pander to their fears. Nostrum manufacturers like Samuel Lee Jr. boasted that there was no harsh mercury in their formulas. Samuel Thompson, another purveyor of the day, wrote, "Physicians learn nothing of the nature of the medicines they prescribe, except how much poison could be given without causing death."

Suspicion of regular physicians and their "heroic" therapies grew deeper with the rise of Jacksonian democracy. The upsurge in anti-intellectualism of the day imbued the citizenry with a belief they had an innate common sense that was superior to that of supposedly trained experts. Lemuel Shattuck, in 1850, in a pioneering report on public health, in Massachusetts wrote, "Anyone, male or female, learned or ignorant, an honest man or a knave, can assume the name of physician, and 'practice' upon anyone, to cure or kill as either may happen without accountability. It's a free country!" (Shattuck, 1860) Into this willing world, the patent medicine manufacturer strode confidently, preaching to his dutiful choir that his remedies, and only his remedies, would set them free from all manner of afflictions.

As patent medicines expanded across the nation, they became the first products reliant on national advertising and marketing campaigns. American newspapers owe much of their growth to the rise and largess of the patent medicine manufacturers. By the middle of the nineteenth century, many newspapers owed their very existence to patent medicine, both directly, as many were started by the manufacturers as nostrum sell-sheets, or indirectly, as over 80 percent of most newspaper revenues came from the patent medicine industry. It was reported to a congressional committee in 1849 that at least one "pill man" was spending in excess of $100,000 per year advertising his purgative. The provision for free delivery of newspapers by the U.S. post office, in the early 1800s, is directly attributable to the power and influence of these salesmen.

Apothecaries did not weather the storm of patent medicine well. During this period, the classic compounding apothecary soon became replaced with druggists. While many of the new druggists were trained as apothecaries, training as apothecaries was dying out. Unlike the old apothecary who ground and mixed medications in accordance with strict published formulas, many druggists were, content to sell the patent medicine elixirs, sodas, and powders. Soon all apothecaries, except those in hospitals or in physician-owned board and care homes, were plying these dubious nostrums as a matter of economic survival.

There were strong ties among the patent medicine men and the railroad and oil tycoons. In 1860, William "Old Bill" Rockefeller, the itinerant father of John D. Rockefeller, founder of Standard Oil, was one of the first patent medicine showmen. Moving from upstate New York to Cleveland, Ohio, he entered the patent medicine racket and had himself listed as a physician in the city directory. In selling his newfound discovery in a pretty bottle, Old Bill simply followed in the footsteps of those selling their wares from the back of wagons in the Midwest. When oil was discovered in northwest Pennsylvania, the new oil racketeers soon found there was more gold in the pockets of the people working in the fields than there was working, in the fields, to extract it. Old Bill opened up a new field for himself and soon began selling bottled "Nujol" as a cure for cancer. Shortly thereafter, to address a larger market, he began to advertise it as a cure for constipation, liver complaints, cholera, and bronchitis.

As patent medicine manufacturers began to accumulate wealth and power, a distinction became clear between who provided "ethical" medicines and those who operated heavily in the "patent" game. If you look deeper; however, you will see that almost all of the drug companies today had some of their roots in patent medicines. Squibb began the development of drugs in 1858, Pfizer in 1849, and Pitcher's (later Fletcher's) Castoria, now part of Sterling Drugs in 1868. The few that did not manufacture patent nostrums were involved in the industry in other ways, by providing food coloring, citric acid, and other chemicals to the patent medicine manufacturers.

Inevitably, the mid-nineteenth century saw a rising tide of concern from government, at both the state and federal levels, over these developments. Physicians, druggists, patent medicine manufacturers, and the Standard Oil Trusts began to work together to assure continued market viability and to gain political influence. With the support of John D. Rockefeller, several organizations were formed to unite these main cogs, so they could forestall the coming storm. In 1847, Doctor Nathan Davis founded the American Medical Association; in 1852, the American Pharmaceutical Manufacturers and Dealers Association was founded (now the APhA). Much later, in 1881, a group of the largest patent medicine manufacturers formed the Proprietary Association of America. These groups formed an uncomfortable alliance. Each of these organizations, initially supportive of the same objectives, began actively to shape the practice of medicine, influence legislation, and gain control of the business and delivery systems of healthcare.

They ushered in an unprecedented period of profligate profiteering and fraud perpetrated upon the American people—with disastrous results for many innocent victims.

Going Under

In 1846, Dr. William Morton demonstrated his method of using ether gas to provide a "pleasant stupor" for patients undergoing surgery at the Massachusetts General Hospital. Most hospitals prior to this time rarely provided surgical intervention, due to the barbarous nature of surgery without anesthesia and the inordinately high death rate from surgical infections. The hospital board of directors played a key role in what became one of the first major inflection points that fundamentally changed healthcare practice in America—a role for which the hospital's board of directors would defend Morton's right to the patent of this invention.

The creation of painless surgery with ether allowed the physician the ability to conduct longer and more precise surgical procedures, which resulted in better outcomes. This fact posed a problem for physicians, because ether was not easily deployed in patients' homes. Larger rooms were needed to provide ventilation for the powerful anesthetic. It would do little good for the physician ministering to a patient in the sick room of his private home to pass out alongside the patient. Ether vapors were also extremely flammable. A burning candle or lit fireplace could cause an explosion. Surgeries moved to special rooms in hospitals, where ether could be safely administered. This simple, practical requirement for a controlled environment for ether gas was a pivotal factor in the development of medicine. It changed the role of the hospital from a place of dying to a place of healing.

Then, in 1867, Joseph Lister published *Antiseptic Principle of the Practice of Medicine.* (Lister, 1909) Within five years, surgeons using Lister's antiseptic techniques were able to reduce the surgical mortality rate from nearly 60 percent all the way down to 4 percent. Not only was this a revolution in the well-being of patients, it marked a second revolution for hospitals too. After Lister, hospitals began to gain stature as *the* center for medical education and, moreover, as the central place for receipt of that day's critical healthcare services. No longer, did "extraordinary" citizens dread the hospital now they began to regard hospitals as the go-to place for complete healing.

Thanks to anesthesia and antiseptic surgery, hospitals rose rapidly in power and status. Their staffs were training many of the new doctors and the paying patients of private physician's began to go to hospitals for care. Along with the rise of Homeopaths, Eclectics, and the patent medicine manufacturing industry, another blow was delivered to the Allopathic physician in terms of business prospects.

The decline in the reputation of the private physician and the apothecary and the corresponding rise in the status of the hospital and the patent medicine manufacturer set the stage for battles over control of medicine in the late 1800s. These battles would alter the basic practices of medicine and help lay the haphazard groundwork for the healthcare system that we know today.

III. (1850 – 1899)
Medicine Becomes an Industry

Imagine . . .

Leonardtown, December 14, 1872

Master William Alexander Loker
Bards Fields
St. Mary's, Maryland

Dear Father,

I am most proud to inform you, that you are yet again a grandfather, as to my wife Eliza, and I, was born a son, on the 11th of February. Eliza and I have decided to name him after you and great-uncle Mev. I have recorded his name at Aloysius Church as William Meverell, and I pray he lives up to both of your characters.

The birth was most difficult and laborious. Eliza is still in bed with fever. She is weak, and I fear we could lose her just like as happened with her sister in '68 and our cousin in '71. The doctor has been to the apartment and, provided the powder medications, but they seem to just stupefy her. They do nothing to reduce the fever.

Little Robert is now 2 years old. His teething has caused many agonizing, and sleepless, nights these past few months. We are still living in the Sterling house, and as there are so many families roomed here we are most grateful for "Mrs. Winslow's Soothing Syrup" as it is the only remedy to quiet Robert's cries of pain. Your recommendation on this matter has helped greatly. I rushed out and purchased this wonderful elixir yesterday as Eliza lay with fever. Upon one teaspoon, Robert was, like magic, immediately calmed and shortly asleep. He has slept the full night, these past few days, much to the relief of all of us housed here. I expect William will also benefit from this nostrum. I intend to ask the druggist at what age we can administer it, although I see no limitation on the printed label in the box. I don't know why I, simply, did not take matters into my own hand earlier, as we would all have been the better for it.

Leonardtown is growing rapidly as the new county seat, and the wharf is becoming the economic center of St. Mary's County. It is stiflingly hot here in the summer, bitter cold in the winter and always damp. In the worst of the summer, the cool breezes seldom make their way this far up the bay. Because of the heat and humidity, every little scratch can turn septic, so we must always be vigilant for infection.

The store I am building with your Cousin Elizabeth's son, Bessen De Wall, will be open soon. Along with sundries, linens, hardware, fuel oil, dry goods and nails; I have arranged with our distributor out of Baltimore to sell patent medicines, as well. I am sure Mr. Greenwell, the druggist, will not like it one bit, but the Baltimore man who is our distributor of products said Greenwell simply did not have enough footage in his store to serve the demand in the town.

Now, that the war is over, many of the newly emancipated colored workers at the wharf have become regular customers of these nostrums, as the rigors of moving heavy hogsheads of tobacco onto the ships are quite acute. Old Mr. Greenwell seems to have no interest to serve colored men at his drugstore, bul Bessen and I do not feel we should restrict our clientele in such a manner. Instead, we have constructed a back door for colored patrons so they, and our white patrons, will feel they have comfortable access. The Baltimore man assures us these people will continue to give us a brisk trade, which we intend to do. With the Negro P. B. Pinchback, just *elected Governor of Louisiana, we suspect this discomposure to the African race will soon end.*

We have been able to secure a bit of credit for stocks, but Bessen does not think it wise to use it, as the money we have seems to be more worth less each day. I, on the other hand, have convinced him in the short term if we buy on credit when the value is high, we will be able to pay the debt in fewer dollars than it will take to buy the replacement stock. I believe, we should be able to grow our business just like the government is growing theirs!

The man of the family in the room next to ours is the preacher for the town's new Methodist church. They are of the temperance mind, and he openly preaches the evils of liquor to all that will listen. Some of the good Catholic women of the community have persuaded their men to join his congregation, as a result. Leonardtown's women reformers, the "suffragettes," as they are called, want to remove from men not only our perquisite to vote, but they would deprive us of our indulgences, as well. They claim that the 15th Amendment granting suffrage to Negro men should apply equally to women of all races, and they sermonize that men hold women in both religious and social bondage. Many Protestant churches are springing up around this part of the county as a result of the guile and temptation wrought by these kinds of women. I read one of their principals, Susan Anthony, was arrested for trying to vote for President Grant. Can you imagine?

Times are changing, for sure, though some changes are not for the best. Perhaps you have read about the woman doctor recently graduated from Geneva Medical School. Father, I ask you how, on God's green earth, can a woman do such work, ably, as they just don't have the strength or constitution for it?

And, what man in his right mind would seek treatment from a female doctor?

We presently have no doctor here, since old Doctor Beasley passed away in July. Mr. Cameleer's son, Henry, is soon completing his physician apprenticeship in Baltimore and is supposed to return here to practice. For now, if one suffers an injury, a doctor must be summoned from Waldorf or La Plata, which is over fifty miles away. Few doctors would want to make the two-day ride here, since most people here still pay by barter instead of cash. Imagine traveling two days on horseback, and then have to carry a bushel of oysters, crabs, some chickens or side of beef back with you. Those who have broken bones or other serious injury don't usually do well in the back of a cart or scow if we transport them there, or to Washington, DC. Leonardtown is still without railroad connection, even as we see that the rails are now laid all the way across the nation to the Pacific.

I read each day of new discoveries like the electric light and a device that can send images over telegraph wires. I even hear tell there is a city in Vermont that has put some electric lines to people's businesses and homes that power electric machines that can do the work of men and women. The Washington Post is publishing sections from this British gentleman who is claiming we are all the children of apes. In church, two Sundays ago, our good Father Gallagher was not so kindly to the theories of this man, Darwin. I thought some of the more fervent parishioners would die of prostration as he railed on.

Henry Cameleer, during his last visit home, was telling me that they now cannot only apply surgery painlessly, but they can do it antiseptically, as well. He also told me of a man in Prussia that has an idea that there are small animals called germs that cause infection and disease. And yet of another gentleman in France who has developed a method using heat to kill these little buggers and stop milk sickness and keep wine and beer from going rancid.

We had contemplated putting in one of those newfangled Liquid Carbonic machines like Mr. Greenwell has in his drugstore, so we can draw more clients for the patent medicines. He is doing a brisk business in these medicinal sodas. However, we are not able to afford the machine at this point. It is getting harder and harder to be able to buy some of the medicinal syrups if you are not a druggist due to the new American Pharmaceutical Distributors and Manufacturers Association. They are protecting their own here, and refuse to sell us a number of these items because were not one of their members. You can't fight them as they got the American Medical Association, who Henry tells me now all doctors have to join to get their license, and J. D. Rockefeller backing them, as well.

Bessen has established a contract with the new St. Mary's Beacon newspaper so we may advertise our goods. He tells me that they are quite anxious for us to start, as much of their money comes from the national nostrum manufacturer's advertising dollars and they think that our sales will be supported by what the patent medicine men are already spending.

Some of the drug manufacturers seem to be straddling the fence about an open, free market. With certain of them, we can buy and sell their goods out of our store with no problem. More and more others want to restrict sales only to druggists. They call them the "ethical" manufacturers. All these products seem to work about the same as far as I can see: I just don't see why they need these highfalutin' druggists. Our Baltimore man brought us some catalogues, and Bessen says there are over twenty-thousand varieties we can buy—they can cure just about anything old Doc Beasley could!

Well Pop, it is getting dark. The gas lights in the Sterling house leak and we try not to use them much for fear of consequences. I need to go tend my brood, as Eliza needs her powders, Robert his syrup and Wm. Meverell his sleep. With Mrs. Winslow's around, I am sure the boy will sleep the night. We hope to make the trip home for the Independence Day celebration. We will likely leave July 1st and stop, at Mulberry Fields, to see Cousin Thomas. Since Tom moved down county to live, and was never known to pick up a quill, no one has seen or heard neither hide nor hair of him for years. We hear tell he has added onto Uncle Meverell's home quite extensively since he bought it, in 1832. We hope to spend the night there and then arrive at Bard's Fields on the 3rd, weather permitting.

Affectionately yours;

Thomas Alexander Loker

Physicians Seek Safety in Numbers

By the middle of the nineteenth century, the medical profession in the United States faced a crisis in public confidence. The rise of patent medicines, the expanded role of hospitals (particularly in treating the wealthy), the popularity of less "heroic" Homeopathic and Eclectic treatments, and the general ineffectiveness of the Allopathic "bleeding and purging" treatments all worked together to erode the prestige of the physician profession.

When compared with their European counterparts, American physicians suffered from low status and, for most of them, commensurately low pay. As *New York's Medical Society Journal* reported at the time, "There is a handsome income for a few, a competence for the many, and a pittance for the majority" (Bristow, M.D., 1909). Country doctors were the most impoverished of the lot, since most of their patients lacked the cash to pay them. They were forced to accept bartered farm goods—a brace of chickens, a side of pork or a slab of beef.

It was during this time these growing numbers of people came to rely on home remedies or patent medicines to treat chronic illnesses, aches, and pains. For serious injuries or significant illnesses, patients now sought out the new painless, and antiseptic, procedures offered at hospitals where physicians were still barred from charging for their services. The role of the traditional private physician who treated patients in their homes was shrinking.

At the same time, colonial-era medical licensure laws in most states had been either repealed or had gone unenforced, creating an atmosphere in which uneducated practitioners and charlatans were free to compete with fully-trained physicians. Medical schooling was plentiful and inexpensive. Although some medical schools were connected with respected hospitals, colleges, and universities, many others were simply income-producing ventures run by single practitioners or small groups of physicians.

In 1847, the American Medical Association (AMA) was founded to defend and promote the endangered practice of Allopathic medicine.

The stated purpose of the new organization was to "elevate the standard of medical education in the United States."

Dr. Nathan Davis, a member of the New York Medical Society, led the effort to form the AMA. The New York society had enjoyed some success in taking over formal control of the process of licensing physicians in the state. Dr. Davis proposed that the AMA take the New York model to other states and lobby the legislatures to allow Allopathic physicians to set standards for the licensure of all physicians.

The new AMA developed a three-prong strategy:

- ✓ Assume control over the granting of physician licenses in order to regulate the number of doctors in practice.
- ✓ Open private physician-owned board-and-care homes to compete with hospitals for upscale patrons.
- ✓ Wage a national campaign to convince the public that only AMA-certified medical science could bring real cure and relief to illness, injury, and disease, and that other forms of care were nothing more than "quackery."

The AMA's Committee on Medical Education and its *Code of Medical Ethics* established the first minimal standards for medical education. Proponents of the code of ethics hoped that the public's growing interest in exciting new scientific discoveries at the time would help restore the respect for Allopathic medicine and would reduce the public's interest in non-scientific practice.

The AMA also saw that it could restore both the prestige and the income levels of Allopathic physicians by reducing the number of medical practitioners. At the start of the nineteenth century, there were fifty-three thousand physicians practicing in the U.S., out of a total population of 5.3 million or one physician for every ninety-six people. In 1870, the total number of physicians had grown to 62,000 out of a total population of 38,558,371 or one physician for every 622 people. At the time, about 5,300 of those physicians were licensed as Homeopathic practitioners, and 2,700 of the Eclectic variety. By the end of the century, most non-Allopathic physicians would be out of business. The battle for dominance over the medical business had begun.

Wealth, Power, and Panic

The U.S. during this period was rocked by a pair of financial crises, known as the Panic of 1873 and the Panic of 1893. Despite our modern view that these economic crises are anomalies, the U.S. has had a long and tortured economic history. We are a nation founded on debt and now exist with an economic system predicated on debt. The disconnection between gold and silver reserves and the paper currency, and the lack of commercial controls due to an immature legal system created an environment where vast amounts of wealth were created for a few.

The U.S. had been plagued with a lack of capital its entire existence. The War of 1812, which had served to unite the country behind the cause of preserving its independence, also had two other significant lingering effects. First, the war consumed resources and diverted public attention away from the need to build the country's infrastructure and promulgate laws that were necessary to control commerce and growth. Second, it prompted the federal government to create more currency to fund the war effort by disconnecting paper specie currency from the gold and silver standard. Both changes boosted the economy in the short term, but ultimately caused a shortage of the specie (gold and silver) that underwrote the country's international credit. The specie linkage would not be restored until 1878.

The U.S. was always short of specie to back the paper currency it produced. The value of the American dollar declined from one dollar in 1774 to fifty-nine cents in relative buying power by 1780. By 1790, the dollar had regained part of its value, and risen to the relative worth of eighty-nine cents.

The Civil War not only tore the nation apart, but, like the War of 1812, it also helped obscure the depressed economic conditions in parts of the nation. The consumption of supplies and materials during the war helped the struggling economy recover and to some extent, created a huge demand for raw materials, as well as the need for a rapid expansion of transportation. These took the form of railroads, which further spurred the demand for raw materials like steel and lumber. Then, too, there was manpower in the form of unskilled labor. This particular era marked one of the first examples of this, but not the last, in which a war economy drew America from the brink of depression, spurred technological innovation, and gave the appearance of meaningful economic growth.

Following the war, men who controlled businesses capable of generating large amounts of cash on a national basis had an easier time converting their paper money to gold and silver, and thus were better able to retain their net value as the dollar was again devalued. Others who produced goods from raw, natural resources or who enjoyed massive profit margins in their line of trade also enjoyed a distinct advantage in accumulating vast personal fortunes. These were the men who could exercise true power throughout the economy, and they included the so-called "robber barons" like John D. Rockefeller in the oil industry, Andrew Carnegie (steel) and Cornelius Vanderbilt (railroads). They also included newspaper magnates William Randolph Hearst and Guy Gannett.

The member companies of the patent medicine Proprietary Association represented the single largest and wealthiest group of businesspeople in America at the time, with a firm control over communication media and state legislatures, as well. Purveyors of medical services, patent medicines and the chemical manufacturers (who supplied the patent medicine industry) coalesced into large groups or cartels of collective wealth and consolidated power. The medical industry became a three-legged stool, with the patent medicine manufacturers, doctors, and hospitals each assuming one leg that was interdependent with the other two.

Businesspeople who did not have the wealth and power to shape the nation and its laws found it necessary to come together in associations and develop other forms of control to preserve their respective businesses. They needed to find some common areas where they could gain support from the robber barons. So it happened that, in this era, associations were formed to represent the interests of physicians, apothecaries, medicine manufacturers, and newspaper owners. They all found, they had certain interests in common, with one another, and also with many of the big robber barons of the era.

While it is always easy to look at those who have accumulated great wealth and power as being in some way morally corrupt, such views are often too simplistic. There is little doubt that many that prospered during this time were able to do so with poor ethics and questionable morals. However, the conditions that permitted such abuses were also responsible for creating industries and methods of commerce that helped the country grow beyond many pending catastrophes. The same conditions and opportunities continue today. As a people, we must recognize that we bear a great deal of responsibility for the rise of the morally-corrupt. If we chose to remain uneducated in the areas of personal economics and health safety and to rely on others for our personal prosperity, then we will find ourselves continually taken advantage of by others.

Both the good and bad that we find in current healthcare systems have their beginnings in this narrow window of time. Further, our expectation for what we should gain from healthcare springs from its fundamentally flawed roots here, as well. It was then that we began to develop high expectations for the under performance of our healthcare providers. Said conversely, it is during this period when our method of solving our personal problems related to disease, illness and injury were to *swallow* the advertising, *suffer* the treatment, and *imagine* the results. Very little has changed!

New Medicines: Selling the Cures

The popularity and availability of patent medicines exploded during this era. Their chief attraction was that the consumer could use them to self-dose without seeing a doctor or obtaining a doctor's prescription. In 1857, there were about 1,500 patent medicines listed for sale in New York. By the end of the century, there were estimated to be 28,000 patent medicines advertised, marketed, and distributed all across the nation.

In 1872, the year that little William Meverell Loker (later Judge William Meverell Loker) was born, some of the best-selling brands of these incredible mixtures—based on newspaper advertising in the day—included the following:

- ✓ Mrs. Winslow's Soothing Syrup will "likely sooth any human or animal," and effectively to quiet restless infants and small children. It was widely marketed in the U.S. and in Britain. The company used newspaper advertisements to promote their products, including recipe books, calendars, and trading cards. The primary ingredients of this soothing syrup included morphine sulfate (65mg per fluid ounce), sodium carbonate, spirits foeniculi, and aqua ammonia.

- ✓ Hall's Catarrh Cure was marketed as a remedy for Catarrh, which is better known today as bronchitis. The cure was manufactured by Frank J. Cheney, who would become the largest advertiser of patent medicines and one of the principal leaders of the patent medicine trade group, the Proprietary Association of America. (Primary ingredients: alcohol, potassium iodide, sugar and small amounts of vegetable extracts)

- ✓ Lydia Pinkham's Vegetable Compound for Women was promoted as a women's tonic to relieve menstrual cramps. Its primary ingredient was alcohol.

- ✓ Peruna was introduced in 1890 as another cure for catarrh, but its owner Dr. S. B. Hartman expanded the definition of catarrh, so Peruna could treat catarrh of the kidneys, stomach, bowels, spleen and just about any other organ you can think of. Peruna was very popular and became the main curative enjoyed by many temperance supporters, even though it consisted of 28 percent grain alcohol.

- ✓ Birney's Catarrhal Power competed with Dr. Cloe's Catarrhal

> Cure; Dr. Gray's and Crown powders. All claimed to cure catarrh and asthma, but most patrons of these powders used them regardless of their effect on treating lung ailments, since they contained between 270 and 1,250 (mg) of cocaine per ounce.

These products all had three things in common. Each provided little medicinal value was addictive, and was sold at an extremely high profit margin. Since most medicinal treatments of the day weren't very effective, expectations for these remedies were exceedingly low. If you found that a particular remedy did not provide the cure it claimed, you might likely assume you were suffering from some other malady. Due to the predominance of cocaine, morphine, and alcohol in these elixirs, many users became addicted to them. Then the symptoms *followed* the dosage, instead of preceding it. America was getting hooked.

In April 1885, Pemberton's French Wine Coca hit the market and became an immediate success. This tasty potion contained a high percentage of alcohol, a significant amount of caffeine and 8.46 mg. of cocaine per liquid ounce. Like most patent medicines, the beverage was advertised as a cure for nerve trouble, dyspepsia, mental and physical exhaustion, gastric irritability, wasting diseases, constipation, headache, neurasthenia, and impotence. It also was recommended as a cure for morphine addiction. Company founder John Sith Pemberton marketed his elixir to "scientists, scholars, poets, divines, lawyers, physicians, and others devoted to extreme mental exertion."

Born in 1831, in Knoxville, Georgia, Pemberton enlisted in the Confederate army and was wounded at the Battle of Columbus, Georgia, in April, 1865. Like many wounded soldiers of the day, he rapidly became addicted to morphine.

Pemberton tried various concoctions of coca and coca wines to wean himself off morphine, but to no effect. Desperate to find a curative, he formulated his own remedy by mixing alcohol, coca, kola nut and damiana, a small shrub native to Central America. The damiana plant produces small, aromatic flowers coupled with a strong, spicy aroma, one that had traditionally been used in tea for its reputed relaxing effects.

Pemberton's French Wine Coca was promoted as being "particularly beneficial for ladies, and all those whose sedentary employment caused nervous prostration, irregularities of the stomach, bowels and kidneys, and those who needed a nerve tonic and a pure, delightful diffusible stimulant." It could also cure "neurasthenia" among "highly-strung" Southern women. His colorful advertising campaigns in newspapers of the time played to the widespread concern about drug addiction, depression, and alcoholism among veterans.

In the same year of its introduction, however, Pemberton's magical elixir was banned in Atlanta and the surrounding Fulton County because its alcohol content ran afoul of new temperance laws. Pemberton responded by reformulating his brew, substituting carbonic acid (soda water) to replace the alcohol, and keeping the other ingredients. Having satisfied the chemical requirements of the laws, he came up with a new name: Coca-Cola. The beverage was introduced in May of 1886 at the Jacobs Pharmacy in Atlanta, where it was delivered as syrup and mixed via a soda delivery system (the forerunner of the modern soda fountain). Jacobs sold twenty-five gallons of Coca-Cola the first year and 1,049 gallons the next. In 1888, Asa G. Chandler, along with several other investors, bought the rights to Dr. Pemberton's formula for $2,300. It was Chandler's aggressive marketing that brought real success to Coca-Cola, making him and his investors many, many millions of dollars.

Coca-Cola was not sold in bottles until 1894. Even then, distribution through pharmacies continued to account for most Coca-Cola sales. The company pioneered the development of the soda fountain and patrons enjoyed visiting these establishments for a "fresh, soft drink." This is where the phrase "soft drink" originated. As concern over the addictive contents of patent medicines grew over time, pharmacy soda fountains gradually transformed from providing therapeutic medicines to simple carbonated beverages. "Soft drink" meant it was free of habit-forming drugs, although Coca-Cola continued to contain cocaine, until 1903.

Coca-Cola spawned a large number of competitors, many of whom share the company's roots in patent medicine and survive today as soft drinks. Charles Alderton, a pharmacist at Morrison's Old Corner Drugstore in Waco, Texas, created Dr. Pepper. Others promoted their formulas for their alleged health benefits. Hires Root Beer claimed to purify the blood and make the cheeks rosy. Jamaican Ginger Beer, later known as Ginger Ale, alleged to ease a sour stomach.

Physicians Take Control

In 1883, the AMA created the *Journal of the American Medical Association* (*JAMA*) as a vehicle for promoting "medical science," the treatment of disease with drugs and surgical process through Allopathic medicine.

JAMA was instrumental in the campaign by Allopathic doctors to first gain control of the licensure of physicians, then gain control over the hospitals, and finally force the hospitals to let private physicians charge for services. Soon they realized they could use the same approach to subrogate medicine manufacturers.

Many hospitals were either associated with medical schools or operated as medical schools at this time. A growing number of medical schools were granting licenses to Homeopathic and Eclectic doctors, as well. In 1889, according to a report published by the Illinois Board

Table 2: Point of interest

Retail is a word from Middle English. In the Middle-Ages, transactions in gold and silver became quite inconvenient for the King because he did not have enough supply of the metals to make sufficient coins for his kingdom. Instead, he chose a method by which to measure workers' output using a notched stick, called a tale. When work was completed, the stick was broken, one half going to the person who had done the work, and the other half going to the king's treasurer. The half-tale could be traded to others for goods and services. At any given point, the owner of the half-tail could present it to the treasurer who would provide them with the proper amount of gold or silver. The tale could also be used to pay their taxes. People that were willing to sell goods using this system became "re-tailers." When the use of the wooden stick was changed back to gold and silver and later paper money, the term evolved. Those who bought in bulk and then cut into smaller amounts to sell to others were considered retailers. Actually, apothecaries were some of the first retailers. Those in the medical profession were breaking away from their barter system and drug companies were becoming retailers. Medicine was suddenly becoming a prosperous industry.

of Health there were 179 medical schools in North America. Of these schools, twenty-six were Homeopathic, twenty-six Eclectic, thirteen miscellaneous, and an additional thirteen were condemned as fraudulent. The remainders were Allopathic schools or "regular sect," as the report referred to them.

As a condition of joining the AMA, Allopathic physicians agreed to have the AMA act as their licensing authority, which meant they had to give up their authority to license their own apprentices directly. Homeopaths and Eclectics, however, continued to license their apprentices and the AMA was powerless to stop them. So, the AMA began lobbying efforts in each state, pressing their legislatures to adopt the AMA's standards for licensure of all physicians. The AMA also adopted a publicity campaign to promote the development of "medical science" as the sole legitimate basis for medical education.

For many long-practicing and decent non-Allopathic physicians, this development created significant problems. In 1882, the West Virginia State Board of Health rejected Frank M. Dent's application for a medical license. Dent was a physician of the Eclectic sect, a group which vigorously opposed the excesses of drugging and bleeding, still among the dominant practices used by Allopathic physicians at the time.

Dent had been in practice for six years when he was convicted under a new West Virginia law that required a physician to hold a degree from a reputable medical college, pass an examination, or provide proof that the physician in question had practiced in West Virginia for the previous ten years. The State Board of Health refused to accept Dent's degree from the American Medical Eclectic College of Cincinnati, and Dent was forbidden to practicing medicine in West Virginia.

By 1899, as a result of lobbying by the AMA, most states had reinstituted physician licensing laws like those in West Virginia, which reflected AMA standards and its code of ethics. The days of Homeopathic and Eclectic practitioners were numbered.

The Apothecary's Dilemma

What was an apothecary to do about patent medicines? The historical apothecary, a healer trained mostly as a herbalist—had evolved over time into the pharmacist, a trained and educated chemist. As far back as the 1700s, patent medicines from England gave pharmacists an expanded livelihood. They could buy the pre-prepared medicines in bulk and resell them without prescriptions, which reduced their reliance on physicians. Now, however, with the explosion of domestic patent medicines in the late nineteenth century, pharmacists were facing stiff competition from untrained, uneducated retail druggists.

As physicians began to fall out of popular favor, the apothecary was caught in the middle. Many physicians still had some standing and power in their communities, so the apothecary knew to tread lightly on their turf. However, more and more people were casually bypassing physicians and coming to apothecaries directly for medical advice and to buy elixirs and potions. The trade in patent medicines was too reliable and profitable to resist.

As the practice of apothecaries and druggists started to become one and the same, both knew very early on that many of these nostrums were ineffective and even dangerous. But, there was no legal responsibility imposed on the apothecary or druggist for health problems caused by the medicines they dispensed. *Caveat emptor* (buyer beware) was the rule of the day, and for the most part, the law of the land.

Godfrey's Cordial was one drug widely known by both practitioners to be problematic. Deaths from this concoction had been reported in professional journals as far back as 1825, but both continued to sell it.

In the December, 1872, edition of *The Medical Press, A Weekly Journal*, it was reported, "A child a month old was dosed with two tea-spoonfuls of stuff sold as Godfrey's Cordial, and it died. The Chemist who sold the mixture said he sold about a half a gallon per week; the greater portion went out in cups he did not label, one ounce for a penny."

And yet, druggists were not in a business position to refuse to sell the elixirs and tonics. If they didn't sell patent medicines, others would. Patent medicines could be purchased at many locations including bars, dry-good and grocery stores (like at my ancestor's new general store, Loker & DeWall's, in Leonardtown).

The following side article (Figure 1) from the *American Journal of Pharmacy* (Volume 42, Philadelphia College of Pharmacy and Science, July, 1870) illustrates the pharmacist's conundrum of the period. Mr. Morse advocates a recipe of opium, molasses and sassafras—ingredients also found in the dangerous Godfrey's Cordial. For both the apothecary and the druggist, the dilemma was in determining which concoction would generate more revenue, create less work, and which one will be less likely to cause death or injury.

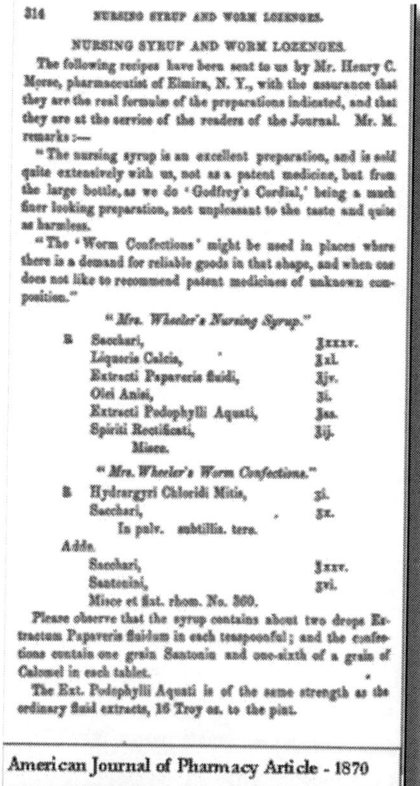

314 NURSING SYRUP AND WORM LOZENGES.

NURSING SYRUP AND WORM LOZENGES.

The following recipes have been sent to us by Mr. Henry C. Morse, pharmaceutist of Elmira, N. Y., with the assurance that they are the real formulæ of the preparations indicated, and that they are at the service of the readers of the Journal. Mr. M. remarks :—

"The nursing syrup is an excellent preparation, and is sold quite extensively with us, not as a patent medicine, but from the large bottle, as we do 'Godfrey's Cordial,' being a much finer looking preparation, not unpleasant to the taste and quite as harmless.

"The 'Worm Confections' might be used in places where there is a demand for reliable goods in that shape, and when one does not like to recommend patent medicines of unknown composition."

"Mrs. Wheeler's Nursing Syrup."

℞ Sacchari, ℥xxxv.
Liquoris Calcis, ℥xl.
Extracti Papaveris fluidi, ℥iv.
Olei Anisi, ʒi.
Extracti Podophylli Aquati, ℥ss.
Spiriti Rectificati, ℥ij.
Misce.

"Mrs. Wheeler's Worm Confections."

℞ Hydrargyri Chloridi Mitis, ʒi.
Sacchari, ʒx.
In pulv. subtillis. tere.
Adde.
Sacchari, ℥xxv.
Santonini, ʒvi.
Misce et fiat. rhom. No. 360.

Please observe that the syrup contains about two drops Extractum Papaveris fluidum in each teaspoonful; and the confections contain one grain Santonin and one-sixth of a grain of Calomel in each tablet.

The Ext. Podophylli Aquati is of the same strength as the ordinary fluid extracts, 16 Troy oz. to the pint.

American Journal of Pharmacy Article - 1870

Figure 1: American Journal of Pharmacy Article 1870

In 1852, the American Pharmaceutical Association was formed "to help provide advance-ment of pharmaceu-tical knowledge and elevation of the professional character of apothecaries and druggists throughout the United States." In reading the Proceedings of the National Pharmaceutical Convention minutes from its inaugural meeting, October 6th, 1852, one is struck by the similarity of constitution, pur-pose, and actions as that of the formation of the AMA five years before, and of the Pro-prietary Association of Ameri-ca in 1881. There is anecdotal and circumstantial evidence that all organizations received en-couragement, support—and likely funding—from J. D. Rockefeller

The apothecaries and druggists of the latter 1800s were in a quandary and needed partnerships with each other and with other powerful entities in order to survive. More importantly, they needed to get some control over the practice of pharmacy to elevate public opinion about them and their goods. They also needed to manage the rise of patent medicine. If not, they would soon be out of business. As the trends within their business came into alignment and the American Pharmaceutical Association gained power and control, the transition from competing interests to a controlled and regulated business for the benefit of all was seen in the rise of the "professional pharmacist" as the epitome of both professions.

Nurses to the Rescue

The history of the profession of nursing is as colorful as that of any other field in medicine. In the early days of the nation, when hospitals functioned as warehouses for the dying and the sick-poor, nursing care was typically provided by men and women serving punishment. Nurses were very often prostitutes and other incarcerated female criminals. Some had reputation for being drunk and obnoxious—a view echoed by the doctors of the time who often let it be known they were not enamored of their services.

The earliest role for nurses in hospitals was to clean up the mess left by staff members as they made their rounds. Since there was little regard or understanding of the role of sanitation in the provision of healthcare before 1857, cleanliness was not a priority in hospitals. With the publication of Lister's theory on the principal and practice of antisepsis, however, physicians suddenly saw the practical role of nursing, despite their dim view, in general, of women in the workplace, and of nurses in particular.

Nursing became a credible profession around 1860, not long after the publication of Lister's theory. Florence Nightingale, a well-educated woman from a middle class family in London, claimed she "heard God's call to become a nurse" and earned worldwide fame for herself and the profession by treating the wounded during the Crimean War. Nursing and antiseptic practice grew together in subsequent years and helped forge the growth of quality of care provided at hospitals. In 1873, Linda Richards graduated from the New England Hospital for Women and Children and became the first professionally trained nurse in the U.S.

Although women like Florence Nightingale, Mary Seacole, Agnes Elizabeth Jones, and Linda Richards continued to expand the role of nursing, acceptance by physicians was slow in coming. As late as 1906, Dr. Gilman Thompson published an article entitled "The Over-trained Nurse," wherein he made the point that, in his opinion, "Nursing is not, strictly speaking, a profession . . . Nursing is an honorable calling; nothing further" (Thompson, M.D., 1906). Another physician of the day, Dr. Robert Abbe, said, "I can teach a nurse in a week all she needs to know."

It is likely that Dr. Abbe and others saw nurses as a threat. At the time, Allopathic physicians were in the middle of a war, with their competitors, to maintain the integrity and viability of their field. The elevation of the role of nursing to a profession was likely considered yet another form of unwelcome competition. This dynamic remains today, as nurse practitioners are taking over many roles—once reserved exclusively for doctors—and some doctors are still pushing back against perceived encroachments on their turf. Old habits do, in fact, die hard!

The General Welfare

The latter half of the nineteenth century was the age of great improvements in medical science. Besides the development of anesthesia, antiseptic practice, and germ theory, there was the profusion of new vaccines for cholera, anthrax, rabies, tetanus, diphtheria, typhoid fever, and plague. Other common causes of death, including influenza, tuberculosis, and diphtheria, were also greatly reduced in impact. The mandate of smallpox vaccination by the states was the first, crucial step in its near-total eradication. The efficacy of these treatments and the great scope of progress they represented measures up impressively against the new treatments we see today. All these developments helped medicine became an industry.

As a society, however, we have been, and will continue to be, vulnerable to many of these diseases. Medical science has only provided us what our bodies need to kill off all, or most of, the germs causing the infections inside us. Even today we see the resurgence of some of these diseases since the public has grown complacent in getting vaccinated. Vaccination does not necessarily prevent all occurrences of death as a result of these diseases.

In later chapters, I will address this conundrum, but for now consider the "cures" we have today. The sad truth is that we have very few cures for any disease. The confusion over what constitutes a "cure" has had its strong tentacles firmly planted in the period between 1850 and 1899. By the early 1900s, with an increase in life span due to vaccination, lethal ailments such as cancer and heart disease became more common, and neither of them can be treated by vaccine.

While there was many impressive scientific leaps in this era, the general welfare of the population during little William Meverell Loker's early years was hardly optimal. While he went onto become a respected lawyer and a renowned circuit court judge, he continued to suffer for most of his life from problems related to his digestive system. His mother told his future wife, Mabel Ford, "Meverell has a weak constitution and always has been subject to periods of illness, and he must eat carefully." It is highly likely that if he had been treated with Mrs. Winslow's Soothing Syrup or another of the opiates widely in use at the time, his parents' decision to medicate him as an infant was perhaps the cause of his lifelong suffering.

IV. (1900 – 1929) The Progressive Era and its Aftermath

Imagine . . .

The covers are pulled tight to your neck, and the featherbed mattress has you deep in its firm embrace. You're traveling in a faraway land, marveling at the sights, sounds, and smells, but off somewhere in the distance you hear someone calling your name . . . "Mev . . . Mev . . . Mev . . . it's time to get up dear . . . Mev!!! Get Up! I am not coming back up the stairs for you!"

Like a shot, you are back in your warm bed at home, and you know it is the start of another day—another sad day! Your wife, Mabel, leans down and kisses you on the forehead and leaves, saying she will go down to prepare your breakfast.

As you rise from your bed, you feel every bit of your fifty-seven years. You slip your robe on over your dressing gown and enter the bathroom. This indoor plumbing is such a handy convenience, so much better than the basin, cold water, and outdoor privy you had just a few years ago. It is a shame all the things that come with this "modern convenience" are not as pleasant.

You turn to push the pearl button that switches on the Edison light. As usual, you hesitate first. Why is it that so many others find this new invention so marvelous? The installation was expensive, and it seems like, every time you turn on the light, there is a spark from the cloth-covered wires. More often than not, you get a shock. If not for Mabel, you would still have the gas lights working. They were cheaper to operate, and you understood how they worked.

You switch on the light and flinch, but today no shock, nor spark that you see. You move to the sink and begin the morning ritual. You dampen your tooth brush, shake out some Colgate tooth powder and brush your teeth. Being able to rinse your toothbrush in the running water seems better than the germ laden water that used to sit all night in the pitcher next to the basin. And, your expectorant just flows down the drain, not into the basin where you washed your face and hands.

You lift the razor strop that is attached to the wall next to the mirror, and put a fine edge on your reliable Gillette straight razor, lather your Burma Shave with your horsehair shaving brush in the ceramic shaving-mug, and begin your shave. As you shave, you think about Ernie Bell telling you that he just bought one of those new Schick electric razors. Who in their right mind would do such a thing? Electricity and water—that's a shock waiting to happen! You know others are using the "safety" razors with the disposable blades. They are supposed to reduce cuts and infections. It is hard to believe that with all this modern technology and advances of medical science, people are still dying from infections from simple cuts. Life is still so fragile, and so much time is still devoted to simply providing for your family. There are still days, like today, that you don't feel well—today, of all days!

You, on the other hand, simply wonder who would give up the peaceful and contemplative ritual of shaving! So much of becoming a man is tied to this ritual. You remember watching your father shave. It is what defined his role as father and provider for you. "Is this not what separates men from women?" you ask yourself.

Completing your shave you wash your face, dress, and descend the back stairs to the kitchen for breakfast. As you enter the kitchen, you remember that all the kids are at home, save one. Susan Elizabeth, eighteen years old, and Robert Leslie (Leck), twenty-three years old, come for their morning hugs just like they used to when they were little. You should really begin to call them by their new names. Now, she's Sister Francis Miriam, still a novice and Leck is Brother Clyde, who has completed his holy orders. Susan says how she and Leck have been praying for Betty, and they know she is with God. You choke back your tears, not just from the words, but the dedication to God that exists in both Little Susie and Leck. For a moment, your sadness has been replaced with pride in your children.

Next is William Aleck (Aleck), nineteen years old and just returned from Europe. He and his new friend, Carl Albert, won the trip for finishing in the top six in the National Oratorical Contest. Aleck looks older than he did when he left, achieving his honor only six days after the tragedy. How strong he was to stand there and orate on the value of the Constitution; in front of the members of the Supreme Court of the U.S. who sat for that day as judges of the contest instead of the law. You remember Justice Sutherland telling you after, "That boy will make as great a lawyer as his father." "No parent should outlive his children," you say to yourself. Daughter, Francis, age twenty, receives her hug and asks you what you said. You mutter, "Nothing dear, just thinking out loud."

Frank Ford, age eleven, and William Meverell, Jr., known as Little Billy, age seven, come up in turn. Ford says, "Pop I have decided I want to be a doctor so what happened to Betty never happens again."

You are proud of all your kids. The older ones are all growing up to be fine young men and women. So far, all the new technologies don't seem to have damaged them. Prohibition and the lawlessness of alcohol do not seem to have captured them either. Maybe one day soon they will repeal this damnable law since the only ones that pay attention are the ones getting caught. Hell, everyone you know is taking a taste now and then, and without some shine once in a while last year, you know you would not have been able to cope. Aleck, Robert Leslie (Leck), and Francis are all old enough to have a drink every now-and-then. As long as they don't end up in front of you in your courtroom, what are you going to say?

Ever the caregiver, Mabel has your breakfast ready. She has been a great wife and partner these twenty-six years and has always taken care of you, weak constitution and all. She always has your "good healthy-start" ready. Since it is May, and the wood stove in the kitchen will be cold so as not to contribute to the beginning summer heat. Today's menu is two raw eggs, one tablespoon of cod liver oil, and a yeast cake. How she came up with this concoction, you will never know, but, since she started serving it to you seventeen years ago, it has saved you from the digestive distress that you used to live with every day of your life.

The new "tele-phone" in the hall rings shaking you from your thoughts. "Mabel, let the damn thing ring! I had it put in for my convenience, not for everybody else's!" Always, considerate of others, Mabel answers it and says she will give you the message.

"I am going to the office," you tell Mabel. Aleck asks if you want a ride. "No," you say. "I don't want to use that infernal machine!" You

think, why do I have that car? I hate them! You bought the Chevrolet AA Capital new from Webster Bell when they came out in 1927 and loved to drive it up till last year. Now you don't want to be in it, and you don't like your kids in them, either.

As you walk out the screen door onto the porch, you yell back in; "Aleck, I want you and Jim to take the horse and wagon out to St. John's Farm, and make sure things are OK. Since your grand-ma has died, we need to keep an eye on the tenant farmer. He doesn't take as good a care of the farm as I wish he would. And bring back some clabber, side of bacon, some eggs, a good ham for Sunday, and a tin of lard." Aleck objects. "It will take all day with the horse, and we can be there and back in the car in an hour!" he says. Nevertheless, you are adamant—No car! "I don't care how long it takes! You and Jim take the cart! I don't want you in that damn car!" You say as you head down the steps and to your office.

It is a one-mile walk from your home down the walnut and oak tree-lined main street of Leonardtown and along the way; you can't help thinking about Little Betty. Your baby girl died today one year ago to the day, on May 21, 1928. For five days, she lingered after the car struck her, finally succumbing to the infections that they could not fight. You used to think, this science stuff was bringing great things, electric lights, central heating, telephones, automobiles, medical science. But, what good has any of it accomplished? Who can you blame? Your little girl is gone, and you have to live with the grief. You can't blame the driver of the car. There is no way he could have seen Little Betty running out from behind the fence into the road! Even if, he had seen her, he could never have stopped that thing in time. A horse would have reared when it saw the child, but not a car—the damn car, It is just a soulless, murderous machine. And now she is gone . . .

As you are walking lost in your thoughts, Mrs. Cameleer's daughter calls out to you from behind their front pickets, "Good Morning Judge, how are you today!" About Betty's age, the little sweetheart seems to have greeted you each morning since the accident. The ravages of polio have left her in leg braces, but the girl's indomitable spirit never ceases to elevate your heart. "Good day, Emily." You say "I hope you are well and say good day to your mother!"

A few blocks later, you begin your walk up the steps to the old courthouse. Cold and drafty, and built in the 1833, its charm is in its history, not its conveniences. Only in the last twenty years, has the outdoor privy been replaced with indoor plumbing. The courtrooms are grand and reflect more the English form of design than the modern American and that, in itself, is part of its charm.

At the top of the steps, you turn right at the end of the hall and proceed down the interior corridor to your chambers. You remember when you were first appointed Circuit Court Judge; how you had literally to ride a circuit of courthouses on your horse and buckboard. Today, you still travel, but it's not like the old routine. Most of the cases you hear now are held right here in town.

Your office is spartan, keeping with your penchant for austerity, but over your desk, you have kept the old painting of an English barrister that was once your father-in-law's favorite. Seeing this each, and every, day, reminds you of your duty to the people of the county. Your robes hang near the door to the courtroom. You have just two hours to prepare for your first case. You open the folders of the handwritten briefs on your desk. As is the new custom, some of the briefs are typed, and easier to read. Most of the old-timers still inscribe their briefs by hand, which brings, in your view, some of their character and passion into the written arguments. Again, you think, even as technology brings some benefits, it seems that it also removes a bit of our humanity.

At ten minutes to ten, the clock on the wall chimes. You rise from your briefs and notes, put on your robe, and you walk down the hall to the privy. Court appearances are long, and you hate to interrupt a good argument from either side for nature's call. Precisely at 10:00am, you walk through the door, just as Mr. Jarboe, the bailiff, announces, "This court is now in session, the Honorable Judge William Meverell Loker presiding, all with business before this court, come forward and be heard!"

"Call the first case, please Mr. Jarboe," you say. Promptly, the bailiff responds in a loud and commanding voice, "The case of The

Government of the United States vs. Archibald Paul Bell is called." The government prosecutor introduces himself as John Paul Bailey. The defendant Archie Bell stands. "Mev, I am representing myself," he says.

You are not shocked by his familiarity, but you reply, "Mr. Bell, while you and I have known each other for many years, and our families have known each other for many more, I want you to understand in this court you are to refer to me as Judge or Your Honor. Any other way, and I will find you in contempt. Further, I know you will understand that I am here impartially and that our familiarity with each other brings neither benefit nor contempt in regard to this matter before me. Unless either of you objects, I will hear this case. If one of you does choose to object, I will recuse myself. So is there an objection?"

There is no objection. Mr. Bailey says, "Heck, Judge, if we had to ask any Judge to recuse himself in St. Mary's County because they know one of the parties in a suit, we would never hear any of the darn things."

You ask for the nature of the complaint. Mr. Bailey responds, "Mr. Bell is charged with illegally running a distilling operation and producing and selling alcohol from said still without the proper medicinal production licenses. And, since said alcohol was not sold for medicinal purposes and, in fact, made its way into a series of "underground" establishments including his own located at Abell's Wharf, he is further charged with distribution,"

"Mr. Bell, how do you plead?" you ask.

"Not guilty Mev . . . Sorry, I mean Your Honor. Hell, I am just selling the same stuff that they sell in those Peruna medicine bottles at the drug store. A man's got to make a living, and I don't see why this is any different. I thought this was a free country, I mean, if a man wants to take a drink now and then, why does the government tell him that he can't . . ." As Archie drones on, you realize this is going to be a long day.

CRACKKK! The sound of your gavel hitting the bench shocks the court, and quiets Archie in mid-syllable.

"Mr. Bell, I advise you to get counsel for representation. If you choose not to do that, go see Lemuel Guyther and ask if you can read his law book on court procedure. And additionally Mr. Bell, if you can't understand the book, pay him ten dollars and ask him to teach you what you need to know before you come back to my courtroom!" You close the file in front of you. "This case is continued to next Tuesday 1:00pm. Call the next case, Mr. Jarboe."

"The case of Benjamin Wieland vs. Maryland Hospital, all are present your honor," says the bailiff.

"Gentleman," you begin, "I have reviewed the case as presented, researched your points of authority and reviewed your summaries. To recap for the record, Mr. Dorsey, the plaintiff, claims that he was admitted to the hospital, June 19, 1927, after he fell from scaffolding. He was transferred to Maryland Hospital.

"The Defendant showed that it is a public institution incorporated in June of 1906, specifically for the public good, and its funds originate predominantly from grants, devises, donations bequests, and subscriptions of money and other property contributed by the state and benevolent persons, to be used for the erection, support, and maintenance of a general hospital to treat sick and insane persons. A small percentage of their funds originated from the board of paying patients.

"Upon arrival at the hospital, the attending surgeon examined Mr. Wieland and determined that he had broken his upper arm. Mr. Wieland contends at this point that he informed the attending surgeon that he did not want any student to treat him. Mr. Wieland and the hospital records, both reflect that the attending surgeon assigned the case for treatment to another physician, who at the time of his treatment of Mr. Wieland was a student. Mr. Wieland further contends, that the setting of the arm was improper, he has suffered physical and emotional distress since the incident, and he wishes this court to award him a judgment in his favor, and against the hospital.

"Additionally, and most relevantly, Mr. Wieland was admitted as an 'ordinary' patient and as such he was not charged for the services he received. The Tort claimed, is for the injuries sustained by reason

of neglect and unskillful treatment of the plaintiff by the defendant's servants."

You continue, "In my ruling, I have looked at several cases cited in your briefs. While a number of the citations reflect in some manner on the arguments at hand in your briefs, I am relying heavily on my review of 'McDonald vs. Massachusetts General Hospital, 120 Mass. 432, Suffolk County, Mass. 1876.' In this case, we have an identical set of circumstances. Mr. James McDonald fell from a building on which he was working, fractured his thigh bone, occupied a free bed, received admittance from the attending surgeon, and was treated by a student. The hospital is also a public institution funded for the public good. I see no reason for my decision to deviate from Judge J. Allen's ruling in this matter. He found that even if the plaintiff should be able to prove that the fractured bone was not properly set in consequence of the incompetency of the treating physician or of the house surgeon, the plaintiff will not be entitled to recover as the bed was provided free. I thereby find for the defendant and against the plaintiff Mr. Wieland. Case dismissed."

"Next case Mr. Jarboe!"

"The case of Copsey vs. Corner Drugs," says the bailiff. "All the participants are present in the courtroom, your Honor."

"Oliver Guyther, representing Mr. Copsey Your Honor," says the plaintiff's lawyer. "James Mattingly, representing Corner Drugs, Your Honor," says the lawyer for the defendant.

"You may begin your opening statement Mr. Guyther," you say. Guyther begins. "Your Honor, the plaintiff will prove that the defendant did with incompetence and willful intent, sell to my client's oldest daughter, Elizabeth Joyce Copsey, fifteen years old at the age of her death, numerous bottles of Birney's Catarrh Cure. Thirty-four bottles were found under her bed after she died of this concoction. We will further prove, that Birney's Catarrh Cure is primarily an addictive mixture of 1,230 grains of cocaine per ounce in 40 percent alcohol solution and that it is widely known, in the druggist trade, to be both highly addictive and subject to rampant abuse by the common folk. Finally, we will prove that the plaintiff was keenly aware of these facts as published widely in the American Druggist Magazine and

the Pharmaceutical Monthly magazine, both of which the plaintiff subscribes to and has admitted under oath that 'My staff and I read these publications religiously.' We will prove beyond any reasonable doubt, that the plaintiff exercised profligate, willful disregard for the well-being of my client's daughter, knew she was, in fact, addicted to the very nostrum that he had sold her originally for her monthly difficulties when she first came of age, that he knew this nostrum was addictive, by his sales to this minor child—made this young, innocent girl a cocaine fiend—and in effect, if not, in fact, murdered this young girl purely to enhance his own profits by the sale of this witch's brew. I have completed my opening statement, your Honor."

"As it is near to noon and supper is upon us," you say, "the court will recess until 1:30pm." You rise and head for your chambers.

As you remove your robe and walk out to go home to your wife and kids for mid-day supper, you wonder at what all this modernity has wrought. Like Mr. Copsey, these supposed scientific or technological innovations have not cured but led to the death of both his and your child. The Daily Record, the trade journal of the American Bar Association, is still full of the impact of the recent "Scopes Monkey Trial." God vs. Science—man vs. gods. None of it seems to make sense. Clearly, there have been marvelous inventions and great strides in healthcare since you were a child, the discovery of germs, painless surgery, and the need for antiseptic process. But, all of these advances are bringing, compounding problems that you seem destined to adjudicate. New drugs are bringing benefits, but right alongside come addictions and dangerous side effects. New technologies like the light bulb were supposed to stop fires, but we still have fires, now mostly they are from faulty wiring. You recently judged a negligence case of a person getting electrocuted from being in the proximity of water and frayed wires and found against the party that installed the electric services.

As industrialization has taken over the country, the cost of products has dropped, but the dangers for workers in these industrial jobs have increased. Just last month you finished such a case at the tobacco warehouse down at the wharf. Vaccines are the new things and apparently effective for those vaccinated, but the diseases are still there for those that aren't vaccinated. They call everything cures, but they don't really cure much at all. Painless surgery makes surgical procedures easier and safer, they say, but now they are doing many more surgeries than they have done before, and many still die from infections. Antisepsis is reducing the infections, but not eliminating them. In aggregate, it seems more people are dying before their time, not less. And, with rare exceptions, the doctors in rural areas continue to be of poor quality and, like Leonardtown, most small towns are thirty or forty miles from the nearest hospital. If there had been a local hospital, maybe little Betty would have survived. For your little Betty and Elizabeth Copsey, what did all this matter? They died. They are gone! Your heart will carry Betty's loss till your death. You wonder why it is that so many innocent children must leave this life so soon.

One thing all this last year has taught you is that the measure of your impact is very small indeed. The largest impact that you can have is not going to come from what you ever do yourself but by what your children become and what character they aspire to project. In that regard, you are starting to feel you are doing what you can. One day Aleck will be a fine lawyer, and he will minister to the inequities wrought upon his neighbors just as you have done, rendering "a pound of flesh" to the injured party where justice is needed. Susan (Sister Francis Miriam), and Robert Leslie (Brother Clyde), will minister to the souls of their neighbors and help prepare them for life everlasting at God's side. Frances will make a fine wife. Perhaps she will marry that Wigginton boy she seems to like. Ford wants to be a doctor so maybe he will bring his skills back to Leonardtown and help minister to the physical needs of his neighbors, and not stay in the city like all the others. For now, Little Billy is your little boy. You have no idea what he will become. You know it is more likely his older brothers will lead the way, more so, then you at this point.

As you finish this thought, you hear your shoes clop up the back steps and across the porch. As you open the door, you see all the family there, along with Father Paul. You move into the dining room where Mabel has spread a fine fare of fresh fried chicken, crab cakes, okra, watercress salad and some fresh afternoon tea. You hope she's sweetened that tea with a bit of Archie Bell's 'shine. This meal will be a special one as you will all come together to end the year of mourning for Little Betty, for Elizabeth West Loker, in celebration of her short life. Perhaps, this one event will be a seminal one for all of your kids, to help them find a reason to dedicate their life to some higher purpose.

You don't know it now, but all your children will go on to fine achievements. Each will live up to your hopes and dreams. Each child will stay true to the character you instilled in their person and their souls. Each will touch so many others—hand linked to others—to help their neighbors rise to new heights.

In the end, you will have made just the difference you contemplated on this day and you will have lived a great life as will your children who follow in your footsteps.

Muckraking

While there is no direct tally available, using a summary of contemporaneous sources like *The Journal of Inebriety,* (Inebriety, 1892 – 1903) other temperance pamphlets, and pharmaceutical association and distributor papers, at the dawn of the twentieth century, an estimated 15 to 25 percent of the population was addicted to alcohol, morphine, cocaine or any number of other narcotics. Frequently, they became addicted to one or more of the above simultaneously. Most of the narcotics were unknown ingredients of the popular patent medicines. People did not know what was in these concoctions, they simply knew they felt good when they drank them, or felt worse if they did not. Even the venerable Sears and Roebuck catalogue—a common fixture in every household, privy and outhouse of the day—offered cocaine and a syringe for $1.50, in its 1890 edition.

The term of the day in general was "inebriant" and the action "inebriety." The term reflected the role that people of the day felt personal choice played in addiction. Inebriety was considered a sign of moral degradation, personal choice, and/or biological determinism. Inebriants were considered to be immoral, derelict of character, and the downfallen by God. The term alcoholic and alcoholism emerge in the middle of the nineteenth century, but it was almost a century before it would be seen as a medical condition. At the turn of the century, habitual drug users were "morphinists," "cocainists," or "dope fiends."

Beginning in October 1905, *Colliers Weekly* ran a series of articles by Samuel Hopkins Adams that promised to provide "a full explanation and exposure of patent medicine methods and the harm they have done to the public by this industry, founded mainly on fraud and poison....The object of the series is to make the situation so familiar and thoroughly understood that there will be a speedy end to the worst aspects of the evil."[1]

Adams was a muckraker, one of a breed of turn-of-the-century journalists who uncovered fraud, waste and corruption. The rise of national magazines like *Collier's* and *McClure's* helped give exposure to scandals of this kind. At *McClure's*, writers like Ray Stannard Baker, George Creel, and Brand Whitlock were active raking muck at the state and local levels, while Lincoln Steffens exposed the corrupt rule in many large cities. Ida Tarbell went after Rockefeller's Standard Oil Company. It was President Theodore Roosevelt who gave these journalists the "muckraker" nickname when he complained that they were not being helpful by raking up all the muck they could find. The term has stuck around to this day.

Adams, for his part, exposed the addictive nature of most patent medicines. His articles illustrated the danger of these drugs and the hypocrisy of many who defended them. He was able to establish clear connections among the various members of the patent medicine cartel and show how they conspired to evade public accountability.

Perhaps most importantly, Adams revealed the shady business practices that the cartel employed to control the nation's newspapers, the supposed "watchdogs" for the public good. In one of Adams' articles, *Collier's* printed verbatim the following, damning statements by Frank J. Cheney, manufacturer Hall's Catarrh Cure and president of the industry trade group, the Proprietary Association of America.

1 Note: You can read the 1905 version or Hopkins book entitled The Great American Fraud on Google Books.

While addressing fellow members at their annual meeting in 1899, Cheney said:

We have had a good deal of difficulty in the last few years with the different legislatures of the different States . . . I believe, I have a plan whereby we will have no difficulty whatever with these people. I've used it in my business for two years and know it is a practical thing . . . I, inside of the last two years, have made contracts with between fifteen and sixteen thousand newspapers, and never had but one man refuse to sign the contract, and by saying to him that I could not sign a contract without this clause in it, he readily signed it . . . This is what I have had in every contract I make:

> *It is hereby agreed that should your State, or the United States Government, pass any law that would interfere with, or restrict the sale of, proprietary medicines, this contract shall become void . . .*

In the State of Illinois a few years ago they wanted to assess me $300. I thought I had a better plan than this, so I wrote to about forty papers and merely said: "Please look at your contract with me and take note that if this law passes you and I must stop doing business, and my contracts cease." The next week every one of them had an article opposing the bill in the legislature.

In the end, Cheney continued to get his way—at least in the short term!

Thanks to this clever contract clause promoted by Cheney, and known as "The Red Clause," any state-level attempt to regulate patent medicines constituted a direct attack on the financial well-being of all the newspapers in that state. Cheney stated that he had contracts with over 14,000 newspapers at the time and estimated the newspapers earned revenues of $20 million per year from the industry, a hefty sum in those days.

Patent medicine was the number-one source of advertising revenue for newspapers of this era. At this same meeting of the

Proprietary Association, Dr. Frederick K. Humphries of Pond's Healing Cream (now sold as Pond's Cold Cream, without the healing) said that "the twenty thousand newspapers of the United States make more money from advertising the proprietary medicines than do the proprietors of the medicines themselves . . . of [the patent medicine manufacturer's] receipts, one third to one-half goes for advertising." And then, adding an almost sinister air to the proceedings, the record showed Humphries was concerned about what the public would think about this blatant form of manipulating the press through The Red Clause. Humprhies said, "Will it not be now just as well to act on this, each and every one for himself instead of putting this on record? . . . I think the idea is a good one but really don't think it had better go in our proceedings."

The *Collier's Weekly* articles were not the first ones to raise the issue of addiction and patent medicines. The AMA had done exposes about patent medicines in its journal, *JAMA*, but these did not have much effect since they were not widely read by the public. The AMA was not completely opposed to patent medicines, either. In fact, the AMA was tightly allied with the patent medicine industry in marginalizing the Homeopathic and Eclectic schools of medicine, since these schools eschewed treatment by patent medicines. For a long time, *JAMA* ran ads for many patent medicines that most physicians suspected were neither safe nor effective. And, while the AMA had set up a committee to test the efficacy of some nostrums on the market, it was widely noted that the medications that *JAMA* found ineffective were those that had *not* bought advertising space in *JAMA*! The AMA and its physician members was not yet in a position to alienate druggists, nor did they wish to alienate the patent medicine men.

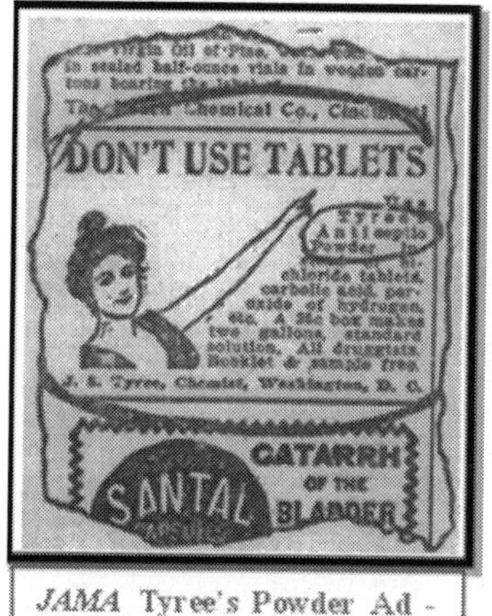

JAMA Tyree's Powder Ad -

Figure 2: JAMA Ad for Tyree's Powders

Following are some excerpts that quote from *The Great American Fraud* (Adams, 1905):

Adam's comment on the effect on the populace

Restrict the drug by the same safeguards when sold under a lying pretense as when it flies its true colors. Then, and then only, will our laws prevent the shameful trade that stupefies helpless babies and makes criminals of our voting men and harlots of our young women.

With pharmacists dispensing some medications based upon a

Adam's quote on the responsibility of the newspaper owners

Every intelligent newspaper publisher knows that the testimonials which he publishes are as deceptive as the advertising claims are false. Yet he salves his conscience with the fallacy that the moral responsibility is on the advertiser and the testimonial-giver. So it is, but the newspaper shares it. When an aroused public sentiment shall make our public men ashamed to lend themselves to this charlatanry, and shall enforce on the profession of journalism those standards of decency in the field of medical advertising which apply to other advertisers, the Proprietary Association of America will face a crisis more perilous than any threatened legislation. For printers' ink is the very life-blood of the noxious trade. Take from the nostrum vendors the means by which they influence the millions, and there will pass to the limbo of pricked bubbles a fraud whose flagrancy and impudence are of minor import compared to the cold-hearted greed with which it grinds out its profits from the sufferings of duped and eternally hopeful ignorance.

prescription and some without, a distinction arose between so-called "ethical" prescription medicines and the suspect over-the counter "patent medicines." The question of whether a drug was "ethical," or not, had little to do with its actual safety and effectiveness, it was more a matter of its mode of distribution.

For instance, the *JAMA* advertisement (Figure 2) for Tyree's Antiseptic Powder and the endorsement that appeared in *The Medical World: A Practical Medical Monthly* in 1919 (Figure 3), would seem to indicate that the medical community endorsed this product and its use because its formulation was advertised and sold as "ethical" to the druggist trade.

Only a year earlier, however, *JAMA* had published an article (dated March 30, 1918) in which the AMA Council denounced this drug and another drug just like it, declaring:

> *. . .both of these twin nostrums are utterly unfit for treating the various conditions for which they have been recommended . . . Do physicians believe that a simple mixture of boric acid and zinc sulfate... is in any way superior to a prescription such as any physician could write?* **The council article continued,** *There is a far more important question to consider than the relative merits of such nostrums and a prescription of the physicians own devising, and that is whether the medical profession is going to help to perpetuate the chaotic conditions that the use of such nostrums help foster.*

The patent medicine industry's Proprietary Association fought back against these and other attacks by the AMA and by *Collier's Weekly* by casting aspersions on the victims of its concoctions. If medicines were being abused, it wasn't the manufacturer's fault. The fault lies with the abuser.

An article representing this view appeared in a 1905 edition of the *Practical Druggist* periodical. It carried the offensive title, "The Niggers in the Wood Pile." The author, Joel Blanc, made a mighty attempt to play down the whole problem of the rising tide of concern about addiction and the problems with patent medicines. The root of the problem was the "fiends who are abusing these harmless medications." The title of the article was more than a curious usage of a pejorative of the day. It was a part of an orchestrated campaign by the Proprietary Association to lay the problem caused by the "fiends" directly at the feet of freed slaves. Blanc never made direct reference to race in his article, but he used certain code words that laid the source of the problem at the feet of the lower classes and the disenfranchised. The Proprietary Association technique, of targeting minorities as the cause of any related issues, had a long history in the patent medicine trade. During this period, the blame not directed to simply the poor classes, it was now seen repeatedly in newspaper articles, often in the south, where it began to attribute the concern to rising violence and rape of "white" women by addicted "Negroes" or in the West as an expected outcome due to the unscrupulous nature of "China-men." While society rejects this type of invective today, race-based execration was all too common in this country's sad history during this period, which directly contributed to the distrust and disaffection among the races for many years.

Wilmington, Del.

Mr. J. S. Tyree,
Washington, D. C.

Dear Sir:—

I wrote you sometime ago as to my experience with "Tyree's Antiseptic Powder."

I was sincere in every word I said in that letter and I will say now while I never had any one use my name in reference to a preparation, you are at liberty to use anything I may write you about Tyree's Powder, for I do not hesitate to cheerfully recommend it in all you claim it will do. I have used it for over 15 years in almost everything it can be used for, as in Gonorrhea in the male as an injection, on tampons for the same in the female, as a gargle and spray in nose and throat troubles, as a wet dressing and in full strength as a dressing. I will continue to use it as I consider it truly reliable and would advise all Physicians who do not know of your liberal samples to have you send them a sample and try it both in the Medical and Osteopathic Profession and I am positive they will become as positive advocates of it as I am.

Sincerely yours,
GEO. W. QUINN, M.D., D.D.

that's the whole story

Figure 3: Medical World Endorsement - 1919

Nonetheless, it was Adams' series of seven articles in *Collier's Weekly* that brought the public out of its stupor, both figuratively and literally. Unlike the articles in *JAMA*, Adams' writings reached the broad public. More importantly, his articles offered fuel for the women's organizations coalescing around the twin causes of temperance and suffrage, led by Susan B. Anthony and others.

A wide variety of temperance organizations had sprung up to rid society of the scourge of inebriation and to address the growing numbers of people falling into moral decay. On the prevention side, a series of actions that began in towns, cities, counties, and states occasionally resulted in temperance laws being passed. It is a result of the passage of local temperance laws that John Pemberton was forced to remove alcohol from French Wine Coca and come up with Coca-Cola.

Nevertheless temperance was not often that popular with the masses. Most temperance movements found their moral calling in the hands of religious belief. Many towns had one or more religious facilities almost singularly devoted to the evils of inebriety and often the inebriates themselves. Saving the souls of the inebriant and rescuing him or her from the clutches of Satan became a major campaign of the day, and quite coincidently, a good fund-raising tool for the sponsoring church or society.

It is at the dawn of this new century that a rising secular opinion began to create a shift from religious, divine action to secular determination. Some began to see indications of more than simply lack of religious devotion or moral decay in the behavior of the inebriant. Across the country, mutual aid societies begin to take root. Having existed since the mid-1800s, entities like the Salvation Army and the Washingtonian Total Abstinence Movement began to gain a foothold as the new, progressive movement and secularization took hold.

The public began to question whether, or not, there was a scientific basis for addiction as traditional religious beliefs started to change from a vision of a wrathful and inscrutable God to a more benign and rationalist understanding. A new scientific perspective on alcoholism, morphinism, cocainism, opiumism, and canibisism [marijuana] stimulated a change in view of addiction, so that the addict was seen less as a moral failure and more, the victim of the drug and its maker.

Disputes of this kind continue to rage between religious believers and adherents to secular scientism. Across all kinds of health-related issues today we see this continued divide, with no room in the middle between belief in religion, and belief in science.

Government to the Rescue

On September 14, 1901, President William McKinley was assassinated, and Vice-President Theodore Roosevelt assumed the highest office in the land. At forty-two, Roosevelt was the youngest American President in history, and his subsequent eight years in office would herald the beginning of the Progressive Era in American politics.

The underlying goal of the progressive movement was to improve the climate of opportunity for the common man. The progressive movement led to the significant changes enacted at the national levels including the imposition of an income tax with the Sixteenth Amendment to the Constitution, direct election of Senators with the Seventeenth Amendment, Prohibition with the passage of the Eighteenth Amendment, and women's suffrage through the Nineteenth Amendment.

The roots of progressivism were, in the 1890s, prompted in part by the excesses of the robber barons. The lack of a uniform set of commercial codes and poor controls in the areas of interstate commerce and inconsistent public education had left the American consumer exposed to fraud, misrepresentation, and manipulation, often with dire and deadly consequences. Progressivism also marked a period of social activism that also helped clean up government by exposing the corruptions of political machines and their bosses.

Thanks to the *Collier's Weekly* articles by Samuel Hopkins Adams and the efforts of the temperance movement, President Roosevelt signed into law the Pure Food and Drug Act in 1906. Also called the "Wiley Act," this was the first federal law to require that certain specified substances—including alcohol, cocaine, heroin, morphine, and cannabis—be accurately labeled, with contents and recommended dosage, on the bottles of patent medicines. All these addictive substances continued to be legal in over-the-counter sales, as long as they were properly labeled. Nonetheless, it is estimated that sale of patent medicines containing narcotics decreased by about a third after labeling was mandated.

> *It would not stretch matters to say that the Pure Food and Drug Act of 1906 . . . (P.L. 59–384, 34 Stat. 768), (the Wiley Act) stands as the most consequential regulatory statute in the history of the United States. The act not only gave unprecedented new regulatory powers to the federal government, it also empowered a bureau that evolved into today's Food and Drug Administration (FDA). The legacy of the 1906 Act, includes federal regulatory authority over one-quarter of gross domestic product, and includes market gate keeping power over human and animal drugs, foods, and preservatives, medical devices, biologics, and vaccines.[2]*
> *— Daniel P. Carpenter (Freed Professor of Government, Harvard University) (Landsberg 2004)*

Carpenter, further noted that while other laws of this general era have received more study, including the Sherman and Clayton anti-trust acts, "the Pure Food and Drug Act has had the longest-lasting and most widespread economic, political, and institutional impact."

And yet, the act did not work all that well. The patent medicine industry, already reeling from attacks by the temperance movement and the press, nonetheless, found it fairly easy to circumvent the act in any number of ways. They also were effective in preventing its expansion. When there was an attempt to outlaw Coca-Cola, in 1909, because of its excessive caffeine (which by 1903 had entirely replaced cocaine by as Coca-Cola's active ingredient), the patent medicine men warned their congressmen and newspaper owners that "this act will practically destroy the sale of proprietary medicines, in the US." The effort to outlaw caffeine in Coke failed.

It would not be until 1938, when the next President Roosevelt augmented the Pure Food and Drug Act with real legislative bite, that government regulation put a severe dent in the patent medicine game. Even still, the patent medicine era didn't come to a complete end until 1963. That was when the FDA finally forced the makers of

2 James P. Gray, a drug policy reform advocate, cites this act as a successful model for re-legalization of currently prohibited drugs by requiring accurate labels, monitoring of purity and dose, and consumer education.

Listerine to retract its claim to be a cure for the common cold and to spend $10.2 million in TV ads to assure the public that "contrary to prior advertising, Listerine will not help prevent colds or sore throats or lessen their severity."

Before the passage of the Pure Food and Drug Act in 1906, there was no legislation other than the Sherman Act that truly attempted to control the efficacy of the items sold to the public. The Sherman Act had passed into law in 1890, but no President had been willing to enforce the law until Theodore Roosevelt took office in 1901.

Despite its name, the Sherman Antitrust Act of 1890 had very little to do with "trusts." It is, in fact, a law against monopolistic business practices, and at the time, trusts were popular vehicles for monopolists to evade trading fairly in the market. According to one contemporary account, the Sherman Act's goal "is not to protect business from the working of the market; it is to protect the public from the *failure* of the market." The act was meant to prevent cartels and other entities from damaging free competition. Nowhere in our history has this been more necessary than during the patent medicine era. The prime motivation for its passage was to break the back of monopolies like the Standard Oil Trust, the railroad cartel and to weaken the market control of the patent medicine Proprietary Association.

One of the first major cases prosecuted under the Sherman Act was that of *Dr. Miles Medical Company vs. John D. Park & Sons.* Miles had sued Park & Sons because they were freely discounting his product in violation of the contract that he had with them. The case went all the way to the Supreme Court, which ruled, in 1911, in Park's favor. A majority of the justices agreed that Miles' contracts were unenforceable since their resale price enforcement provisions violated the Sherman Act. This milestone ruling would set the precedent of prohibiting manufacturers from setting minimum retail prices for the next one-hundred years.

Miles changed the wording in his contracts, but continued to try to sidestep the law. Patent medicine men, in general, became adept at obscuring the price paid by purchasers through various schemes, like spiffs, rebates, and market development funds. These same schemes proliferate today as way effectively to obscure pricing and cost. The Sherman Act continues to be litigated to this day, and in recent years, the Supreme Court has ruled in a series of cases that walk back the basic tenets of *Miles vs. Park.* It is no longer black letter law that a manufacturer was prohibited in all circumstances from establishing minimum price guidelines for their downstream outlets.

Prior to the Progressive Era, laws were more often made to protect monopolistic behavior rather than control it. The Trademark Act of 1870, for instance, was passed with support by the rising cartels of the day who wanted protections for their products without having to meet the disclosure requirements of patent law. Under patent law, details of the invention (including chemical formulations) were mandated for disclosure, and inventors relied, on the government, to protect them from infringement. Many inventors, however, including my maternal grandfather, resisted disclosure of their inventions because there was little federal enforcement of the law. Then, just like now, there were people making a business of reading these patents and reverse-engineering them so as to steal the market from the inventor. The Trademark Act was a way around this problem.

After the original Trademark Act of 1870 was struck down, in 1879, as an unconstitutional expansion of power, a new Trademark Act of 1881 was passed in Congress, conceived as an expansion of the Commerce clause of the Constitution. This Act was also lobbied for by the patent medicine makers' Proprietary Association and by various pharmaceutical and drug retailer and distributor associations.

It was not until the Trademark Act of 1905 these certain restrictions were added to the use of trademarks that discouraged cartel behavior in the marketplace. This act *was not* supported by the Proprietary Association. In fact, the Trademark Act of 1905 marked the first split among the Proprietary Association and other trade groups, including the AMA.

In a story, about the AMA annual convention in Baltimore in 1898, *American Druggist and Pharmaceutical Record* reported:

The trade-mark law should so read as to make it necessary for every article of commerce, when first introduced, to have a name given it, for public use, as a part of the common language, it should also require that the common descriptive name, of each article advertised, should appear in advertisements equally prominent with its brand-name, so that the latter may be used, by the public, for the purpose of specifying a particular brand, when desired, and the former employed to designate the article itself as such, irrespective of who is the maker. In describing trees as to natural order, genera, and species, so is it in describing medicines: every kind of tincture, fluid extract, and pill must have a specific name by which it may be described, and if the introducer does not supply it, he has no reasonable complaint if the name claimed by him as a trade-mark ceases to perform its function as a brand-mark and falls into the public domain as a descriptive word or appellative. The trade-mark law should be so revised that its ambiguous wording will not protect those who desire to create perpetual monopolies of secret medicines by claiming that their commonly-accepted names are trade-marks. The main argument was the Trademark law gave exemptions from protection for words and names of common use. ***The AMA now sensing a shift in the tides against the Proprietary Association supported this legislation.***

Other Progressive Era legislation continued to put pressure on Proprietary Association members, breaking the medicine cartel's stranglehold on the industry and causing schisms in the mutually supportive relationships with the other cartels of the day. The Clayton Act of 1914 directly targeted the abusive behaviors exhibited by the patent medicine industry by prohibiting specific types of conduct not deemed in the best interest of a competitive market. It prohibited price discrimination between different purchasers if it reduced competition. It also forbade sales that are conditioned on the buyer not dealing with competing suppliers, or sales that are conditioning on forcing the buyer to purchase other products if such acts substantially lessen competition. Mergers and acquisitions that stood to reduce competition came under federal scrutiny for the first time, as did the practice of individuals maintaining seats on the boards of competing companies.

This increase in legislative force continued to weaken the control of the patent medicine men and also helped prompt the break between the drug retail and distribution cartels, the AMA cartel, and the Proprietary Association.

The first federal law to deal with the problem of narcotic addiction came with Harrison Narcotics Tax Act of 1914. There were hundreds of thousands of opium addicts in the U.S. at the time. Some were men who frequented opium dens operated by Chinese immigrants, but three-quarters were women. In seeking relief from menstrual pains, women obtained opiates though prescriptions by physicians and pharmacists or through purchase of various self-dosed patent medicines. By 1914, forty-six states had enacted regulations on cocaine and twenty-nine states had put in place laws against opium, morphine, and heroin. The Harrison Act forced manufacturers and distributors to register with federal tax collectors, and pay a special tax on "opium or coca leaves—their salts, derivatives, or preparations and—for other purposes." The courts interpreted this to mean that physicians could still prescribe narcotics to patients during normal treatment but not for the treatment of addiction.

Finally, 1919 saw the passage of the Volstead Act, the popular name for the National Prohibition Act, passed through Congress over President Woodrow Wilson's veto on October 28, 1919. The act established the legal definition of intoxicating liquor, and set down various penalties for producing it. Though the Volstead Act prohibited the sale of alcohol, the federal government did little to enforce it. By 1925, in New York City alone, there were anywhere from 30,000 to 100,000 speakeasy clubs.

Many states had already enacted various temperance laws before the Volstead Act was passed. The effect of these laws on the patent medicine industry was very limited; in fact, the Cullen-Harrison amendment provided a "medicinal use" exception to the law that actually gave to patent medicines a boost during what was the industry's period of general decline.

On December 5, 1933, the ratification of the Twenty-first Amendment by the states repealed the Eighteenth Amendment. However, U.S. law still prohibits the manufacture of distilled spirits without meeting numerous licensing requirements, making it impractical to produce distilled spirits for personal beverage use.

Overall, the various Progressive Era laws enacted by both Congress and by state legislatures provided a series of hurdles for the patent medicine men, the pharmacists and physicians, forcing them to change their business dealings. The realization by the AMA, in particular, that a change was in the wind ultimately opened the door to change. According to the *American Druggist and Pharmaceutical Record* of November 1905, a special closed-door meeting of the Proprietary Association was convened to discuss the loss of a case brought under the Sherman Act.

Ostensibly, the case targeted use of a "triparty" contract between the retailer, the Druggist Association and the Proprietary Manufacturer. In *C. G. A. Loder vs. the Philadelphia Retail Druggists Association, et al*, Mr. Loder, a Philadelphia retailer of medicines, was ejected from the Druggists Association because he failed to hold the prices as established by the association. He was then refused delivery of goods from distributors and manufacturers. The writer in the *Pharmaceutical Record* noted that "The gravity of the situation was reflected in the attitude of the principal members, who showed hesitancy about discussing the business of the meeting with the representatives of the pharmaceutical press which looked like real fear."

Later in the article the writer reports the resolutions as adopted. The report reads as follows:

> ***Resolved,*** *That this association thoroughly disapproves of the effort on the part of any person or firms, members of this association or not, to market as medicines any articles which are to be used as alcoholic beverages or in which the medication is insufficient to bring the preparation properly within the category of legitimate medicines.*
>
> *Resolved, That the Legislative committee be and is hereby instructed to earnestly advocate legislation which shall*

> *prevent the use of alcohol in proprietary medicines for internal use in excess of the amount that is absolutely necessary as a solvent and preservative.*
>
> *Resolved, That the Legislative Committee be also instructed to continue its efforts in behalf of legislation for the strictest regulation of the sale of cocaine and other narcotics and poisons or medicinal preparations containing the same.*
>
> *Resolved, That this association urges upon its members the most careful scrutiny of the character of their advertising and of claims for the efficacy of their various prescriptions, avoiding all over statements.*
>
> *It was learned that two firms occupying a high position in the proprietary manufacturing field, who had become dissatisfied with the policy of the association in the recent past, had tendered their resignations, and one firm in membership, a Western concern, which had been denied the use of the mails by the postal authorities, had been asked to resign. The firms, which resigned voluntarily, are understood to be Fairchild Bros. & Foster, New York, and the Mellen's Food Company, Boston.*

Most of the pharmaceutical retailers and druggist associations began to distance themselves from patent medicines and their manufacturers at this time, and began touting the benefits of "Ethical Pharmaceuticals" instead.

One glaring error in the modern interpretation of progressivism has been that the progressives of that day felt it was the role of the federal government to provide additional rights. In fact, much of the writings of the day indicate an obvious and pragmatic approach to the exposure, understanding, and remediation of many of the problems of the day. They dispel the notion that progressivism was directly or indirectly a movement toward socialism.

For instance, in 1915, the American Association of Labor Legislation (AALL) published a draft bill for the compulsory provision of health insurance by employers. Initially the bill was directed at both the U.S. Congress and the state legislatures. Aggressive campaigns were mounted in many states, and received support by the AMA, as you would expect. However, the effort failed to gain any traction. There was consensus in the U.S. at this time that the government had no role in compelling people to be covered with health insurance. A point of character for a person during this period was to be measured by how well they provided for their family and how it was they protected themselves in the event of an unexpected consequence.

Physicians Rise in Power

In 1900, statistics showed that the average American life expectancy from birth to death was 49.2 years. By 1930, it had grown to 59.2 years. No era in our history has ever seen such an impressive gain in longevity.

There were many reasons for this gain. Indoor plumbing reduced disease caused by community sanitation problems. Surgeries performed in hospitals had now become commonplace. Vaccinations continued to spread. Where they existed, hospitals provided valuable care points for all. The adoption of expanded roles for nurses and orderlies, and extended accessibility by automobile, significantly reduced patient mortality in the face of accident or significant injury.

Hospitals increased in numbers throughout the U.S., growing between 1900 and 1930 from 1,400 to 2,100. By the end of the 1920s, baby deliveries and complications from abortions, adenoidectomies, appendectomies, tonsillectomies, and treatment of accident victims accounted for over 60 percent of hospital admissions. A decade later, in the middle of the 1930s, a third of Americans had begun and ended their lives in hospitals, representing an enormous change from just ten years earlier.

There were technological advances, too, but they proved to be a mixed bag of breakthroughs and quackery. Alongside the technological innovation of Willem Einthoven with his invention of the electro-cardiograph in 1903, for instance, came the claim by Dr. John R. Brinkley that male virility could be enhanced by injecting men with colored water. Brinkley called himself an "Electro Medic Doctor," and claimed to practice "electric medicine from Germany." Brinkley would go on to even greater infamy through the transplant of goat testicles into men's scrotums as a virility treatment—with predictably fatal results.

The overall health of the medical profession, however, was still not very good in the early 1900s. Physician incomes had not improved nor had the quality of physician education improved much, outside a few select East Coast cities.

The AMA, on the other hand, was developing real clout. It began to consolidate its power over the licensing of doctors and physicians by campaigning for control over the licensing of medical schools. In 1870, there had been 474 registered medical schools in the U.S. and Canada. By 1904, the AMA's efforts had reduced the number to about 160.

In 1910, the Carnegie Foundation funded a study of America's medical schools in conjunction with the AMA. The study was led by Dr. Abraham Flexner and the resulting Flexner Report provided the necessary clout to bring the AMA forward as the major arbiter of medical education.

The findings of the Flexner Report allowed the AMA to establish strict guidelines for medical education, defining it almost exclusively as the practice of "medical science" in the Allopathic tradition. In conjunction with the power and influence of the Carnegie Foundation, and with the cooperation of the Rockefellers, the AMA succeeded in eliminating the licensure of Homeopathic and Eclectic schools of medicine. The AMA "Propaganda Department" used the Flexner Report to disseminate information cautioning the public about health fraud and quackery.

In 1914, the AMA further asserted its authority with the creation of standards for hospital internships. Around this time, it published, for the first time, a list of approved hospitals for would-be doctors to intern, pending licensure. In other words, if the hospital were not on the AMA list, a doctor-in-training would be wasting his time. He would not get a license. This was how the AMA was able to assert its power and ultimate control over hospitals in the U.S. In 1927, after continually increasing the requirements for education and training of physicians and effectively limiting the number of physicians licensed to practice, the AMA published the first list of hospitals approved for residency training.

By this time, the AMA had gained all-but-complete control of the practice of medicine in the U.S. The Eclectic and Homeopathic schools were dispensed with, and physicians who practiced within these disciplines were either discredited or re-trained and became practicing Allopaths. Two targeted schools of medicine that survived the onslaught, although not without significant reductions in the public view of their practice areas, were osteopathic medicine and chiropractic medicine.

One additional result of the Flexner report is that medical education became much more expensive under AMA standards. This single fact put the pursuit of medicine as a career out of reach of most people, except for upper-class white males. Some remaining proprietary schools and "land grant" schools continued to admit African Americans and women, but for a period of time, access to the medical profession for these two groups was exceedingly limited.

By extending the pre-requisites for admittance to medical school and the duration of medical education, the AMA effectively controlled the form of medicine taught and type of people who could become doctors. By limiting the number of schools, and, in turn, the number of graduates each year eligible for licensure, the AMA at last found a method for increasing physician incomes by controlling the supply of qualified medical professionals.

Of course, the arguments in favor of AMA control point to improvements in the quality of care provided by doctors to their patients. Based on data and findings, it appears that these actions yielded significant improvements in the education of doctors, along with the elimination of many unscrupulous physicians and charlatans. That said, it is naive to believe these humanitarian motives drove the AMA's efforts. Everything the AMA did was carried out to preserve the incomes and future prospects for Allopathic medical practitioners. One might ask whether the elimination of all other forms of treatment was justified. Did we forsake other pragmatic, effective and less heroic methods of treatments as a result of this process? Are some of the current problems in our healthcare system directly or indirectly a result in whole or in part of these steps?

Pharmaceuticals from the Medicine Men

Table 3: A short sampling of the pages from Squibb's Pharmaceutical Catalog published in 1919, shows an interesting collection of products available to druggists:

Cannabis (bulk)	Extract Cannabis Powder
Extract Cannabis Soft bulk	Fluid Extract Cannabis
Tincture Cannabis	Tablets Acetanilid and Cannabis compound
Tablets Cannabis Extract	Tablets Cannabis and Aconite compound
Tablets Zinc Phosphide, Cannabis and Nux	Tablets Cannabis and Hyoscyamus compound
Tablets Cannabis and Strychnine compound	Tablets Nerve Tonic No.5
Tablets Neuralgic (Dr. Kenyon)	Tablets Neuralgic Brown-Sequard
Tablets Neuralgic Brown-Squard (Half Strength)	Tablets Neuralgic Improved
Tablets Triple Bromides and Cannabis Compound	Tablets Zinc Phosphide and Cannabis Compound

Most of our major prescription drug companies had their beginnings in the patent medicine game; although today, they are generally loath to expose their dubious roots to the public. If you take the time to research the history of drug companies on their corporate websites, and leaf through their publications, you will see few, if any, references to patent medicines, nor will you find listings of any of the fraudulent potions, powders, and elixirs that these now-reputable firms once produced.

Bristol Myers-Squibb, for instance, is a multinational empire today, worth $14 billion with 28,000 employees. It began, however, as a company that dealt in medicines of very doubtful value. The company was founded in 1887 when William McLaren Bristol and John Ripley Myers bought a failing drug manufacturer called Clinton Pharmaceutical Company. They released their first nationally recognized product, Sal Hepatica in 1900. Termed "the poor man's spa," it was touted as a laxative mineral salt that, when dissolved in water, could reproduce the taste and effects of the natural mineral waters of Bohemia.

Around this same period, E. R. Squibb, a U.S. Navy medical officer, set up his own laboratory in Brooklyn. By 1859, his circulars advertised thirty-eight preparations. By 1883, he was manufacturing 324 products *and* selling them all over the world—many of them contained cannabis (Table 3).

Warner Lambert sprung from similar origins. In 1879, Dr. Joseph Lawrence and his partner, Jordan Wheat Lambert, came up with a formulation of menthol, thymol, methyl salicylate, and eucalyptol dissolved in a solution of 21.6 percent alcohol. The combination, they felt, had a significant antiseptic effect, and they also believed that the methyl salicylate had an anti-inflammatory effect.

They initially marketed their product as a surgical antiseptic, but it met with little success. Still searching for that magic market, it was next sold as a floor cleaner and as a cure for gonorrhea. Next, in 1895, the pair started to sell it to dentists for oral care. In 1914, it became the first "over-the-counter" mouthwash, sold under the name of Listerine.

It was Jordan Lambert who hit on the idea that in order to sell a new cure, one must identify a new ailment. By the 1920s, he came across the obscure medical phrase "halitosis" as a description for bad breath. Listerine was the cure for this horrid condition that the manufacturer claimed that if left untreated, could "blight anyone's chances of succeeding in romance, marriage or work."

This was the first example of the now-universal technique of inflating a common everyday condition to the level of a pathology that will simply destroy your chances of ever _________! (Feel free to fill in the blank with whatever comes to mind. That is what Lambert and his partner did!)

Along that line of thinking, some of the illnesses we see advertised today for prescription treatments include erectile dysfunction, female sexual dysfunction, attention deficit hyperactivity disorder, restless leg syndrome, social shyness, osteoporosis, bipolar disorder, balding, enlarged prostate, irritable bowel syndrome, high cholesterol, and mildly excess weight (not clinical obesity). This is not to say these conditions don't exist. As with many of these modern cures, the underlying disorder is problematic for some people. The problem is the extent of the illness, the relevance of the issue to the life and health of the individual, and the effectiveness of the treatments, which are wildly exaggerated.

Johnson & Johnson now owns the Listerine brand name, while the Warner Lambert enterprise is now part of Pfizer. Founded, in 1849, in Brooklyn, Pfizer was one of the few pharmaceutical companies that did not dabble in the patent medicine racket directly. Instead, the company was hugely successful in supplying chemicals for the industry. Beginning with the production of iodine, boric, and tartaric acid, Pfizer went on to pioneer the production of citric acid. In later years, many of the original nostrum makers became part of the growing Pfizer empire.

In 1884, Dr. Franklin Miles founded what is now the Miles Laboratories division of the Bayer AG group. One of first curatives produced by the Dr. Miles Medical Company was Dr. Miles' Compound Extract of Tomato. Many of us have this medicine in our refrigerators today and routinely use it at cookouts and ballgames. We call it ketchup.

The industrious Dr. Miles also developed a drug, called "Nervine," as a cure for nervousness, nervous exhaustion, sleeplessness, hysteria, headache, neuralgia, backache, pain, epilepsy, spasms, fits, and St. Vitus' dance. Nervine would eventually be reformulated into an effervescing tablet called Alka-Seltzer.

The Law and Malpractice

Those who suspect that physician concern over malpractice litigation is a modern phenomenon should consider this insert (Figure 4) from the January 1919 *Medical World* magazine:

In response to our request, in the April, 1915, World, page 148, for copies of a blank agreement releasing a surgeon from claims for damages that might ensue upon the performance of a surgical operation, Dr. E. B. Lambert, of Port Jervis, N Y, sent us the following form:

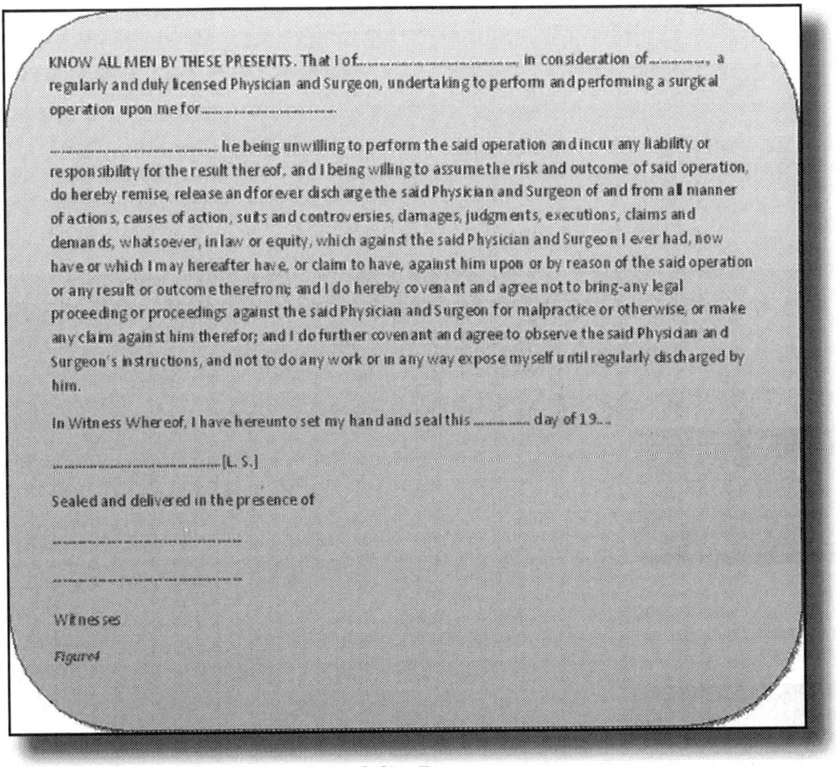

KNOW ALL MEN BY THESE PRESENTS. That I of.............................. in consideration of............, a regularly and duly licensed Physician and Surgeon, undertaking to perform and perfoming a surgical operation upon me for..............................

.... he being unwilling to perform the said operation and incur any liability or responsibility for the result thereof, and I being willing to assume the risk and outcome of said operation, do hereby remise, release and forever discharge the said Physician and Surgeon of and from all manner of actions, causes of action, suits and controversies, damages, judgments, executions, claims and demands, whatsoever, in law or equity, which against the said Physician and Surgeon I ever had, now have or which I may hereafter have, or claim to have, against him upon or by reason of the said operation or any result or outcome therefrom; and I do hereby covenant and agree not to bring-any legal proceeding or proceedings against the said Physician and Surgeon for malpractice or otherwise, or make any claim against him therefor; and I do further covenant and agree to observe the said Physician and Surgeon's instructions, and not to do any work or in any way expose myself until regularly discharged by him.

In Witness Whereof, I have hereunto set my hand and seal this .... day of 19...

..............................[L. S.]

Sealed and delivered in the presence of

....

....

Witnesses

Figure4

Figure 4: Medical World Sample Liability Form

> *This form is a leaf torn out of a book. Another leaf accompanied the agreement, on which a record of the case is made. The following is a copy:*
>
> *Memoranda to form.*
>
> *Note.—Full particulars, complications, if any, and condition when discharged. If patient neglects to observe instructions or does anything to hazard recovery, a record of same should be made here.*
>
> *It is better to have an understanding and execute the release soon after the operation is performed than before.*

There were further instructions, not reproduced here, on how to create a post-surgical record in order to protect the surgeon from the patient and his lawyer. Before this period, surgical notes were not taken routinely and few, if any, were designed to protect the doctor from a lawsuit. It is obvious these physicians were being alerted to the rising tide of litigation, for mistakes real or imagined, as a result of their attempts to provide relief to the suffering of others.

While there was ample justification for lawsuits that targeted known charlatans and quacks, all physicians quickly became at risk. Physicians provided services in a discipline that was based more in art than science, despite marketing their profession as that of medicinal *science*. In the diagnosis and treatment of disease, in that period, the number of potential causes for the symptoms presented was even larger than the suspected causes today, given the advances in knowledge have been made over the past one-hundred years. Physicians then, as now, were wise to make a series of step-wise decisions in order to narrow down the root-cause and treatment. Each step can present the physician with a potential second guess later. Even in 1910, the issue of "hindsight is 20/20" for liability was an ugly specter. Like the sword of Damocles, this risk started to hang oppressively over the heads of practitioners during this period, and its size has continued to grow ever since.

The Life and Death of a Patent Medicine King: Dr. Morse's Indian Root Pills

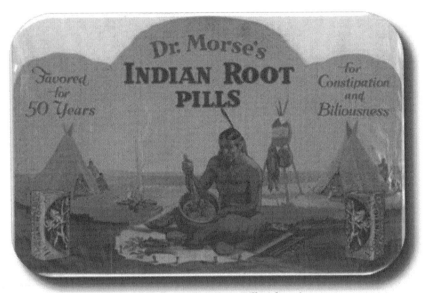

Figure 5: Dr. Morse Indian Root Pills Advertisement

Picturesque Morristown lies on the banks of the St. Lawrence River in northern New York. Few visitors to this sleepy town, organized in 1871, would suspect that it once been home for over a century to one of the most famous and infamous purveyors of patent medicines of the late nineteenth and twentieth centuries: the W. H. Comstock factory, better known as the manufacturer of Dr. Morse's Indian Root Pills.

Morristown had been a quiet backwater, 280 miles from New York City, before the Comstock brothers relocated their operations there in 1867. They moved there, in part to jettison some of their notoriety for a series of lawsuits between the family members in the business and many others in New York City. Dairy farming was the main economic activity in the area prior to the arrival of the Comstocks. Lacking a powerful water flow at this part of the St. Lawrence, Morristown never developed as a major haven for mills. It was the arrival of the Comstock operation that spurred a significant period of growth in the town.

Besides its isolation, what attracted the Comstock brothers to Morristown was its proximity to Canada and access to land immediately across the river. It was also the perfect location for shipping. At the time of the relocation of the W. H. Comstock factory, the railroad was just beginning operations in the area, making travel back-and-forth to New York simple and convenient. Comstock not only developed a factory in Morristown but developed a similar operation directly across the river in the Canadian town of Brockville. It was this dual production and distribution system that helped the Comstocks become one of the dominant players in the patent medicine game.

Like many in others in the same game, the Comstocks were hard men in a hard business. Founded by Edwin Comstock in 1833—along with numerous other brothers and sons—their business evolved as a result of a number of questionable and contentious events in its early history.

Table 4: Comstock sold many more products other than the signature Root Pills. In 1854, Comstock & Company—then controlled by Lucius Comstock, listed nearly forty of its own preparations for sale, namely:

Oldridge's Balm of Columbia	George's Honduras Sarsaparilla
East India Hair Dye, colors the hair and not the skin	Acoustic Oil, for deafness
Vermifuge	Bartholomew's Expectorant Syrup
Carlton's Specific Cure for Ringbone, Spavin, and Wind-galls	Dr. Sphon's Head Ache Remedy
Dr. Connol's Gonorrhea Mixture	Mother's Relief
Nipple Salve	Roach and Bed Bug Bane
Spread Plasters	Judson's Cherry and Lungwort
Azor's Turkish Balm, for the Toilet and Hair	Carlton's Condition Powder, for Horses and Cattle
Connel's Pain Extractor	Western Indian Panaceas
Hunter's Pulmonary Balsam	Linn's Pills and Bitters
Oil of Tannin, for Leather	Nerve & Bone Liniment (Hewe's)
Nerve & Bone Liniment (Comstock's)	Indian Vegetable Elixir
Hay's Liniment for Piles	Kline Tooth Drops
Tooth Ache Drops	Carlton's Nerve and Bone Liniment, for Horses
Condition Powders, for Horses	Pain Killer
Lin's Spread Plasters	Carlton's Liniment for the Piles, warranted to cure
Dr. McNair's Acoustic Oil, for Deafness	Dr. Larzetti's Acoustic Oil, for Deafness
Salt Rheum Cure	Azor's Turkish Wine
Dr. Larzetti's Juno Cordial, or Procreative Elixir	British Heave Powders

The Comstock family came from a medical background, and many of them were, or had worn, the moniker of physician. More interestingly, and likely very telling, is that the Comstock family home was in Connecticut only a few miles from the maker of the first American patent medicine, Lee's "Bilious Pills." "Bilious Pills" both from Lee and many other imitators, found such public acclaim and rapid success that it certainly must have had a profound impact on Edwin's decision to venture forth in the same line of business.

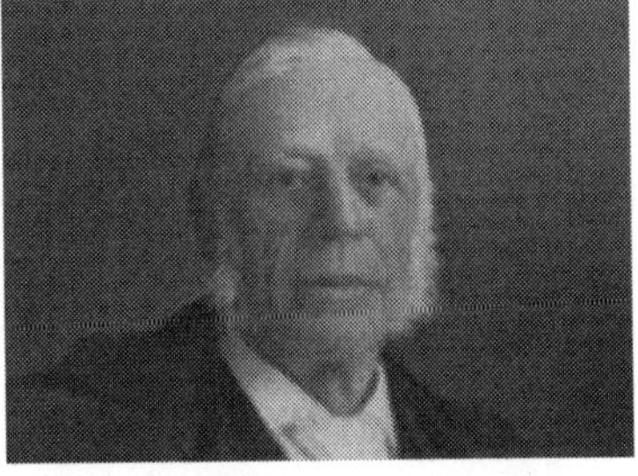
Figure 6: William H. Comstock - 1910

Clearly, Edwin was not a novice when he established his business in 1833 at New York City. As the years progressed, he would bring his brother Lucius into the business and also other brothers: Albert Lee, John Carlton, and George Wells. He later took on his son William Henry, who ultimately succeeded him and who was the Comstock who brought the factory to Morristown (Figure 6).

Like many of the patent medicines of the day, none of the Comstock's products were patented. Instead, they relied on the new trademark laws for protection. Also like many others, they had numerous unscrupulous counterfeiters—including members of their own family.

A great book for those who would like to learn more about the tortured history of the Comstock family along with the development of the patent medicine business might be obtained in the *History of the Comstock Patent Medicine Business and Dr. Morse's Indian Root Pills* by Robert B. Shaw[3].

Because of its diverse inventory, Comstock became one of the major patent medicine companies during this period.

As Comstock began to develop its product line, the patent-medicine era was entering its golden years. As Shaw states in his book, "Improved transportation, wider circulation of newspapers and periodicals, and cheaper and better bottles all enabled the manufacturers of the proprietary remedies to expand distribution—

3 The book was published in 1916, and still available from Google Books.

the enactment and enforcement of federal drug laws was still more than a generation in the future. So patent medicines flourished; in hundreds of cities and villages over the land enterprising self-proclaimed druggists devised a livelihood for themselves by mixing some powders into pills or bottling some secret elixir—normally containing a high alcoholic content or some other habit-forming element—created some kind of legend about this concoction, and sold the nostrum as the infallible cure for a wide variety of human (and animal) ailments. And, many conservative, old ladies, each one of them a pillar of the church and an uncompromising foe of liquor, cherished their favorite remedies to provide comfort during the long winter evenings. But, of this myriad of patent-medicine manufacturers, only a scant few achieved the size, the recognition, and wide distribution of Dr. Morse's Indian Root Pills and the other leading Comstock remedies."

Comstock took the lead as one of the leading pioneers of the almanac—a sales brochure phenomenon of the day. Almanacs were so popular and so widely distributed that it was typical for a person to walk into any drugstore and pick up three or four of them. Some of these publications grew rapidly from just a few pages, to over sixty-four pages by the mid-1800s.

Stories published in the almanacs of the discovery of these nostrums, and on the wrappers of the elixirs themselves, provided great reading and were the story-board commercial of their day. Mr. Shaw relates in his book some examples of such inventive pitches,

---

Before 1900, the detailed story of the discovery of Dr. Morse's pills was abridged to a brief summary, and during the 1920s, this tale was abandoned altogether, until the end the principal ingredients were identified as natural herbs and roots used as a remedy by the Indians. In more recent years, the character and purpose of Dr. Morse's pills also changed substantially. As recently as 1918, years after the passage of the Federal Food and Drug Act of 1906, they were still being recommended as a cure for the diseases listed in Table 5:

Further, two entire pages in the almanac were devoted to explaining how, on the authority of "the celebrated Prof. La Roche of Paris," appendicitis could be cured by the pills without a patient having to resort to the surgeon's knife.

In another segment from the book, Mr. Shaw relays information mainly directed to the female health problems of the day.

THE GREAT FEMALE MEDICINE the almanac read:

The functional irregularities peculiar to the weaker sex are invariably corrected without pain or inconvenience by the use of Judson's Mountain Herb Pills. They are the safest and surest medicine for all the diseases incidental to females of all ages, and more especially so in this climate.

Table 5: Dr. Morse's list of diseases cured	
Biliousness	Dyspepsia
Constipation	Sick Headache
Scrofula	Kidney Disease
Liver Complaint	Jaundice
Piles	Dysentery
Colds	Boils
Malarial Fever	Flatulency
Foul Breath	Eczema
Gravel	Worms
Female Complaints	Rheumatism
Neuralgia	La Grippe
Palpitation	Nervousness

Ladies who wish to enjoy health should always have these Pills. No one who ever uses them once will ever allow herself to be without them. They remove all obstructions, purify the blood and give to the skin that beautiful, clear and healthful look so greatly admired in a beautiful and healthy woman. At certain periods, these Pills are an indispensable companion. From one to four should be taken each day, until relief is obtained. A few doses occasionally, will keep the system healthy, and the blood so pure, that diseases cannot enter the body.

Watch any television show, listen to any radio broadcast or read any periodical or newspaper and one of the most prevalent areas of medicinal support will point to the area of sexual dysfunction. Viagra and Cialis are boldly marketed for the treatment of men's lack of "libido" or rigor in performance. Only slightly more discreetly advertised are products for women related to dryness, libido enhancements or other more prurient pursuits. While we think these issues are a modern connivance, they are not. Again Mr. Shaw's excellent history provides valuable insight to back up this assertion. It reads:

Over on the Canadian side of the river, where another plant approximately the same size as the Morristown facilities was in operation, the Comstock Company had assimilated the Dr. Howard Medicine Co. Dr. Howard's leading remedies were his Seven Spices for all Digestive Disorders and the Blood Builder for Brain and Body. The latter, in the form of pills, was prescribed as a positive cure for a wide array of ailments, but like many other patent medicines of the era, it was hinted that it had a particularly beneficial effect upon sexual vitality.

They have an especial action (through the blood) upon the ***Sexual Organs*** *of both Men and Women. It is a well-recognized fact that upon the healthy activity of the sexual apparatus depend the mental and physical well-being of every person come to adult years. It is that which gives the rosy blush to the cheek, and the soft light to the eye of the maiden. The elastic step, the ringing laugh, and the strong right arm of the youth own the same mainspring. How soon do irregularities rob the face of color, the eye of brightness?*

Everyone knows this. The blood becomes impoverished, the victim ***Pale****. This pallor of the skin is often the outward mark of the trouble within. But, to the sufferer there arise a host of symptoms, chiefest among which are loss of physical and nervous energy. Then Dr. Howard's* ***Blood Builder*** *steps into the breach and holds the fort. The impoverished Blood is enriched. The shattered nervous forces are restored. Vigor returns. Youth is recalled. Decay routed. The bloom of health again mantles the faded cheek. Improvement follows a few days' use of the pills; while permanent benefit and cure can only reasonably be* *expected when sufficient have been taken to enrich the Blood.*

Before the Blood Builder pills were taken, all their users were advised to have their bowels thoroughly cleansed by a laxative medicine and, happily, the company also made an excellent preparation for this purpose—Dr. Howard's Golden Grains. While the good doctor was modern enough—the circular quoted from was printed in the 1890s—to recognize the importance of the healthy activity of the sexual apparatus, such a suggestion should not be carried too far—so we find that the pills were also unrivaled for building up systems shattered by debauchery, excesses, self-abuse or disease. Along with the pills themselves, was recommended a somewhat hardy regimen, including fresh air, adequate sleep, avoidance of lascivious thoughts, and bathing the private parts and buttocks twice daily in ice-cold water.

Certainly during the early days of the "Victorian" era these findings did not soften the ardor of the general populace who took to these remedies nor did the nature of these times force subtlety in the description of the cures available. Today, the main findings we see pushed down our throats, very often literally, are cures for sexual dysfunction, "female problems," constipation, the common cold or flu, mental stimulation, and my favorite compensating for loss of energy. If one looks at the advertising for Comstock's products one will see a historical mirror illustrating the sale of exactly the maladies and remedies for them, sometimes by the use of blunt and bold copy. Most of the messages were communicated via the almanacs, product wrappers and newspapers. It would not be unlikely for all concerned about the evolution of healthcare not to wonder how much longer the patent medicine men would have held sway if radio and television had also been mediums to reach the gullible public. Then again, who is to say these purveyors of the quack and addictive have disappeared?

In a final section from the book, Shaw cites two other main points of interest during this period in which Comstock stands out as a solid illustrative member of the illustrious patent medicine industry; the use of testimonials in advertising its products and the lack of hard money in communities (important later relative to understanding the issues physicians faced in their practice, in rural communities). The use of testimonials was critical in the sale of these nostrums. The experience of the everyday user was what rung most true to consumers, again just like today. A great deal of newspaper ink was devoted to the publication of the merits of this nostrum or that elixir. On rare occasions, they showed up as advertisements. More often than not, they also appeared as articles and letters to an editor. Mr. Shaw summarizes these issues as follows.

> *Testimonials submitted voluntarily by happy users of the pills were always widely featured in the almanacs, newspaper advertisements, and handbills. Although, the easy concoction of the stories about Dr. Morse and Dr. Cunard might suggest that there would have been no hesitation in fabricating these testimonials, it is probable that they were genuine; at least, many have survived in the letters scattered over the floor of the Indian Root Pill factory. In some cases, one might feel that the testimonials were lacking in entire good faith, for many of them were submitted by dealers desiring lenient credit or other favors—witness, for example, the enclosed letter (reproduction) from B. Mollohan of Mt. Pleasant, Webster County, West Va., on April 16, 1879. (Figure 7)*

June 18, 1861

Please find here enclosed Two dolars & 50¢ for wich pleas Place to my credit and return receipt to me for same. I can't praise your Dr. Morse Pill two high never before in all my recollection has there been a meddeson here that has ~~done~~ given such general satisfaction. I hope the pills will always retain their high standing and never be counterfitted. I could sell any amt Pills almost if money wernt so scarce. I have to let some out on credit to the sick & poor & wait some time though I am accountable to you for all I recd and pay you as fast as I collect. I have about 1 Doz box on hand

Signed:
B. Mollohan

Figure 7: B. Mollohan Letter – 1861 (reproduction)

> *Mollohan's complaint about the shortage of money and the long delay in collecting many accounts reflected a condition that prevailed throughout the nineteenth century. Money was scarce, and the economy of many rural communities was still based largely on the barter system, so that it was very difficult for farmers to generate cash for store goods. Consequently, country storekeepers had to be generous in extending credit, and, in turn, manufacturers and jobbers had to be lenient in enforcing collection.*

Contrary to popular perception, and in spite of many government regulations and actions taken, by numerous associations, to curtail the business of patent medicines, the W. H. Comstock enterprise continued to thrive long after World War II. The company reached its heyday shortly after World War I, but continued to sell many of its nostrums to retailers and distributors until March 31, 1960, when the last shipment of Dr. Morse's Indian Root Pills left the building. One, one-dozen box of pills was sent to Gilman Brothers of Boston, and two, one-dozen boxes were sent to McKesson & Robbins of Mobile, Alabama on April 11, of that year. With this final consignment, the factory closed its doors, ending ninety-three years of continuous operation in the riverside village of Morristown.

In many ways W. H. Comstock was a true representative of the rise and decline of patent medicine manufacturers of the early twentieth century. I use the term decline, as opposed to death. It will be left up to the reader to determine if the patent medicine era has died or if the leopard has simply changed its spots. Later in this section, and in the others that follow, the reader will note that most of the companies are still with us, they have just changed their tactics or abandoned the "medicine" market for what is now referred to as "ethical pharmaceuticals" and/or the consumer product category. Perhaps as a reader, you may come to the conclusion that "ethical" is a very flexible word when it comes to the acceptance and approval of pharmaceuticals. After almost one hundred years, the last true survivors of the original patent medicine era went out of business. Many others continue to survive, to this day, but they long ago gave up the "patent medicine" game. Today they continue to present their suspect wares as nutraceuticals, consumer products, drinks, candies and confections or have morphed into "ethical" pharmaceutical companies.

Final Thoughts

As Judge Loker was contemplating the relative benefits of new technologies as they applied to his daily routine and the culture around him, so did many others just like him. In this short period, more than any other time in our history, the role of technologies in the public's general welfare showed dramatic changes.

Air conditioning was invented, in 1902, by Willis Carrier as a way to gain productivity in factories, during the hot and humid summer months. Dave Lennox's invention of the riveted steel stove in 1850 for industrial use gave rise to home furnaces, replacing fireplaces as the main source of heat. Extending the gains of gas lighting; gas kitchen stoves begin to replace kitchen wood stoves improving the convenience and availability of well cooked food.

By 1903, when Judge Loker was thirty-one years of age, Ford Motor Company incorporated. Henry Ford introduced the assembly line to lower the cost of automobiles, so the common man could readily afford one. In that process, Ford introduced the Model 'A' automobile. It was reported, that 1703 cars were made the first year which revolutionized transportation and which also reduced the role of the horse (thus the death of the buggy whip!) Within a few years, people were able to travel farther over distant terrain opening access to goods and services that were otherwise not available. Rural communities now had better access to hospitals in nearby cities—facilities that were not accessible before the popularity and affordability of the automobile.

By 1914, there were fifty-five electric grids available in the US; more and more people were replacing expensive and dangerous oil, kerosene, and gas lamps with the electric light which created an opportunity for a more productive day. Previously, days were shortened by darkness since homes and factories would close for the day when the sun went down. Now they could stay open and work into the night. Soon factories were running twenty-four hours a day due to this marvelous invention.

In 1917, air conditioning made a huge leap from the factory floor into commercial venues debuting at New Empire Theatre in Montgomery, Alabama. Today, it is hard to imagine going to watch a movie in the summer without air conditioning.

Like the Judge, some in this period were not immediately enamored by "modern conveniences." While it is obvious that advances in technological and medical sciences brought substantial gains to society, many worried and questioned the unintended consequences brought on by their use. For Judge Loker the car, at first, was a wondrous invention, but the loss of his daughter to the contraption changed his perspective. Historically, we can see by the comparison of culture, modernity, and technology coming together simultaneously, these factors can have both positive and negative effects.

While science was taking a strong foothold in society, science was also used, as a method, to attack opposing views in many areas deemed a threat. The AMA used the rising interest in science, against the other forms of medical practice, thereby making the public increasingly more skeptical of the results emerging from the use of technologies. For others, just like Judge Loker, the advent of electricity, the light bulb, radio, medicines, surgeries, telephone, and automobiles were double edged swords. The public had only recently been made aware of the destruction, to society, caused by the medicinal nostrums where they had put their faith. And, with only small change, distrust of scientific and medical advancements remains today.

Chapter 4 Addendum
Medical Advances 1900 – 1929

- Smallpox vaccination became mandatory and widely available, which drastically reduced the incidence of this killer.

- 1901, Karl Landsteiner described the cause of blood transfusion failure by identifying 4 blood groups. His findings greatly reduced deaths and aided in surgical procedures and treatments.

- 1907, the first successful transfusion, based on Landsteiner's ABO typing system was performed.

- 1907 – 1909, Dr. David Marine, a young doctor from Cleveland, OH, began working explicitly on using iodine-fortified salt to prevent goiter.

- 1913, Dr. Paul Dudley became one of America's first cardiologists and pioneered the use of the electro cardiograph in the diagnosis of diseases of the heart.

- 1917, The American Pharmaceutical Association, proposed that the six national associations, including the patent medicine Proprietary Association, work as one because the six organizations had not yet been effectively organized and unified. They were not analogous to other organized professions such as dentistry, law and medicine. This laid the modern groundwork for the APhA powerhouse organization that still controls Pharma today.

- 1922, insulin was used to treat diabetes.

- 1923, vaccine for diphtheria became available.

- 1924, iodized salt was commonly available in the U.S., Goiter incidence plummets. Incidence of goiter in Detroit went from 9.7 percent to 1.4 percent within six years.
- 1926, the vaccine for pertussis (Whooping Cough) was discovered.
- 1927, the vaccine for tuberculosis developed.
- 1928, Alexander Fleming discovered penicillin
- 1920s buffered aspirin becomes widely available.

V. (1930 – 1949)
New Depression, New Deal, New War

Imagine . . .

Judge William M. Loker
Leonardtown-Hollywood Road
Leonardtown, Maryland

July 10, 1947

Dear Pop,

I hope you and Ma are doing well. Katie, the children, and I will see you on the 26th for the one-year anniversary of Brother Clyde [Leck's] passing. We will leave Baltimore about 7:30AM and should arrive at about 11:00AM. Tell Ma, that little Sissy can't wait to have her hushpuppies and gravy.

She loves her grandparents so much, and she tells Katie and me that she wants to spend the summer with her Ma and Pop in Leonardtown. We keep trying to tell her, that at four years old, she is too young and, at seventy-four, you are too old, but she won't hear of it. You know you brought this on yourself the last visit, when you told her to, "come visit and stay a while next time." I am going to ask Aleck and Margaret if she can stay with them next summer.

Since the government is funding the expansion and development of rural hospitals, two of my friends here at Mercy hospital and I are working with Dr. Guyther to help him get St. Mary's Hospital off the ground. I have agreed to help them secure their surgery licensure by becoming the surgeon of record. I finally will be able to bring part of my practice back to Leonardtown and help our neighbors, just like you always wished. I told Ma on the phone this morning, you really should use it, you know;

I will be coming down every week on Tuesday nights and staying at the house with you. I will get up early Wednesday and go to St. Mary's and operate all day on those that need it and return home to Katie and the kids Wednesday night. Dr. Guyther will do all the follow up.

Both Dr. Guyther and I have agreed we will accept as payment whatever the people of St. Mary's can pay or provide. I know that cash is scarce, so perhaps Ma can teach my New York City wife how to make preserves and can goods. I am sure we will be getting a lot of produce, crabs, and oysters very soon. In speaking to Aleck, he said half of his law practice income is paid with hams, bacon, crabs, oysters, and tomatoes. At least, we can bring some better hospital services closer to those that need them.

Truman's Hill-Burton Act should really help grow rural hospitals around the country, just like it is doing in the county. A number of my colleagues are also starting to go back to their home towns and foster the development of their own hospitals. When Congress and the President were talking about a national insurance policy, the AMA was dead set against it as they felt it would give the government too much say in our practice. Privately, many felt that it would also restrict incomes and as you know many of us are not getting rich.

There is a growing trend among doctors who seem to think medicine is simply about money. I recently sponsored an exchange student from Sweden, so he could come to the U.S. as a resident and ultimately open a practice here. His education is outstanding, he is very bright, and I think he will become a gifted surgeon in his own right, but time and again I have to counsel him to stop thinking of the money and to focus instead on providing care and relief of suffering. The livelihood would then simply come. Sadly, most of this "new batch of physicians" looks at the profession more as a path to riches, not as a calling to care for their neighbors.

It is hard to believe Leck has passed. I know it has been yet another tough year for you and Ma. Forty is simply not the age we expect anyone to die these days, although, when you were born it was the average lifespan for your generation. I fear these cancers will be the deadly plague that we suffer, for generations yet to come. I know to most, medicine over the past few years seems like it has discovered one miracle after another. The newspapers seem to report new "Miracle Cures" like penicillin, streptomycin, sulfa-drugs, and others every day. The National Cancer Institute, started 10 years ago, is helping identify the various types of cancer; but the truth is, we still know almost nothing about the causes and preventions of what we treat.

Cancer seems the most mysterious of all. As one of the chief surgeons at Mercy, I am now doing cancer surgeries on a regular basis. Many of my patients, of late, are women suffering from cancer of the breast. I am rapidly becoming the surgeon with the most experience, and I see, every day, more and more women suffering from this disease. Unlike other tumors, it is clear that in many cases simply taking out the breast does not stop the disease. In at least half the cases, I remove what appears to be the entire diseased breast, a painful and humiliating experience for the poor woman, only to find the cancer reappears in either the other breast or somewhere else in the body. The survival rate for a breast cancer diagnosis is not good. So far no one seems to know for sure, either how this spreads or the best way to treat it. Surgery remains the only, and very poor, option.

More and more, my colleagues are concerned over the increasing number of lawsuits for "malpractice." Clearly, when an ill-trained or incompetent physician causes harm to a patient that individual should receive some form of compensation; and if the cost drives them from the practice I say good—they deserve it. But, more and more, in my view, the doctors have been neither negligent nor incompetent. They are following good sound diagnostic principles and the available protocols.

Despite what most doctors seem to indicate, medicine simply does not have all the answers. The lawyers want to make the public think that a doctor should cure anything the first time and every time. This is simply not reasonable, as often many symptoms can sometimes be caused by countless different reasons. If they continue to bring good doctors up on charges because they followed a series of steps to find and help the patient, and in the end, no cure was available, and then who will risk their livelihood to treat the risky diseases. I worry more and more I will get sued for trying to help a patient, who without any intervention, will die, and who dies regardless of my best efforts and I then lose my home, my family's savings and my livelihood in the process. Perhaps you, Aleck and I can discuss this on the 26th after Leck's memorial. I feel that I have to find some way better to protect my family, and continue my "Good Samaritan" practice.

I am very happy to gain the ability to come back to the county weekly and finally be able to help my neighbors as a result of the deal with Dr. Guyther. Katie and I have built a successful and wonderful life in Baltimore, but as I said to you before; I have always felt guilty for not being able to bring my skills back home sooner. While the restrictions on licensing and standards of practice have been necessary and have really cleaned up the practice of medicine and, provided tremendous advancements in the quality of care for people in the cities, the same regulations have, up until recently, made it difficult for doctors to build practices in rural communities. It has been hard enough for general practitioners and, until recently it was almost impossible for surgeons.

Leck's passing reminds me of when Betty died. I remember at that time deciding to become a doctor and in my childish way deciding I was going to learn all I could and come up with ways to fix anything that got broken in people. While I have spent many years in school and in my practice, sometimes I feel I have learned so much, and I often have the satisfaction to know I have made a real difference to this one or that one. But, overall, more often than not, I feel I have learned nothing! With the exception of small things like antibiotics for infection, vaccination as preventatives for many diseases, and numbers of surgical procedures, I still can't fix many of the things that break in people. I wonder if we ever will!

Despite the somber circumstance of our gathering ten days hence, Katie, the kids, and

I look forward to seeing you, Ma and the rest of the family soon. I will talk to Aleck and see if we can arrange, for Sissy to stay with them next summer. In the meantime, I may bring her down home with me on occasion to visit, with you and Ma, while I am at the hospital.

Lastly, Ma tells me you will finally retire next year. We should start to plan that party. I think most of St. Mary's County will want to come.

Love from all of us!
Your loving son;
Ford Loker, MD

The First Great Depression

Perhaps it was our long history of recessions and depressions that focused the moderated responses to signs of economic problems prior to, and throughout, the Wall Street collapse of 1929. There are many theories and few clear-cut answers. The Great Depression not only had a significant impact on the economy. In violent ways, it illustrated the need for an effective safety net for healthcare, housing and the general welfare of vulnerable groups such as children and the elderly.

The issues that we have with our healthcare system today, continue to be sociological, political, economic, and medical-science related. In this chapter, we will spend some time on the economy and War that characterize much of this period. As we slog through this history, please note that many of the weeds that now plague our healthcare system got

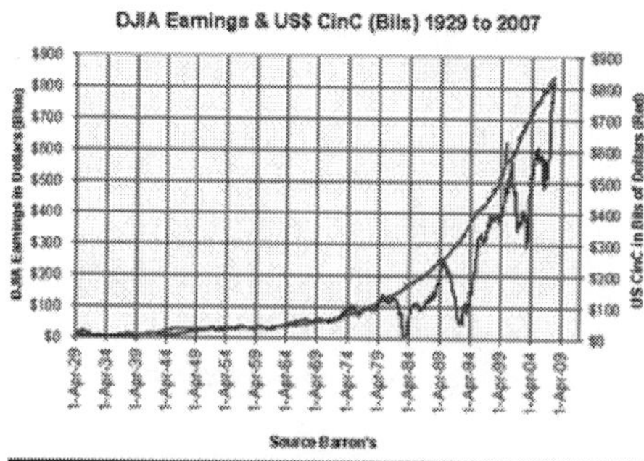

Chart 1: Dow Jones Industrial Avg. vs. U.S. CinC

planted, and laid down strong roots, as a result of the decisions made to address the economic issues resulting from the Great Depression or to prosecute World War II—often intended as short term solutions that later became permanent.

The Great Depression followed closely by World War II, fostered a new set of expectations for government. These events forever altered the idealistic and self-focused, traditionalist understanding of whom we are as U.S. citizens, what we as people expect from ourselves, and what we expect the government to provide to us or do for us. This period is defined by the rise of "American Exceptionalism," the idea that the United States is qualitatively different from all other nations of the world.

Many historians see the cause of the Great Depression as the sudden collapse of the U.S. Stock Market. More and more modern economists see the 1929 Stock Market collapse as a symptom rather than the cause. In 1929, as the Market was crashing John D. Rockefeller said,

> *These are days when many are discouraged. In the ninety-three years of my life, depressions have come and gone. Prosperity has always returned and will again.*

In fact, the market actually turned upward again in early 1930 and returned to the early 1929 levels by April of 1930. Together, both the U.S. government and business spent more money in the first half of 1930 than they had in the same period, in 1929. So then, from a purely market perspective, despite the wide spread panic of the days immediately surrounding the crash the Stock Market itself, much of the market began to recover and did so relatively quickly. The collapse of the banks, on the other hand, had much greater impact. The chart illustrated in Chart 1 shows the Dow Jones Industrial Average (DJIA) compared to the U.S. Currency in Circulation (CinC) from 1929 to 2007. You can see a huge correlation between the amount of currency injected into the economy and the rise in the DJIA.

The next chart, Chart 2, shows the relationship between the Dow Jones Industrial Average during the period of 1900 to 2010, but it has been adjusted to account for inflation in the currency during these years. What is shocking to see is that when you correct for inflation, the DJIA in 1995 is below the peak of 1929. Further it shows that the bear market of 1966 to 1982 was almost as severe as that of the early 1930s.

There were multiple causes for the first downturn in 1929. These include structural weaknesses and specific events that turned a recession into a major depression. Further complicating the issue was the dominance of the U.S. in the world market and the manner in which our downturn spread from country to country.

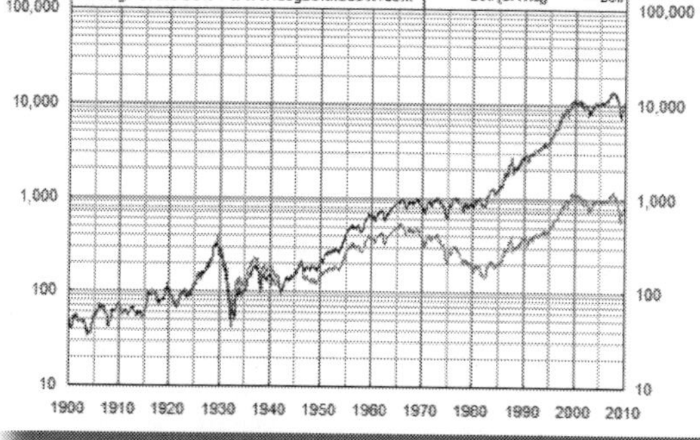

Chart 2: DJIA & Inflation Adjustment

Relative to the 1929 downturn, historians emphasize structural factors like massive bank failures and the stock market crash. In contrast, economists (such as Barry Eichengreen, Milton Friedman, and Peter Temin) point to monetary factors such as actions by the U.S. Federal Reserve that contracted the money supply, as well as Britain's decision to return to the Gold Standard at pre-World War I parities—the U.S. dollar to the English Pound ratio of $4.86 : £1.00.

Two primary and historical factors likely caused the Great Depression. First, since the founding of the country, America had remained a highly debt-laden country and was often subject to wide swings of inflation followed by deflation. Historically, we have seen these boom and bust swings over and over since our very inception as a nation. A look at any history book written prior to 1930 shows numerous and regular national cycles of boom and bust. Second, the mechanics of our economic system, based on its fractional reserve debt structure, and, at the time, the dependence on sufficient specie (gold reserves) to back our currency, once again the country had simply run out of the ability to print money without significantly devaluing the currency because of imbedded regulations on the percentage of gold reserve (40 percent). By not acting to break the tie to specie-backed currency and issue more dollars, the Federal Reserve did nothing, so its policy of monetary contraction reduced the available currency by over one-third thereby transforming what would have been a normal recession into a full on depression.

As cash and gold supplies dried up, banks failed, gold became hoarded as the value of the U.S. dollar dropped and less gold was in the government's vaults. In order for the Federal Reserve to stay within the 40 percent regulation standards, this action caused more contraction of the currency, and as a result, a rapid and severe downward spiral ensued. Americans were no longer simply circling the drain; collectively the country was firmly caught in the suction of the whirlpool effect as it slipped categorically and rapidly down the tubes.

It is now easily understood why President Hoover's protectionist actions like the Smoot-Hawley Tariff Act hurt the economy more than it helped it; his policies failed miserably to reverse the downturns.

Historically, it is also clear that while the market crash and failed economic policies had a severe effect on the American economy and the average American, the Dust Bowl crop failures in the early 1930s contributed to

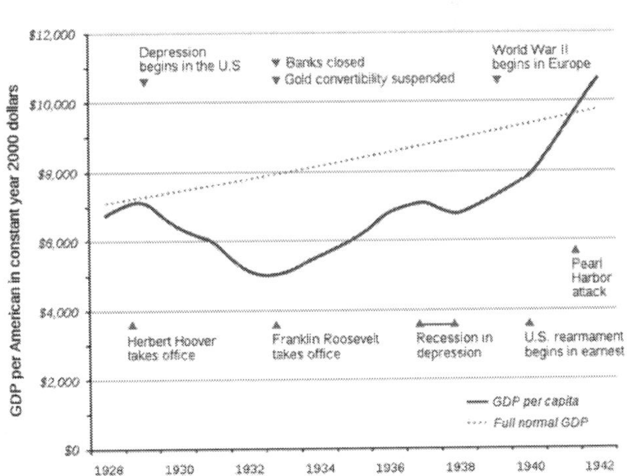

Chart 3: Chart of GDP during the Depression - by William D. O'Neil

the problem. The drought of 1933 and its effect on the erosion of the topsoil caused the Dust Bowl in the Midwest, an event that exacerbated the problem in scope and scale. It soon became even more of a national, and ultimately an international, crisis.

Shortly after having been elected in 1932, Franklin D. Roosevelt argued that a restructuring of the economy would be needed to prevent another depression or avoid prolonging the current one. New Deal programs sought to stimulate demand and provide work and relief for the impoverished through increased government spending and the implementation of financial reforms. (Chart 3)

Following those pivotal moves, the Securities Act of 1933 comprehensively regulated the securities industry. This was then followed by the Securities Exchange Act of 1934, which created the Securities and Exchange Commission. Federal insurance of bank deposits was provided by the FDIC, coupled with, the Glass-Steagall Act. Additionally, the establishment of the National Recovery Administration (NRA) brought about a series of wage and price controls. Today, it remains one of the most controversial actions taken during that period. The NRA made a number of sweeping changes to the American economy until 1935, when its provisions were deemed unconstitutional by the Supreme Court.

President Roosevelt enacted several early changes in what is now called his first "New Deal" including:

- ✓ Establishing regulations to fight deflationary "cut-throat competition" through the NRA.
- ✓ Setting minimum prices and wages, labor standards, and competitive conditions in all industries by NRA regulations.
- ✓ Encouraging unionization, but excluding public employees, as a method by which it could raise wages, in order to increase the power of working people
- ✓ Forcing businesses to work with the government to set price codes, through the NRA

- ✓ Cutting farm production and forcing a rise in food prices through the Agriculture Adjustment Act.

In his Second New Deal, Roosevelt also brought into play the Social Security Act, an initially short term limited social insurance program designed to protect senior citizens, whose lives had been devastated by the Depression. The Works Progress Administration (WPA), introduced as a government jobs program, was also a new face in the economic landscape. It proved to be a strong stimulus to the growth and power of labor unions.

In 1929, total federal expenditures had constituted only 3 percent of GDP. The national debt as a proportion of GDP rose under President Hoover from 20 percent to 40 percent. President Roosevelt kept it at 40 percent until 1941, the start of World War II. By the end of the war in 1945, the national debt had soared to a whopping 128 percent of Gross Domestic Product.

The earlier ringing hopes brought of science and technologies were beginning to echo across the nation as dull thuds. The gulf between those who had, and those who had-not, was never wider. Class envy, long a festering problem, was rising into a tide of discontent. Demands for restitution epitomized by chronic protests, violence, suicides, and rise of the power of the working class through unionization became problematic. The current issues inherent in our healthcare system were the result of many of the short term fixes applied by government in order to arrest these issues. The unintended consequences of their historic fixes continue to plague us today. One may ask has anything really changed.

Henry J. Kaiser's Health Solution

In 1931, the construction firm of Henry J. Kaiser became one of six prime contractors responsible for building the Hoover Dam on the Colorado River. Kaiser was a gifted and creative industrialist who was destined for fame as a prodigious shipbuilder during World War II. During the construction of the Hoover Dam, however, Kaiser's pragmatic talent for logistical problem-solving was challenged by the question of how to provide decent healthcare for the dam's construction workers and their families. He had no idea at the time that his improvised efforts would yield one of the only truly integrated healthcare systems of our age.

> *In the 1940s, the name Henry J. Kaiser was magic. A relatively obscure construction entrepreneur before World War II, Kaiser blazed like a comet across the national sky during wartime. Based on the success of his shipyards, the American media – particularly Henry Luce's Time/Life magazines – hailed Kaiser as the force behind a "can-do" production miracle. Subsequent polls found that Americans credited him with doing more to help President Roosevelt win the war than any other civilian. Roosevelt himself was also impressed, confiding to his cousin in 1944 that he thought Kaiser would be the best man to succeed him.*
>
> **Mr. Kaiser Goes to Washington**
>
> **The Rise of the Government Entrepreneur**
>
> By: Stephen B. Adam - 1997
> (Adams S. B., 1997)

Born in 1882, in Sprout Brook, New York, Kaiser had begun his entrepreneurial rise early in life. He started as an apprentice photographer and by the age of twenty he was running the company. He used his initial earnings to finance a move to Washington State where he started a construction company that fulfilled government road building contracts during the "Good Roads" movement, a turn of the century program to increase the mileage of paved roads in the country. (Figure 8)

Several years after moving to the West Coast in 1906, Kaiser founded his road paving company in 1914. Early on, Kaiser displayed the practical temperament and fondness for productivity-improving innovation that would characterize his life. He was one of the first in the nation to use heavy construction equipment like the steamroller in road construction. His company expanded rapidly and by 1927, Cuba had awarded him an island-wide road-building contract worth $20 million—an unbelievable sum at the time.

After the Stock Market Crash of 1929 and the Dust Bowl crisis that began in 1930 much of the population of the Midwest and Great Plains migrated west. The influx of displaced families created a surplus of workers in West Coast cities, making it easier for Kaiser and his partners (together called the Six Companies) to recruit prospective

Figure 8 - Good Roads - Good Business

The Good Roads Movement occurred in the United States between the late 1870s and the 1920s. Advocates for improved roads originally led by bicyclists turned local agitation into a national political movement. At the turn of the century the interest in the bicycle began to wane and automobiles truly began to supplant the accepted mode of transportation, the horse.

The movement gained national prominence when President Woodrow Wilson signed the Federal-Aid Road Act on July 11, 1916. During that year, the Buffalo Steam Roller Company of Buffalo, New York, and the Kelly-Springfield Company of Springfield, Ohio, merged to form the Buffalo-Springfield Company, which became the leader in the American compaction industry. Buffalo-Springfield enabled America to embark on a truly national highway construction campaign that continued until the end of the 1920s.

employees to the remote and desolate Hoover Dam construction site.

Soon after the dam's funding was authorized, families headed by jobless men descended on southern Nevada. Between 10,000 and 20,000 people migrated to Las Vegas, which had been a small town of some 5,000. The government camp established for surveyors and others near the dam site was soon surrounded by a squatters' camp known as McKeeversville. Another camp on the flats along the Colorado River was officially called Williamsville but became better known by its inhabitants as "Ragtown."

The Six Companies put more than 3,000 workers on the dam construction payroll by July 1932 and then nearly doubled that number by 1934. The project far exceeded the scope of the building of the great pyramids of Egypt. It was a dangerous, risk-filled adventure, plagued by accidents, illness, and disease. There were 112 deaths associated with the dam by the time it was completed, ninety-six of which occurred at the site during the construction phase. Many other workers and their family members died of heat stroke, carbon monoxide poisoning, pneumonia, and other health-related problems that never were officially recorded as work-related fatalities.

The camp, called Ragtown, consisted of tents, cardboard boxes, and anything else families could get their hands on. Health conditions there were deplorable. Temperatures, on the floor of Black Canyon where Ragtown was located often soared to well over 120 degrees during much of the year. Conditions were so severe that Helen Holmes, a Ragtown resident, was quoted as saying, "You really just existed—you would go down to get a pail of water, and then it would settle, and there would be sediment in the bottom, so it would be clear . . . That is why there was quite a lot of dysentery. Everyone was busy lining up to go to the Maggie and Jigs (outside toilets) at that time." Families in the Hoover Dam squatter camps had no access to pediatric and obstetric care. Storage caches that dug into the earth offered no protection from the heat, so essentials like fresh milk were not an option. Lunches packed for husbands often spoiled under the intense and smothering heat.

Kaiser was horrified by what he witnessed when he visited the camps, but the Six Companies were unprepared and ill-equipped to deal with these problems. Kaiser came to realize that in order to maintain productivity and reduce the risk for families at such a large and isolated project, it was necessary for contractors to provide healthcare services for the workers no factory owner in a city would ever consider. True to his pragmatic thought process and his style of resolution, Kaiser set about developing an industrial solution to his healthcare problem. Before starting work on the Grand Coulee Dam project in 1933, Kaiser reached out to a California doctor, by the name of Sidney Garfield.

Years earlier, Dr. Garfield had helped provide medical care for the thousands of men involved in building the Los Angeles Aqueduct. He borrowed some money and built a facility called Contractor's General Hospital, a twelve-bed institution in the Mojave Desert, and six miles from the Aqueduct project. Financing was difficult during the Depression, workers had little money after payday and very few had insurance. When his patients were insured, Dr. Garfield found that his insurance companies were very slow to pay for his services. Often, he was left with no payment at all for the care he rendered. Also, the hospitals expenses were rapidly far exceeding his income.

Harold Hatch was a savvy insurance agent who recognized that the cost per claim from death and injury to the insurance companies was a significant, ongoing expense, and suggested that the companies he represented pay Dr. Garfield an up-front, fixed, price each day for each covered worker. The system not only solved Dr. Garfield's cash flow problems, but it allowed him to focus his efforts on the maintenance of the workers' health and safety, rather than merely treating illness and injury. At the rate of five cents a day, a worker received coverage for any injury or work-related illness, and for the additional five cents per day, a worker could receive coverage for all his other health problems, as well. Thousands of workers enrolled in the then-innovative program and Dr. Garfield finally began to experience a modicum of financial success.

By 1935, the Aqueduct project was winding down. Dr. Garfield was considering a move into solo practice in the Los Angeles area when he received the call from Henry J. Kaiser that would change the healthcare industry forever.

Garfield and Kaiser turned an existing run-down hospital near the Grand Coulee Dam work site into a state-of-the-art treatment facility. They recruited a team of doctors to work in what was called a "prepaid group practice." At its peak, the Grand Coulee project employed and housed over 6,500 workers and their families, all of whom enjoyed access to healthcare that few other workers of the time period had ever experienced.

With the advent of World War II, Kaiser went into the shipbuilding business and brought his innovative form of healthcare to the shipyards. With 30,000 workers now working round the clock in the shipyards of Richmond, California, and Vancouver, Washington, health coverage was offered to them by a new company Kaiser established called Kaiser Permanente.

The only obstacle that the new company faced was that Dr. Garfield had been drafted into active duty with the U.S. Army Reserve. Kaiser reached out to his friend and partner in the national war effort, President Roosevelt, who quickly released Garfield from his service obligation. As a result, America's indomitable entrepreneur and his equally innovative surgeon friend, found a cost-effective and efficient method by which to deal with the ongoing healthcare needs of tens of thousands of wartime workers. In the coming decades, the rolls at Kaiser Permanente would expand to millions of workers and their families.

World War II

To understand where we are now with our current healthcare system, a short review of the History of World War II is necessary to get be able to frame the mind set and the economy as we move to current times. This world conflict, in conjunction with the Great Depression and the Dust Bowl, set the stage for a series of decisions that both brought us unprecedented economic growth and prosperity for 20 years, and also propagated the mindset that justified what heretofore were otherwise unimaginable measures that plague us to this day.

In the January 1919 edition of Medical World magazine, the publisher wrote in his "Business Talk to Doctors" column that, "the War is over–unless there should be a 'flare-back,' which is not likely; and if there should be it would be in vain."

This was the prevailing sentiment after World War I. Most people felt the horror of the trenches was so severe that no one would ever go to war again. However, nothing could have predicted that the economic depression in the U.S. that spread to Europe. It was most pronounced in Germany, because of the post-war restrictions and reparations imposed by the victors in World War I, which led to the rise of Adolf Hitler and the National Socialist German Workers' Party, the Nazis.

From late 1939 to early 1941, in a series of campaigns and treaties, Germany conquered or subdued much of continental Europe. Amid Nazi-Soviet agreements, the self-proclaimed neutral Soviet Union fully or partially occupied and annexed territories of its six European neighbors. France and Britain declared war on Germany just two days after the initial invasion of Poland, but soon Britain and its commonwealth of nations remained the only major force that continued the fight against the Axis in North Africa and in extensive naval warfare.

"Power tends to corrupt, and absolute power corrupts absolutely. Great men are almost always bad men."

John Emerich Edward Dalberg Acton, the first Baron of Acton (1834-1902)

In June 1941, the European Axis powers launched an invasion of the Soviet Union, beginning the largest theater of land war in history. From that moment on, the major part of the Axis military power was tied down on the Eastern Front. In December 1941, Japan, which had been at war with China since 1937, and hell bent on dominating Asia, attacked the United States and European possessions in the Pacific, quickly conquering much of the vast region.

Throughout this period, the neutral United States took measures to assist China and the Western Allies. In November 1939, the American Neutrality Act was amended to allow 'cash and carry' purchases by the Allies. In 1940, following the German capture of Paris, the size of the United States Navy was significantly increased, helping to boost our national economy and, after the Japanese incursion into Indochina, the United States embargoed iron, steel and mechanical parts against Japan. In September, the United States further agreed to send Great Britain American destroyers in exchange for possession of British military bases around the world. Still, a large majority of the American public continued to oppose any direct military intervention into the conflict well into 1941.

In September 1940, the Tripartite Pact had united Japan, Italy, and Germany and formalized the Axis Powers. The Tripartite Pact stipulated that any country, with the exception of the Soviet Union, not engaged in the war that attacked any Axis Power would be forced to go to war against all three. During this time, the United States continued to support the United Kingdom and China by introducing the Lend-Lease policy authorizing the provision of materiel and other items and creating a security-zone that spanned roughly half of the Atlantic Ocean. In that region, the United States Navy protected British convoys. As a result, even though the United States remained officially neutral, by October 1941 Germany and the United States found themselves engaged in sustained naval warfare in the North and Central Atlantic.

Meanwhile, Japan seized on the diversion of the attention of world elsewhere to Europe and began a series of military actions to expand its empire. The United States, United Kingdom, and other Western governments reacted to the seizure of Indochina with a freeze on Japanese assets. The United States, which supplied 80 percent of Japan's oil, embargoed further. Japan was essentially forced to choose between abandoning its ambitions in Asia and the prosecution of the war against China, or seizing the natural resources it needed by force. The Japanese military did not consider the former an option, and many officers considered the oil embargo an unspoken declaration of war.

Japan's plan was rapidly to seize European colonies in Asia and create a large defensive perimeter stretching into the Central Pacific. The Japanese would then be free to exploit the resources of Southeast Asia while exhausting the over-stretched Allies by fighting a defensive war. This had the added benefit of aiding Germany by reducing the men and materials that could be brought to bear in the European theater. To prevent American intervention in either the Europe or the Pacific Theater while securing the Japanese perimeter, it was further planned to neutralize the United States Pacific fleet from the outset. On December 7, 1941, Japan attacked British and American holdings with near-simultaneous offensives against Southeast Asia and the Central Pacific. These included an attack on the American fleet at Pearl Harbor, landings in Thailand and Malaya, and the battle of Hong Kong.

These attacks led the U.S., Britain, Australia, and other Allies formally to declare war on Japan. Germany, and the other members of the Tripartite Pact responded by declaring war on the United States. In January, the United States, Britain, the Soviet Union, China, and twenty-two smaller or exiled governments issued the Declaration by the United Nations, which affirmed the Atlantic Charter. The Soviet Union did not adhere to the declaration. It maintained a neutrality agreement with Japan and exempted itself from the principle of self-determination. From 1941 on, Stalin persistently asked Churchill, and then Roosevelt, to open a "second front" in France. The Eastern front became the major theatre of war in Europe. The many millions of Soviet casualties dwarfed the few hundred thousand of the Western Allies. Churchill and Roosevelt said they needed more preparation time, leading to claim by Stalin that they were stalling to save Western lives at the expense of Soviet lives. Much of the actions between the Allies and Russia during this period kicked off the mutual distrust that led the United States into the "Cold War" shortly after World War II.

The U.S. formally entered the war in Europe in 1942. In Europe, before the outbreak of the war, the Allies had significant advantages in both population and economics. In 1938, the Western Allies (United Kingdom, France, Poland, and British Dominions) had a 30 percent larger population and a 30 percent higher gross domestic product than the European Axis (Germany and Italy); if colonies are included, it then gives the Allies more than a five to one advantage in population and nearly two to one advantage in GDP. In Asia at the same time, China had roughly six times the population of Japan, but only an 89 percent higher GDP eventually this is reduced to three times the population and only a 38 percent higher GDP if Japanese colonies are included. In large part, it was these economic advantages that led both Germany and Japan to foster conquest and war as a way to alleviate their domestic economic strains.

Though the Allies' economic and population advantages were largely mitigated during the initial rapid blitzkrieg style attacks of Germany and Japan, they became the decisive factor by 1942, after the United States and Soviet Union joined the Allies, as the war largely settled into one of attrition. While the Allies', mostly America's, ability to out-produce the Axis are often attributed to the Allies having more access to natural resources, other factors such as Germany and Japan's reluctance to employ women in the labor force, Allied strategic bombing, and Germany's late shift to a war economy contributed significantly. Additionally, neither Germany nor Japan nor much of the rest of the world believed the U.S. would enter the conflict. As such, they had not planned to fight a protracted war and were neither financed nor equipped to do so. To improve their production, Germany and Japan used millions of slave laborers. Germany used about twelve million people, mostly from Eastern Europe, while Japan pressed more than eighteen million people in Far East Asia into slavery.

For almost all the countries of Europe and Asia, the economic damage caused by the war was devastating. For the U.S., on the other hand, World War II was a fiscal godsend. The Depression had brought the nation to its knees. The Dust Bowl, and later New Deal agricultural restrictions, had restrained the over capacity of food production in the U.S. Many remained homeless and unemployed in the years leading up the war. After Pearl Harbor, however, the focus on the war and the rise of American Exceptionalism provided an impetus for recovery via war production.

World War II put most of the men and women in the U.S. either in uniform or in gainful employment. It opened up a large demand for war materials—oil, steel, clothing, coal, and food. It increased the U.S. gold reserves because many countries paid gold for American exports. It united the country in the war effort and redirected the anxious energy of the nation from that of a country in decline to one with a noble purpose and a common goal of world freedom.

The Second World War also spurred developments of new techniques in surgery, the development of a usable form of penicillin and other drugs, improvements in the delivery mechanisms for drugs into the body—injectable, liquid, and pill form—and the, development of methods for rapid diagnosis and treatment. One notable discovery that remains a boon to medicine today was the discovery of the use of preservatives to keep blood readily available for transfusion, as well as the newly discovered usage of plasma as a replacement to help reduce mortality. All these advances sowed the seeds for what is now commonly referred to as the practice of emergency medicine.

During World War II, research efforts produced miracle drugs such as penicillin and sulfonamides. Penicillin was the miracle drug of its day. Common causes of death during this period included lung disease as a result of occupational hazards (industrialization and large scale building outpaced safety standards at the beginning through the middle of the war) and acquired infections, which were greatly lessened by the arrival of penicillin. The miracle drug also staved off infections from dental illness or injuries sustained from war combat and environmental accidents. One of the most significant causes of death in the 1940s was due to influenza; an epidemic in 1943 and 1944 caused many to lose their lives. By 1945, however, availability of penicillin and the new influenza vaccine greatly reduced the escalating numbers.

Sadly the war precipitated the frequency of venereal disease in the U.S., primarily because war veterans would return home infected, spreading the horrific disease to those on the home front. Arsenic compounds developed in the 1890s were still the preferred treatment until the stepped-up research of World War II made penicillin the major weapon against syphilis. By 1949, the incidence of syphilis was still high, but sufferers no longer needed to fear its ravages. Disability from venereal disease was dramatically altered by new methods of treatment with these new drugs. Nationwide public-health programs, long focused on the issues of sanitation, brought the new treatments to the attention of the public through public-relations campaigns designed to entice venereal disease victims to come forth for treatment.

Mental health issues were also exacerbated by the war. Increased attention to the treatment of mental illness in the military brought about an enhanced public image of psychiatry. Psychiatry made a marked shift away from rural-based institutions warehousing the mentally disabled, to that of a more proactive treatment of mental illness. As a result, government involvement in all of medicine took the form of increased support for medical research and the development of new federal agencies, including such groups as the National Heart Institute, the National Institute of Mental Health, and the Center for Disease Control, headquartered in Atlanta, Georgia.

And, as we have seen throughout American history, war more than any other factor, helped to pull the country out of the Depression and set the stage for a robust economic boom that lasted well into the 1960s.

The war also fundamentally changed the ideals of America and the people. The country ended the war with a strong sense of pride in America and its accomplishments. These feelings were prominent, partly based on a deserved respect for the country's collective sacrifices along with the freedom that America was so instrumental in perpetuating for most of Europe. But, much of America's new found patriotism was also driven by the propaganda machine within the government as it attempted to motivate a tired and dejected people to step up to the challenge of facing down the Axis Powers and their goal of world domination. It is from this need of the U.S. government, to motivate its people to rise together in sacrifice for the good of the world, that the concept of "American Exceptionalism" was born.

Propaganda was not just an artifice of posters and advertisements. The tenets of American Exceptionalism were broadcast in magazines and newspapers, radio broadcasts, movie newsreels, and communications of all kinds. With the suspension of the first Amendment, all communications were censored by the government. Committees were formed, in towns across the nation, to root out potential threats and conspirators. In some cases, neighbor turned against neighbor. Out of fear, the country saw whole ethnic groups of people displaced and sent to internment camps.

During the war, government intervention in education was deemed to be justified and necessary for national security, and curricula were altered to build national pride and emphasize America's success as a free nation. History books were altered to stress the nature of our "Democratic" form of government, as opposed to the historical "constitutional republic," in order for the U.S. to gain more tolerance from displaced governments abroad. To instill the concepts necessary for the total national commitment to the war effort, the concept of American Exceptionalism required that we de-emphasize our historical struggles in our economy, our unity or our veracity. Instead, America chose to instruct succeeding generations in a history that was based on the vision of America as a perpetual economic powerhouse, a shining star of unity, freedom and opportunity for all. As we were drawn into the war, much of the propagandist's focus shifted to recruiting young, patriotic Americans to stand together and enlist to fight the war against evil. The campaign of American Exceptionalism was highly successful.

While it can be rightly argued that, during this war above all others, these changes and actions were necessary and without them, the outcome for the world and America could have been vastly different, I would argue that we have now come far enough that we should again take a hard look at the contemporaneous histories of the past, and again help the current generation find more truths about our real history. The belief in American Exceptionalism has yielded great things since 1942, but like the continual pattern of all things governmental along with the benefit, it has also brought some harm. Harm has come in the form of the perception of many in the world that America is arrogant. That America believes itself to be supreme. And, that America thinks that it is the sole arbiter of what is right and wrong in the world.

It is also likely that the change in the progressive movement coinciding with the rise of the Bull Moose Party of Teddy Roosevelt focused then on rooting out corruption, fraud, and abuse in the government and the free market began its own change. The term progressive had fallen from favor during the Depression. The new "liberal" philosophy began its development as the original progressives began to find, as a result of the Depression and the war, that regardless of the vigilance and actions taken to clean up government, it was the innate nature of the free market to leave the working class at risk. Many felt that the unions would protect the working class, but the rising power of the unions also brought problems. Some scholars argue that it was the rise in the power of the unions, in conjunction with the actions taken during the war, that were formative in the growing belief in the expanded role of government, as a provider.

The year 1947 also brought forth the beginning of the Cold War. The effect, of the war, on the morale of the country, and the development of a number of government programs to fight this "un-fought" battle, began a series of expenditures that still plague the country today. President Harry S. Truman began Voice of America, The Truman Doctrine (that appropriated $400 million in aid to Greece and Turkey); signed the National Security Act into law creating the CIA, the Department of Defense, the Joint Chiefs of Staff and the National Security Council. He also formally established, the Air Force as a separate branch of service (it had been previously part of the Army), and Congress voted to override President Truman's veto of the Taft-Hartley Act.

Immediately after V-J Day signaled the end of World War II, more than five million American workers engaged in vigorous labor strikes, which lasted, on average, four times longer than any held during the war. The war and the release of the atomic bomb—and its devastating effect—had a drastic effect on the American psyche. Rising union radicalism and increasing cold war hostilities tried the patience of the American people and congress. More than 250 union-related bills were pending in Congress by 1947. The Taft-Hartley Act was developed to demobilize the labor movement, imposing strict limits on labor's ability to strike. Further, the act prohibited radicals from holding union leadership.

The amendments enacted in Taft-Hartley added a list of prohibited actions, or "unfair labor practices," on the part of unions to the National Labor Relations Board, which had previously only prohibited "unfair labor practices" committed by employers. The Taft–Hartley Act also prohibited jurisdictional strikes, wildcat strikes, solidarity or political strikes, secondary boycotts, secondary or "common situs" picketing *(common situs means picketing by a labor union of an entire construction project as a result of a grievance held against a single subcontractor on the project)*, closed shops, and monetary donations by unions to federal political campaigns. It also required union officers to sign non-communist affidavits with the government. Union shops were heavily restricted, and states were allowed to pass "right-to-work laws" that outlawed these union shops. Furthermore, the Executive Branch of the federal government was now able to obtain legal strikebreaking injunctions if an impending or current strike "imperiled the national health or safety" of the country—a test that has been interpreted broadly by the courts and that was aptly utilized by President Ronald Reagan during the Air Traffic Controllers Union Strike, in the 1980s.

The Push for National Healthcare Insurance

In 1934, FDR's Committee on Economic Security made its recommendation for a "State-Run" healthcare system with compulsory health insurance for all state residents. In its proposal, states would be able to choose whether to participate or not. As the problem of the Dust Bowl compounded the Great Depression, concern across the country about the rapid expansion of government programs and expenses brought forth a sentiment in Congress that was no longer supportive. Wage and price control were seen as mixed blessings and as some of the principal legislations attached to the New Deal fell by rulings of unconstitutionality by the Supreme Court, the concept of "National Insurance" was dropped from the Social Security Act. It did not help that the AMA was strongly set against this approach. They had the foresight to note that such reform was limiting to physicians' practices and their profitability.

After FDR's death, Harry Truman, still facing a nation in crisis and deeply embroiled in a world war, revived FDR's National Health Insurance initiative when he endorsed the Wagner-Murray-Dingle bill of 1946—a bill that still managed to gain little traction among a nation of the war weary, who was rationed out and economically struggling.

In a secondary effort, Truman endorsed the Hill-Burton Act, also known as the Hospital Survey and Construction Act. This bill targeted the specific issues of improvement in access to care and development of more hospitals, as well as development of desperately needed rural hospitals. Unlike proposals for national health insurance, the bill quickly gained the required support and was passed.

The Hill-Burton Act became landmark legislation during this period, and more than anything else made a huge difference in access to care in rural communities. Many physicians like Dr. Ford Loker finally found a way to bring their skills back to their home towns. From 1941 to 1950, the number of hospitals in the United States doubled from approximately 3,000 – 6,000. This legislation also prohibited discrimination in the application of services based on race, religion, or national origin. It also required hospitals to provide a "reasonable volume" of charitable care.

By 1948, the National Health Assembly convened in Washington DC under the auspices of the Federal Security Agency. That entity issued a final report endorsing voluntary health insurance. It also reiterated the need for all people to be covered. In the very same year, the AMA launched its own national campaign in opposition, to the various national insurance proposals, and began to work with regional groups of physicians, to bring about a market driven alternative. For the time being, the push for a national governmental insurance program died and the nation began to see the rise of a variety of regional physician association insurance plans.

As the nation began to purchase these new policies, many in the government viewed unions as a major vehicle to encourage health insurance plans paid for by employers. This remains one of the main factors that led to the rapid rise of the unions during that period, and later fostered some of the legislation limiting the power of unions.

The AMA was still actively restricting the numbers of physicians who could graduate and be granted their licenses, partly to ensure quality, but chiefly to assert control over the rules of supply and demand. Many of the newly "ordained" physicians were now able to move back to their hometowns and practice in newly created hospitals. Prior concerns over the cash-strapped nature of rural economies were being supplanted with employer-provided insurance plans, or individually purchased policies from either Blue Cross, Blue Shield or one of the other emerging insurance companies now offering such coverage. In the coming decade, doctors would enter a golden age of medical practice.

Hospital stays decreased from 13.7 days in 1940, to 10.6 days in 1950. While the government, through the Hill-Burton Act and other legislation, increased the number of hospitals and fueled research, the AMA, and the country in general, veered away from focus on medical education. Since most physicians were off fighting the war, the shortage of physicians was not seen as a problem that would sustain itself. The decision to expand hospitals without expanding medical-school enrollments led to an acute shortage of interns and residents in the nation's hospitals.

Since the founding of America, both physicians and hospitals had always been in short supply. This particular war further complicated the situation. In 1940, there were 133 physicians for every 100,000 Americans—about one doctor for every 752 people. By 1944, with so many physicians in active military service, civilian doctors saw on average 1,700 people per year. By decade's end, the country began to awaken to the seriousness of the doctor shortage. Between 1925 and 1950, the population of the United States increased from 115 million to 151 million, but only six new medical schools had been established, which was not nearly enough to address the population's demands. In 1949, eighteen states were still without medical schools.

This was the beginning of what has been termed the "golden age" for physicians and the business related to their work, doctor's salaries had increased dramatically. An average gross income of $7,632 was recorded in 1940, and by the end of 1949, it had risen to $19,710. This increase paralleled an equally dramatic rise in total medical-care expenses, in the nation, from $3.018 billion in 1940, to $8.11 billion in 1949. While it may be easy to chalk up this increase to greed, that is not the case today. Physicians then were making more money, but during that period, the standards by which they practiced; their cost of operations and the large increase in the volume of services they administered, due to the shortage of doctors, contributed greatly to those numbers.

With the benefit of effective new methods developed to reduce infant mortality and to prevent or cure infectious diseases, came the continued rise in the average age of the population. From 1940 to 1950, for instance the percentage of the population over age sixty-four increased from 6.9 percent to 8.2 percent. The diseases of the elderly—cancer, heart disease, and stroke—rose proportionately. However, concurrently, with the number of the elderly population rising, there was also an increase in deaths from these diseases.

The Nation Gets the Blues

In the 1920s, the rudimentary state of medical technologies meant that most people had relatively low medical expenditures. A 1918 Bureau of Labor Statistics survey of 211 families living in Columbus, Ohio found that only 7.6 percent of their annual medical expenditures went for hospital care. For instance, the biggest cost to these people was not the medical care costs but the loss of wages when they could not work. A 1919 report from the State of Illinois stated that lost wages due to sickness were four times larger than the medical expenses associated with treating the illness. In 1926, the average cost of a private room was $2.50 per day according to a *Farmers Bulletin* issued by the U.S. Department of Agriculture.

As demand for care increased the cost of supplying care rose along with increases in standards for both physicians and hospitals. In 1947, according to a survey conducted by the American Hospital Association (AHA), the average daily rate, most commonly charged to private patients for single rooms in 1,645 reporting U.S. general hospitals, was $8.57 plus extras. The average daily income was only $7.27. This did not include the cost of tests, medications, or physician charges. By 1949, the average life expectancy had increased to 67.5 years from 59.2 in 1929.

Facing new legislation and narrowly avoiding the implementation of a national single payer health insurance plan as proposed by Roosevelt, in 1935, and then later by Harry Truman, the AMA and many physicians felt the need to respond to the national cry for access to affordable care. While, both Roosevelt and Truman proposed legislation that would open up access to affordable care to all Americans the underlying issues for much of their push was the lack of trained physicians coupled with the lack of hospitals and physicians in rural areas. While the Hill-Burton Act stimulated the rise of rural hospitals and industrialists, like Henry J. Kaiser, who found ways to provide workers care cost-effectively, much of the rest of the country was caught by the rising cost of food and staples both during the war and after it as the country struggled to recover.

The benefit of healthcare as seen by Henry J. was not simply in a boost in the productivity of the worker, and gains in the efficiency of production. Kaiser soon realized that due to price and wage restrictions—set and enforced by the National Recovery Act—that it would be hard to recruit and keep workers in steel mills and shipyards when they could also earn fair wages in less risky and harsh working environments in other industries, like clothing factories or food production. Since he was restricted from augmenting the wages of employees, the offset of the cost of healthcare became a very effective way for Kaiser to recruit employees. As most of the men went to off to fight the war, the women workers, who began to dominate the nation's and Kaiser's workforce, were especially savvy in understanding the value of the additional benefits of working for Kaiser.

I am not attempting to suggest in any way that Henry J. Kaiser was not sincere in his concern for his workers. In fact, nothing could be further from the truth. Kaiser was a man of strong principles and strong, progressive values. Actually, it was the national Democratic Party's concern for his strong, progressive stance on workers' rights and strong support of unions that precluded Kaiser from being considered for the presidential ticket as a candidate for vice president and paved the way for Harry S. Truman to become the candidate for vice president with Franklin Roosevelt. After Roosevelt's death and as the nation mourned, Truman ascended to the presidency. This turn of events leads many scholars to ponder where the nation would be had Henry J. Kaiser and his "Find a Need and Fill It" philosophy, become FDR's vice presidential candidate? One can only wonder!

When Truman took office, Kaiser persuaded Truman's administration to provide an exemption for employer-provided insurance taken from employee's taxes. As the war wound down, and Kaiser's employee count dropped rapidly from 90,000 to 13,000 in just a few months, once again Kaiser, ever the problem solver, opened Permanente's internal healthcare practice to the public at large. This was in October, 1945. Within ten years, enrollment surpassed 300,000. The first integrated model for healthcare in America began its singular existence.

As hospitals were being built in rural communities and qualified doctors were starting to provide improved quality of care and better services to those geographical areas, both the focus on rendering care and the cost of it began to rise. For many, care was available, although most of the diseases of the day still had a devastating impact on people's financial status. Routine illnesses, like appendicitis, tuberculosis, and asthma, could severely cripple a family's economic viability. The diagnosis of cancer, polio, and many other severe ailments would often leave them destitute.

Two primary paths for care soon developed; care provided by employers and care purchased through insurance plans. Along with the Kaiser Permanente model, other employment based programs developed during the first part of the twentieth century. First in lumber and mining camps, in the Pacific Northwest, employers began offering medical care by paying fees to medical service bureaus composed of groups of physicians who were eager to care for their employees. These plans covered physician's services, but they did not provide for hospital services. The first official Blue Shield Plan was formed in California in 1939. By 1949, the Blue Shield symbol was formally adopted by nine plans, which were formally dubbed the American Medical Care Plan. The name was later changed to the National Association of Blue Shield Plans.

What is now known as Blue Cross began as a plan guaranteeing teachers access to hospital-based services that were available from Baylor University in Dallas, Texas. In 1929, the first plan provided to teachers offered up to twenty-one days of hospital care for six dollars per year. Soon the service was expanded to other employee groups in Dallas. These plans paid for hospital-based services but did not cover the cost of private physicians. While employers paid Blue Shield medical groups to provide healthcare, the employee paid Blue Cross. In 1939, the American Hospital Association adopted the Blue Cross Symbol and, provided this as an emblem for other plans that soon sprung up across the country–plans that met the specific standards based on Baylor's pioneering model.

With the exception of Kaiser Permanente, few insurance plans of this period covered routine visits or preventive care. Most plans were in place for catastrophic coverage protection. Many citizens of the day saw these plans as a form of mortgage protection. If they suffered a catastrophic accident or illness, the supplemental monies to pay for the hospital or doctor would allow them still to be able to make their mortgage payment, thus holding onto their most prized possession: the family home.

All in all, as the country moved into the 1940s, several historic advances contributed to a significant decline in mortality. New medications began to arrive in droves—ones that were designed treat chronic conditions like heart disease and cancer. Penicillin significantly reduced death and amputations stemming from infection during the war. As America emerged from the war, Penicillin began to work its miracles on the population.

Final Thoughts

While the period, from 1900 to 1929, saw many advances in medicine and changes in the structural relationships among the various players in the healthcare system, as the country entered this period the continued medical and technological discoveries prompted huge gains in the provision and access of quality care to Americans. But, more importantly, these advances brought a peace of mind, that is until technological gains were overshadowed by, the despair caused by the collapse of the stock market and the banks, the drought associated with the "Dust Bowl," and ultimately, the Great Depression. Immediately following those fiascoes, both the trauma of Japan's attack on Pearl Harbor and the war the country had to enter in Europe served to emphasize the rise of American Exceptionalism.

In the end, these events left us with a combination of boundless hope for many, and desperate desolation for others. The mood of the country was both buoyed by the war and our great victory and concerned about what could happen next. A nation long unable to focus on the effects of the collapse of our economy and loss of faith in our economic systems and the government had been circumvented by the need to win the war. This event, however, tragic and nerve racking elevated the people's morale and instilled a tremendous can-do drive, spirit of patriotism, and belief in our world leadership role. The incongruity of the lingering doubts that remained, and the afterglow of the positive effect that the war had on our economy, would bring us the prosperous gains of the 1950s, and set the stage for the radicalization of the subsequent era of massive change of the 1960s and 70s.

Chapter 5 Addendum
Medical Advances 1930 – 1949

- 1930s, Werner Forssman uses a catheter to inject opaque dye into his heart in an attempt to outline the organ's chambers on X-Ray photographs.
- 1931, Dr. John H. Gibbon, Jr., Massachusetts General Hospital, Boston, conceived the idea of the heart-lung machine for extra-corporeal circulation to remove pulmonary emboli from moribund patients.
- 1935, first vaccine for Yellow Fever.
- 1935, Dr. John Gibbon, Jr. successfully uses a heart lung machine to keep a cat alive.
- 1937, first vaccine for Typhus.
- 1937, Bernard Fantus starts the first Blood Bank at Cook County Hospital in Chicago.
- 1939, Charles Drew, a Ph.D. candidate at Columbia University reports to the National Blood Transfusion Committee that the use of plasma is preferred over whole blood for the treatment of shock, burns, and open wounds.
- 1940s, O. H. Robertson, a Canadian medical officer during World War I, discovered that a solution of citrate glucose could preserve blood for as long as twenty-one days.
- 1943, Selman A. Waksman discovers the antibiotic Streptomycin.
- 1945, first vaccine for influenza.

- 1946, Penicillin becomes available to the public and infection diseases rapidly decline.

- 1946, Cortisone produced by the cortex of the adrenal glands was synthesized and proved to have therapeutic value in rheumatoid arthritis and a variety of inflammatory diseases.

- 1948, National Heart Institute enacts the Framingham (Massachusetts) Heart Study. Initial enrollment of 28,000 subjects to study the effects of factors influencing coronary artery disease. The project is ongoing.

- 1949, IBM develops the Gibbon Model I heart-lung machine, delivered to Jefferson Medical College, Philadelphia, PA. It consisted of DeBakey Pumps and a film oxygenator.

VI. (1950 – 1979)
Hearts, Minds, Government vs. Ourselves

The rise of the disaffected, disillusioned, entitled generation

Imagine . . .

The swish, swish, swish sound of water from a hose hitting the concrete floor has a calming effect on you, as does the cigarette hanging from your mouth. As you clean out the dog pound, you fill your lungs with tobacco smoke and exhale a satisfying cloud.

Like all your friends, you have been smoking since you were twelve years old, when you and your buddies used to save your pennies to buy cigarette papers at your cousin, Bessen's "Loker and DeWall's General Store" and unable to afford tobacco—smoked corn silk out behind the barn.

Here, it is 1968, just forty-six years later, and cigarettes are again starting to cost too damn much. Ever since the Surgeon General made them post the warning that smoking may be hazardous to your health on the package, more and more people are suing the tobacco companies and the cost of cigarettes keeps rising. Every time the government gets involved, the price of stuff . . .

"Aleck! Aleck!" Your wife, Margaret is calling. "You need to come in here and get cleaned up! Everyone will be here in a few hours, and you need a bath and a shave! It would not be good for a prominent member of the local bar association to look like he has actually been hanging out in a bar!" You continue the task at hand, more to allow time to finish your quiet smoke and to figure out what you need to get done for today, than actually to accomplish much more cleaning of the pens.

The Fourth of July annual gathering of the Loker clan is about to tick off another year. In recent years, these gatherings have been very festive occasions, and as the family has grown ever larger, now you need the entire lawn area to accommodate all of them. Buying old Joe Gough's run down farm and rebuilding, was the best thing that you ever did—even if finding the building materials during the war was so difficult and expensive. Overlooking Breton Bay, with a large, expansive front lawn running all the way down the hill to the water, and an inviting large pond for swimming to the right of the house, it is a perfect spot for all the family to come get together. The other twenty acres make a respectable farm, and Leo Pilkerton is a good tenant farmer and has made the farm quite productive with good yield in tobacco, soybean, lespedeza, corn, pigs, cows, and chickens. But, this year, the 4th festivities will surely be less so. Ford's wife, Katie, and her kids will be here from Baltimore and with your brother, Ford's, death just last October; it will be the first time that the family will have gathered since his funeral in Baltimore. Unlike your long family tradition, you will use this occasion and not the annulus to make the celebration of his life.

Ford's oldest daughter, Sissy, will be coming with her new husband. She is almost like your own daughter, having spent all those summers here while Ford practiced at St. Mary's Hospital. Aleck, your oldest son, will be here with his new wife and Peggy, your oldest child, will be here with her husband, Jackie, and their three boys.

Your sister, Francis,' and her husband, your wife's brother, George Wigginton's son, Peter, will pick up Pop (Judge William Meverell Loker) and drive him down. Peter loves Pop's old Chevrolet, and it seems only Peter can get him to ride in the car after all these years. How he got that old thing running again, is in itself a miracle.

It has been seven years since Mother passed away in 1962, and Pop is really getting frail. As strong as Mother was, and Pop with his "weak constitution," who would have thought he would outlive her? She was such a strong and proud woman, but the stroke took her just like Margaret's father in 1940. Here one minute—and gone the next. Literally, just one step and they were gone.

"Dad! Dad!" Drawn back from your thoughts, your youngest son Tommy approaches. "Mom says to come out here and help you." You tell him to roll up the hose as you light up another smoke. "Then, take that gunny-sack of copper sulfate in the garage," you say, "and spread it in the pond over on the far edge by the trees. Try not to breathe in the dust. Then go next door to your sister Peggy's and ask Jackie if he will bring over his propane steamer."

Bessie Biscoe paid you to do her will in exchange for three bushels of nice Chesapeake Bay oysters. They will go well with that old ham from the back corner of the meat house that's been curing for a couple of years—it should be perfect now.

You tell your son to get the ham, but offer a caution about your tenant farmer. "Make sure you tell Leo Pilkerton before you get it. I don't want you coming home with a load of rock salt in your rear end like the last time. I will have your mom make some biscuits and slice the ham thin, so people can make sandwiches. Also, get the three fifths of Old Setter bourbon and the two cases of beer, out of the back of my car and bring them in the house. And hurry it up; everyone is getting here at noon."

Steamed oysters from Bessie, six bushels of steamed hard crabs from Dick Able, home cooked fried chicken from Mrs. Stauffer the Amish-man's wife—well, you still may not be the richest lawyer around, but your family always eats well. You got the beer, you got the whiskey. All that is left on your list is ice. Aleck Jr. is supposed to stop at the ice plant, and get one-hundred pounds of crushed ice before he comes over. That should do it!

You are glad that the new town doctor, Dr. Gill, is joining the party. It will be good for him, and his practice, for you to let him meet the family and introduce him to the other people of Medley's Neck who are coming today. Old Cuthbert Fenwick's eldest son, John, will be coming, as well. Soon he will complete his residency, and has already told you, he will come back to Leonardtown to practice. It is amazing what the new doctors can treat today, but, like cigarettes, the cost of healthcare seems to keep going up. Every time you get some money saved up for a rainy day, rain always seems to fall!

Margaret's first two pregnancies ended in miscarriages, and that sapped your small savings; even though in the '40s things were much cheaper. Then along came Peggy, happy and healthy but still the cost of the hospital birth again depleted the savings. It would have been cheaper at home with Mrs. Swales working as mid-wife, but Margaret would not hear of it. "Babies are now born in the hospital," she said. Then your first son was born and that nurse, poor Mrs. Ridgel, goes crazy and takes the baby out of the incubator and like a doll, plays dress up–by morning, your first born son had died. Pop was right when he said not to sue the hospital. That would not have made anything better, and it would have probably destroyed the institution. They had no way of knowing she would do this. Responsibly, they covered the costs. What else could they really have done that would have eliminated the pain? Pay money? As Pop, the Judge, said, "This new inclination to sue for money, pain, and suffering yields nothing but blood money—and such is always tainted and infectious!"

A year later, Aleck, Jr. was born. His childhood arthritis treatments cost a hell of a lot, and his asthma compounded the problem, but at least by then you had some insurance. Lucy came later, and fortunately she was relatively healthy. With the exception of her broken arm, which was partially covered with insurance, you have had little more than vaccinations and routine doctor's visits to pay for. Finally, Tommy, your premature mid-life surprise child, came along. His birth by caesarian section, only partially covered by insurance, also cost a lot. It seems like he has always gotten into mischief! You would never know the dog ripped Tommy's throat apart. Dr. Sammadi, the surgeon, did a great job, but again insurance did not cover all of it. "It is a good thing Pop taught us all to focus on saving, or I would have been up the creek years ago," you think.

And, even though the government now has Social Security & Medicare, you don't see how it will be there in the future. With healthcare treatment options increasing in numbers, basic costs going up, the population increasing as more babies survive and people living longer; how does this system work in a way that the money needed is assuredly there? There is simply no way the money Pop paid in, would offset his health costs if he really got sick. Hell, even if Medicare started in the 1950s, instead of 1965, he simply did not make much money then on which even to pay taxes. His salary as a circuit court judge was $9,000 per year plus mileage. If you add in that he got a 7 percent raise each year, the tax rate of 5 percent and an earned interest on the balance he had of 8 percent per year; he simply would only have accrued $35,750, not enough to cover care for cancer, or a heart attack, or much else, at today's healthcare prices. How does this system ever grow to afford tomorrow's costs at today's earnings? Increasingly, it looks to you like there will be more people drawing benefits and less, and less, money to pay for them, unless we really borrow from future generations. Then who will pay for them? And, it's only been four years since they passed Medicaid; and they already have expanded it to offer extra benefits and cover *more people. You have told all your kids that they need to save, and not count on Social Security or Medicare to take care of their old age needs. When you last spoke to your old friend Carl Albert, now a congressman and U.S. House of Representatives majority leader, he was still unable to explain how it was going to work. He said, Wilbur Mills was the resident expert, and he really did not support the bill enthusiastically.*

Bang! You here the side screen door and see your middle daughter, Lucy, walking out the front of the house toward the pier on the bay. "Lucy, come here and help me set up the folding tables under the weeping willow tree," you call. "OK dad, be right there!" She calls back. You walk to the front, stand on the large porch, and look out across Breton Bay. The deep blue sky, the rich green grass lawn sloping down to the water's edge, the magnificent old weeping willow cascading down, the blue-green water of the bay in the background—there is a nice breeze coming down the bay from Leonardtown to the north. It is neither too hot nor too humid very unusual conditions for July 4th in St. Mary's County. It is a marvelous day, and a wonderful place to remember family and country.

Father Gallagher promised to come and say a prayer for Ford, Little Betty, Mother, and Leck. Hopefully, you can get some private time to talk with Katie and make sure that all is OK with her and the kids. She knows how much the county meant to Ford and today she will see how much Ford meant to the county.

Margaret hovers over the help in the kitchen slicing the old ham nice and thin just like you like it. As you look out the back window, you see Pop's old Chevy driving down the long lane between the fields. As you watch, and blow out some soothing smoke, you see Peter pull into the circular driveway. The old tires crunch as the car winds around the crushed oyster shell road bed, recently raked nice and smooth by Leo's son Leroy. You walk out the back door, onto the porch, and open the door to help Pop out of his old car. Still ramrod tall, and sickly thin, he looks just like he did when you were a kid. He never took to smoking tobacco and only occasionally did he take a drink of whisky. At ninety-seven, who would have thought he would still be here, and still sharp as a tack.

"Hi, Pete! Hi, Pop!" You call as they get out of the car. "Aye, Aye!" the Judge returns, with his trademark hello. You remember him telling you, years ago, that the phrase was an expression used, in Old English, to commit one's devotion to service of the group or to the people. It always seemed fitting, as your father spent his whole life in service to his neighbors.

"How are you, Pop?" you ask.

"Son, my days are getting long without your mother," he says. "And I miss Ford and Leck and little Betty. Parents should not be forced to outlive their own children!"

"Well Pop, everyone is coming today to celebrate Mother, Ford, Leck, Little Betty, and the good old U.S. of A. The days may be getting long, but the night is young." Your reply gets a chuckle from the old man.

Soon, the others arrive. Later, as you sit on the back porch; the kids, at least twenty-five or thirty of them are swimming in the pond. Pop is down at the edge of the bay wading in his suit and tie with his pants rolled up to his knees. Some of the older boys are playing horseshoes, smoking, and drinking beer—others are out at the end of the pier fishing, drinking, and smoking. Aleck Jr. is pulling his cousin, Skip, on water skies as their two new wives sit in the boat and watch. Margaret and the ladies are in the living room with young Ted White playing old songs on the piano, drinking cocktails, singing, and smoking.

"Up the Lazy River" is pleasantly drifting to your ears, as you sit back in an Adirondack chair puffing on your cigarette—sipping a bourbon and water—thinking about how far everything has come during your father's lifetime; gas lights, then electricity, and light bulbs—automobiles, paved roads, painless surgeries, sanitation, antibiotic, electric washing machines, the new clothes dryer—four wars exhibiting both the dizzying heights of national patriotism to the heartbreak of antiwar protests—the first intercontinental train was completed just three years before he was born, moving pictures when he was twenty-two, talkies he was fifty-one, telegraph, telephone, television, now color television, air conditioning, central heating, typewriters, electric typewriters, adding machines, and now

computers—the Wright Brother's first air-o-plane when he was thirty-one, next came commercial air travel, then jet aircraft, now rockets, and men in space. In sixteen days, Pop will see American astronaut Neil Armstrong become the first man to walk on the moon. You and he will watch it as it happens on the new color television in your own living room. All the things the Judge has seen in his life! Almost all things he could never have imagined. What will it be like for your own children? What will they see? Will the quality of their lives actually improve or will they just think it does?

As Ford said many times sitting right here; medicine has come far but, no matter how far people are still dying before their time. Leck died of cancer, mother of a stroke, and now Ford of scleroderma. Dr. Guyther told you Ford disclosed to him that he had diagnosed his disease almost 6 years ago, but with no cure, he decided to say nothing to anyone till he was at its end. "We expect so much of medicine, but in the end we simply do little things that slow down the inevitable," Ford told you a few years ago on a fourth of July as the two of you sat right here in these chairs while the kids played in the yard just like today. You now realize, he knew then and there he would soon be gone. His sacrifice for his family and his community simply overwhelms you. You take another sip of your drink and breathe in the smoke and try to find some calm about it all.

"Daddy, Father Gallagher is here," calls Peggy. "Please get your sister Lucy, and let's get everyone gathered together in the living room for the convocation. Tommy, go down to the beach and get your grandfather and help him back up the hill," you say as you get up and walk into your house and prepare for the convocation . . .

You don't know it, at the time, but the coming months will be months of grief and tragedy. Within a year, and just two days shy of his ninety-eighth birthday, Judge William Meverell Loker, will join his beloved wife, Mabel Ford Loker, two sons: Robert Leslie and Frank Ford and his youngest daughter Elizabeth (Little Betty) in paradise. He will pass quietly in his sleep. The man with the "weak constitution," will have outlived all of his contemporaries, and while he did not see the birth of his country, he has watched the rise of a nation, modern healthcare, technology, and his fellow Americans walking on the surface of the moon.

In the end, his "weak constitution" was one of the only maladies he ever suffered. In his lifetime, patent medicines like Mrs. Winslow's Soothing syrup gave way to wonder drugs like penicillin. Machines could now keep people alive replacing at least temporarily, hearts, lungs, and kidneys. Polio, long one of the worst scourges of America had finally been almost eradicated with vaccination. The forests of iron lungs that used to keep those afflicted with polio alive were fading into the scrap heap of history. All of these great and wonderful discoveries, and yet the Judge outlived three of his own children and his beloved wife by many years. As Ford said after the passing of his mother, "Nothing we ever learn, will give us everlasting physical life. For that to happen it would have to consume our very soul and its potential reward, immortality, would itself become an affront to the Almighty! So, we, as doctors, need to be content just to reduce suffering where we can and let faith handle the rest!"

As the Judges Grandson, and the nephew of Dr. Frank Ford Loker, what I learned from both of these men, is that we will neither know what it is that will finally take us nor when that event will occur! It is incumbent upon us, alone, to make our time here among our friends and neighbors as valuable as we can for those that remain after we are gone. This is the only measure of a life that truly matters!

The End of Polio

Throughout the presidency of Franklin D. Roosevelt, many elaborate schemes, and devices, were employed to keep the public from finding out about the "secret" illness that left Roosevelt unable to walk—polio.

Geoffrey G. Jones, the Isidor Straus Professor of Business History at Harvard Business School, published a paper entitled "Restoring a Global Economy, 1950-1980" in that academic institution's "Working Knowledge" series. In it he states:

The 1950s onwards saw the beginning of the reconstruction of a new global economy. Between 1950 and 1973 the annual real GDP growth of developed market economies averaged around 5 percent. This growth was smooth, with none of the major recessions seen in the interwar years. World War II left the United States in a uniquely powerful position. While Europe and Asia had experienced extensive destruction and loss of life, no battles had been fought on the soil of the United States. The U.S. dollar became the world's major reserve currency. U.S. corporations assumed leading positions in many industries. Europe and Japan had to spend the immediate postwar decade undergoing extensive reconstruction, heavily dependent on official aid from the United States, yet over time Europe and Japan closed the technological and productivity gap with the United States. The emergence of a U.S. deficit on its balance of trade in the 1960s, and the devaluation of the U.S. dollar and the end of its convertibility into gold in 1971, provided symbolic signs of the ending of an era.

Polio was without a doubt the scourge of the modern era. Also known as poliomyelitis or infantile paralysis, it had been thought of primarily as a children's disease until the army discovered during World War II that its troops were sometimes struck down by it. A polio epidemic swept the nation in 1949, claiming over thirty thousand victims.

Polio had no cure. Treatment was focused solely on providing relief from symptoms and attempting to prevent the disease's many complications. The available treatment for polio during this period, often required long-term rehabilitation, including physical therapy, braces, corrective shoes and, in some cases, orthopedic surgery. Children, of the

1950s, who succumbed to this disease were sometimes faced with Iron Lungs and portable ventilators, both of which were required to support breathing. While, for some of those afflicted, this support lasted one or two weeks as they dealt with active infections, for others the result was permanent respiratory paralysis which seemingly sentenced them to a lifetime of incarceration. Other historical treatments for polio included hydrotherapy, electrotherapy, massage, and passive motion exercises. Surgical treatments such as tendon lengthening and nerve grafting were also thought to be therapeutic. Devices such as rigid braces and body casts were also proscribed which tended to cause muscle atrophy due to the limited movement of the user.

In 1950, William Hammon, from the University of Pittsburgh, was the first to suggest that a component of blood plasma taken from polio survivors could actively be used to halt the poliovirus infection, preventing the disease and reducing its severity in patients already afflicted with polio. His early results were promising, but widespread use of purified gamma globulin was found to be impractical.

The first candidate polio vaccine, based on one serotype of a live but attenuated (weakened) virus, was developed by the virologist, Hilary Koprowski. Koprowski's prototype vaccine was given to an eight-year-old boy on February 27, 1950. Between 1958 and 1960 Koprowski's vaccine was given to seven million children in Poland. Despite the early use of this vaccine, its lower level of effectiveness and much more complicated production made it obsolete as a public health measure.

In April 1955, Jonas Salk at the University of Pittsburgh announced a polio vaccine developed from a poliovirus grown in monkey kidney tissue and inactivated with formalin. Salk's trial studies showed that after two doses given by injection, 90 percent, or more, of individuals developed protective antibodies to all three serotypes, of polio. He also found that at least 99 percent of them became immune after three injections.

Later, Albert Sabin developed an oral form of the polio vaccine which, by 1962, became the only polio vaccine in use worldwide. The incidence of polio in the United States was reduced to almost zero by 1970. Iron lungs, once a common sight in every hospital across the country, disappeared from view.

War, War, and More War

When the Communist North Koreans invaded South Korea on June 25, 1950, President Truman declared the U.S. intervention in the conflict a "police action" rather than attempt to sell yet another war to a war-weary populace. That simple declaration became a poor descriptive to what was not only the first major conflict of the "Cold War" but also America's longest-running and most-expensive conflict. By the time the stalemate at the 38th parallel drove all parties to seek an armistice, signed on November 1954, the United States Forces had suffered 36,516 casualties in comparison to the total U.S. combat casualties from World War I which totaled 53,402 lives lost. Korea ranks above the Vietnam War in number of casualties suffered per day with forty-five per day for Korea while Vietnam sustained twenty-six.

Once again, America would be paying a price for problems in other parts of the world. The Korean War would bring additional benefits to the U.S. economy, as with other wars, but the Cold War logic that sustained the war created a sense of national paranoia about Communism, and gave birth to a strong and growing distrust of government and the United States' role in the world.

Also like the other wars, the Korean War brought certain health-related gains. Many lessons learned by surgeons during this conflict formed the foundation of emergency room practice in domestic hospitals. The concept of "triage," for instance, came into practical application with the Mobile Army Surgical Hospital (MASH). The MASH units' use of rapid transport to cut the time between injury and treatment, particularly by helicopter, led directly to the current emergency transport system in which injured individuals are flown to Level 1 Trauma Centers. In his paper, "Medical Advances as a Result of War," James P. Cole, Jr., notes that,

> *Perhaps the greatest medical contribution of the Korean War came from World War II-era surgeons, like Army Surgeon Michael DeBakey, who had dabbled with repair of damaged arteries during the previous war so as to minimize the need for amputation. During the Korean War, military surgeons like DeBakey began even repairing complex arterial wounds of the extremities and abdomen preventing countless amputations and deaths. (James P. Cole Jr., Nair, MD, FRCS and Rosen, MD, FACS 2008)*

In order to fully appreciate this philosophical shift among the public, it might be worth considering the enormous economic and cultural changes that took place during this period.

The era between 1950 and 1979, witnessed the restoration of a global economy, which caused a significant rise in American prosperity. But, with the expansion in prosperity came increases in military and medical expenditures as a percentage of GDP—Gross Domestic Product.

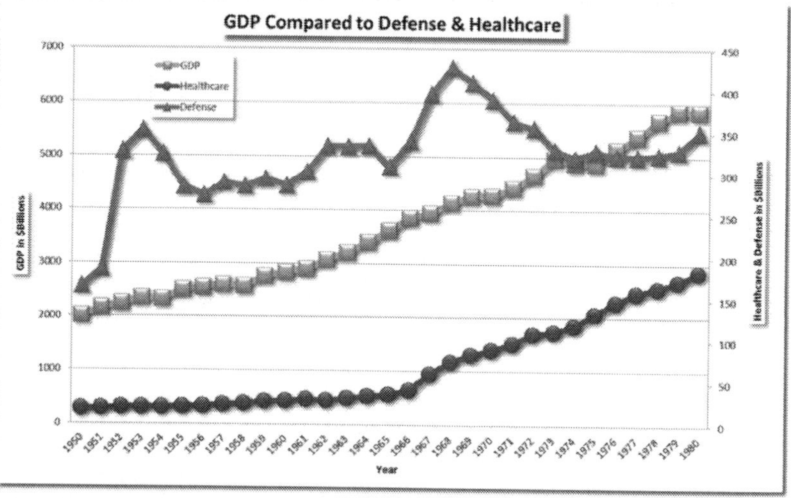

Chart 4: GDP to Defense & Healthcare Costs

A look at Chart 4, the square line shows the steady rise of GDP from 1950 to 1980. The triangle line shows a consistent rise in military spending, beginning with the Korean War and continuing through the Vietnam War. This table then shows a slightly slower growth after

1973. Unlike prior wars, Vietnam was funded almost entirely by the U.S. taxpayer. By its end, the effect on our economy was decidedly negative, and the political and social effect was devastating.

Health expenditures, represented by the circle line, as a percentage of the GDP remained relatively constant at about 0.93 percent of GDP until 1965. Expenditures increased rapidly in 1966 is the direct result of the adoption of the Social Security Act of 1965, which introduced—Medicare and Medicaid as healthcare programs for the elderly and poor, respectively. In 1966, the first year of Medicare payments, health expenditures rose to 1.08 percent of GDP and grew to 3.14 percent by 1980. The CBO estimates that 1 percent of GDP was spent on healthcare in 2010, and projects that with no changes to the system healthcare costs will grow to 31 percent of GDP within twenty-five years.

Television: the People's Medium

In 1927, the Federal Radio Commission (now the FCC) granted the first television broadcast license to Charles Jenkins of W3XK in Wheaton, Maryland, near Washington DC. By 1946, there were approximately 6,000 TV sets in America. By the end of 1949, there were 10 million.

People in the range of the growing number of TV stations could tune into newscasts from *CBS TV News* with Douglas Edwards (1948) and NBC's *Camel News Caravan* (1948) with John Cameron Swayze, who was required, by the tobacco company sponsor, to have a burning cigarette always visible when he was on camera. By the next decade (the 1950s), there would be almost continuous programming from 8AM until 11PM, including many radio shows which were converted to TV format. Some included *Amos and Andy* (1951), the *Jack Benny Show* (1950), and *Your Show of Shows* (Sid Caesar, 1950) as well as many other comedy, variety, and drama shows. In 1947, the children's TV show *Howdy Doody* (NBC) was first aired; as did the show *Meet the Press* (NBC). The *Texaco Star Theater* (NBC) starring Milton Berle followed on the heels of those successes, in 1948.

Television opened the world to everyday people. It changed forever the delivery of information by replacing the second-hand written or spoken word with first-hand imagery that left little to the imagination. Seeing, after all, is believing, which is why television is the most effective advertising medium ever devised. Advertisers' control over the impulses of the American public expanded exponentially, as with John Cameron Swayze's smoldering cigarette. Many of the old patent medicine companies were early patrons of television, offering products relabeled now, as consumer goods or as "ethical" pharmaceuticals. Cleansed of their strongly addictive and self-dosed compounds of the past, these relabeled products continue to consume much of on-air advertising.

This was the heyday for tobacco companies and for the distilling and brewing industry. The 1950s had a rising drug culture (there were still significant amounts of opiate and methamphetamine addiction, as well), but the king of the hill for addiction, during the 1950s, was the combined culture of alcohol and nicotine. They were often delivered in the form of cigarettes, the two-martini lunch, cocktails in the afternoon, cocktails before dinner, cocktails and cigarettes after dinner, and alcohol-based sleep remedies to prepare for bed. The recent TV hit, *Mad Men,* which chronicles the life in the 1960s Madison Avenue advertising industry, offers a very accurate depiction of corporate life in the late 1950s and early 1960s. Few people in those days were ever seen without cigarette burning, smoke wafting from their mouths. Professional offices came, complete with bar sets for executives, fifths of liquor in the bottom right desk drawer, highball glasses in the top left for middle managers. Members of the working class had their hip flasks.

Smoking and drinking was so ingrained in American culture at that time, that to see one *not* smoke or drink in public often aroused suspicion and called attention to their other behaviors. This was the era of "The Man" (meaning powerful establishment figures in government and industry) and the rugged cowboy Marlboro Man! Three of the actors who starred in the famous Marlboro ads: Wayne McLaren, David McLean and Dick Hammer, would all eventually die of lung cancer.

Interestingly, the culture of social drinking and smoking during this period was mostly confined to Caucasians. African Americans of the period were far less likely to use tobacco on a regular basis, and while many whites regularly began drinking at lunch and had several drinks during the day, alcohol consumption by blacks tended to be on weekends and at occasional social gatherings.

The nineteenth century temperance movement had looked upon tobacco use as another form of inebriety. In the great temperance upsurge of the early twentieth century, more than twenty states passed tobacco prohibition laws, but most of them were quickly repealed. As far back as the 1890s, advertisements for patent medicines claimed to help people break the tobacco habit. But, tobacco enjoyed a period of public acceptability from the 1920s through the 1950s. Cigarette smoking grew steadily among women and became a normative habit among men, largely displacing smokeless tobacco, pipes, and cigars.

The beginning of the end of social acceptance for smoking came with the 1964 report of the U.S. Surgeon General that linked cigarette smoking to cancer. Since then, growing attention has been paid to preventing children from smoking and treating those afflicted with tobacco dependence, one of the strongest of all the many addictions. Pharmacological treatments, such as nicotine chewing gum and skin patches, have been used, as have acupuncture, hypnosis, mutual aid, aversive electric shock, and other techniques. While many people advocate that government or private insurance should pay for treatment of this addiction, to date there have been no suggestions that tobacco addicts should be treated on a compulsory basis, even though the places where it is legal to smoke have diminished.

Treatment for alcoholism has followed a different path. In 1970, Congress passed the Comprehensive Alcohol Abuse and Alcoholism Prevention, Treatment and Rehabilitation Act, known as the Hughes Act. Iowa Senator Harold Hughes was a recovering alcoholic and a persuasive speaker. He became the conscience of Congress in developing support for a more humane and decent response to people with alcoholism and related problems. He was supported in these efforts by Senator Harrison Williams, Congressman Paul

Rogers, and several advocacy groups led by the National Council on Alcoholism and the North American Association on Alcohol Problems. President Richard M. Nixon signed the Hughes Act into law in 1974. Federal funds were made available for the first time, specifically for alcoholism treatment programs.

The Hughes Act accomplished three goals of the modern alcoholism treatment movement. First, it effectively redefined alcoholism as a primary disorder, not a symptom of mental illness. Second, it established the National Institute on Alcohol Abuse and Alcoholism (NIAAA) that would *not* be dominated by the mental-health establishment competing for the same resources. Finally, and of great practical importance, the Hughes Act established two major grant programs in support of treatment. One authorized NIAAA to offer competitive grants and contracts directly to public and nonprofit agencies. The other was a formula-grant program, which allocated money to states based on a formula accounting for per capita income, population, and demonstrated need.

Other laws and regulations were passed to try to reduce the attractive image of smoking and drinking in the media. The consumption of alcohol was banned from television. Some TV shows got around the restriction by mixing pseudo drinks with a watered down mixture of Coca-Cola and water to simulate the ever-popular bourbon and water. Advertisers were banned from advertising alcoholic beverages during the family hours of viewing. Eventually, smoking on television, and the advertising for it, was banned outright.

Clearly, there was some effect seen by those who experienced the "*Mad Men* years." But, by the 1970s, little had really changed. Tobacco and alcohol were still significant problems. As their usage waxed and waned during this period, their effects on the nation's health and the national cost of care continued to skyrocket.

Kennedy and Johnson

The 1950s – 60s were also an era of slow-growing disaffection, as the rising generation was encouraged to think critically—to investigate, innovate and question authority. A distrust and disbelief in American Exceptionalism grew as a result, and this group, which had experienced such rapid gains in prosperity without the actual experience of the poverty, and despair, of the Depression, began to feel their country owed them more, and then even much more.

John F. Kennedy's inaugural address widely is considered to be one of the best presidential addresses in history, makes a direct appeal to the nation to attempt to reverse this trend. Kennedy beseeched the youth of America to rise above what they felt was owed to them and to think about what they could achieve for the good of all. *"Ask not what your country can do for you, ask what you can do for your country!"* is perhaps one of the most memorable lines of any presidential speech. Yet, there are others, that President Kennedy also delivered, that helped to reframe the hope this country had seemingly lost from the prior forty years.

Figure 9: A few more inspirational quotes from JFK continuing the same theme:

. . . the belief that the rights of man come not from the generosity of the state, but from the hand of God."

"Let the word go forth . . . that the torch has been passed to a new generation of Americans."

"Let every nation know . . . that we shall pay any price, bear any burden, meet any hardship, support any friend, oppose any foe, to assure the survival and the success of liberty."

"The world is very, very, different now. For man holds, in his mortal hands, the power to abolish all forms of human poverty and all forms of human life . . ."

"Let us never negotiate out of fear. But let us never fear to negotiate."

"For only when our arms are sufficient beyond doubt can we be certain beyond doubt that they will never be employed."

"All this will not be finished in the first one-hundred days. Nor will it be finished in the first 1,000 days, nor in the life of this Administration, nor even perhaps in our lifetime on this planet. But let us begin."

". . . let us go forth to lead the land we love, asking His blessing and His help, but knowing that here on earth God's work must truly be our own."

Kennedy's message on that cold Friday, January 20, 1961, was meant to reach all Americans—whether Democrat or Republican, progressive or conservative—and summon the country once more in pursuit of American Exceptionalism. With his assassination on November 22, 1963, the genie could not be put back in the bottle. The dejected, disaffected nation was dealt another blow.

There are numbers of events that plagued Americans through the 1960s, but the war in Vietnam was clearly the biggest blight. The Vietnam War became for many, the public face for all that was wrong with America. However, it may be too simplistic to believe that it was Vietnam that led the disaffection of the 1960s and 1970s. Vietnam codified a schism of our collective psyche that began in the late 1930s and culminated at the end of the 1950s. This end-point began a new generation that by the 1970s, believed that you could not trust anyone over thirty years of age and that protest and insurrection were the only means by which to achieve happiness and prosperity.

As the country's mentality began to change, other movements gained steam. The Civil Rights Movement took hold; slavery, had given way to segregation, and segregation gave way to integration. *Amos and Andy,* a 1950s television show depicting a crude stereotypical view of African Americans of the day, gave way to *Julia*, a show debuting in 1968 with an African American woman in the lead role playing an educated nurse living a decidedly non-ethnic life compared to her non-African American counterparts.

Homosexuality long a practice repressed, hidden, and derided inside American culture began to appear in public view. *Faggot*, a derogatory pejorative for males who are attracted to other males gave way to *Gay*. *Dyke*, a derogatory pejorative for women attracted to their same sex gave way to *Lesbian*. The long and strong foothold that religious doctrine and institutions held over society began to yield to more secular views. Atheism, long an unarticulated belief in much of polite society began so seek freedom of expression.

As the shackles of prior oppressions began to fall away from these groups, these newfound freedoms gave rise to a burst of radical expression that, just like everything else we have seen over the decades, brought benefit, relief, satisfaction and self-awareness. Yet the downside was of a rise in drug addiction, sexually transmitted diseases, a breakdown of the family unit, health related consequences, increase in poverty, pronounced fear, additional racial tension, growing phobic disorders, and more distrust of authority, government, and one another. At the same time, there was an increase in government intervention and the development of more and expanded government programs, all of which intended to offset these rising issues.

As early as 1964, the unpopularity of the war, the rise in student unrest, fears of the middle class and particularly the elderly, many of whom were too old to benefit from the boom years of the 1950s—the advent of another economic downturn, along with the continuation of the Cold War, and more radicalization of the youth prompted President Lyndon B. Johnson to announce his Great Society initiatives to provide for social reform and eliminate racial injustice.

In such a turbulent time of rising public dissatisfaction, politicians struggled to figure out why the old political games were no longer working and to understand what was driving the increasingly angry and distant new generation of Americans.

As the situation became more and more unpredictable, President Johnson went back to the tried and true axiom of politics, "a chicken in every pot." President Johnson felt that giving the people the new Social Security Act of 1965 would help restore the popularity of government in general and of Johnson and his Democrats, in particular.

There should never be any doubt that the motivation for the Social Security Act of 1965 was predominantly political appeasement. An interesting historical record is available thanks to President Johnson's desire to have everything that transpired in meetings and on the phone recorded in the Oval Office. Now available online, these tapes offer very interesting and revealing insights into the battle over this legislation in 1964 and 1965. As Congressman Wilbur Mills commented to Johnson in a taped private conversation,

. . . I think we've got you something that we won't only run on in '66, but we'll run on from hereafter.

Mills and Johnson were responding to the rise in expectation among the disaffected and disillusioned that the government was there to give us "stuff." One of our longest standing debates, about healthcare, is based on a lack of agreement on where government benefits should end and personal responsibility begin. From Teddy Roosevelt to Truman the debate was never about the provision of free government paid healthcare. It was about every person's right of access to good quality healthcare. While in the prior period this debate clearly was focused on the access part of the equation, by the time we arrive at 1965 the vision has shifted from the government assuring access to good quality care and affordable insurance; to governmental provision of insurance through the expansion of the Social Security Act of 1935 with the revised Social Security Act of 1965.

Couched in President Johnson's rhetoric of the Great Society, this second major expansion of Social Security was signed into law with the simple words, "Care for the sick—Serenity for the fearful!" Former President Harry S. Truman and his wife Bess were at his side as the next chapter of the national dialog between "An unearned entitlement, or a contribution based insurance paid over your lifetime" was begun. Truman received the first Medicare card and his wife Bess the second; both enrolled by President Johnson right after he signed the legislation into law. Like the enactment of Social Security in 1935, many of the first recipients like Truman and his wife had not paid in anything to the system but still they were immediately eligible for some of its benefits. Unlike Ida May Fuller—the first Social Security beneficiary, who, in 1940, received the first payment under the Social Security Act of 1935, and who by the time she died at the age of 100 had received a total of $22,888.92 after paying in a total of $24.75 by the time she was eligible to claim benefits—we do not know how much the Trumans actually received in benefits but it was clear they received more than they paid in and again, with microscopically few exceptions, that has been the case for all beneficiaries since it was signed into law.

In the early 1960s, few elderly had health insurance. Due to the mores of this generation, it was not a purchasing habit. During most of their lifetime, the elderly had not experienced a healthcare system that had many real cures. For most of their life, like that of Judge Loker, medicine had few tricks up its sleeve and the few that they did have were painful, often risky, and mostly unavailable. People relied more on home remedies than trips to the physician, and the allocated cost of care in the family budget was relatively low. The task of daily existence took most of what they could produce or earn and what little extra they had, they saved for later life or unplanned catastrophes.

As medicine expanded their ability to fix, cure, repair, and prevent; the cost of garnering these new services rose accordingly. As more people found treatments for the maladies of life that before would have been fatal, they lived longer. As they lived longer they experienced additional maladies, particularly as they became aged. Soon their rainy day savings, modestly adequate for shorter life spans and fewer things to spend it on became woefully inadequate in the modern age.

As stated before, the economic boom of the post war years arrived too late for the elderly of the 1960s to receive adequate benefit. Those who were approaching the end of their productive years in the 1940s, were now living longer and in greater numbers. The economic demand that they faced was now orders of magnitude greater than they could ever have foreseen.

Into this mounting problem, for the elderly, and on top of the political problems of poverty, civil rights, and an unpopular war; Johnson's Great Society initiative seemed the prescription the nation needed. While Congress was bitterly divided over the issues and many were concerned over the expansion of government entitlements, few truly understood the issues.

The original purpose of the Medicare extension of the Social Security Act was to provide hospital insurance for the aged. Wilbur Daigh Mills, Democratic member of the U.S. House of Representatives and the chairman of the powerful Ways and Means Committee, was considered, by many, to be the only person in Congress who truly understood the actuarial basis of Social Security and was recognized as the Congress's primary tax expert. Mills had serious doubts as to the affordability of the existing Social Security Act, let alone any extensions to the current benefits.

Mills had additional doubts as to the ability of the nation's tax system to fund the liability of Medicare. In his paper, "The Origins of Medicare," Robert B. Helms writes,

> *Even in the face of strong political pressure from other Democrats, Mills had been so consistent in his opposition to adding a medical benefit to Social Security that many suspected him of being sympathetic to the AMA's socialized medicine arguments. He used his detailed knowledge of Social Security to question both the Kennedy and Johnson administrations' cost estimates and to point out that estimating future medical costs was a much more difficult task than estimating the future costs of a cash benefit.*
>
> *In a 1964 speech, Mills said: "In practical terms, this meant that if the hospital insurance system which would be created by the bill was to remain sound, the taxable wage base would have to be increased by $150 each year. Clearly, this would be a case of the tail wagging the dog." (The taxable wage base increased an average of $46 per year from 1959 to 1964)*
>
> *In that same speech, he pointed out that hospital costs were increasing at a rate of 6.7 percent, while average earnings were increasing at only 4 percent (1955 – 1963), and that he saw no reason to assume that the situation would change. His support for the final version of Medicare in 1965 was apparently due to the effects of Democratic gains in the House in the elections of 1964, President Johnson's personal appeals for support, and the many technical changes that he was personally able to insert into the bill during its various stages of development.*
>
> *We now know that Chairman Mills' skepticism was justified: In 1964, the administration projected that Medicare, in 1990, would cost about $12 billion in 26*

years (which included an allowance for inflation); the actual cost was $110 billion. We may not know until the year 2025 if today's actuaries are any more accurate than those in 1964 in making twenty-six-year projections, but at least the current crew is leaving no stone unturned to tell everyone who will listen that the Medicare Part A trust fund does not meet their standards for short-term or long-term actuarial soundness. (Helms, Health, 1999)

Johnson felt, he was swept in with a clear mandate from the people due to his landslide victory in the 1964 election. He made the push for Medicare one of his primary goals. Johnson was so focused on getting Medicare pushed through congress he was willing to leverage anyone, and everyone, with every tool he had, at his disposal, to get this divisive legislation approved. The following transcript, of a taped meeting with his Vice President Hubert Humphrey in the first days after the election, is telling.[4]

Johnson: "They are bogged down. The House had nothing this week-all god-damn week. You and Moyers and Larry O'Brien have got to get something for them. And the Senate had nothing . . . So we just wasted three weeks . . . Now we are here in the first week in March, and we have just got to get these things passed . . . The ones that I'm really interested in . . . one of them is education, one of them is Medicare, and one of them is Appalachia . . . I think the medical care will go through like a dose of salt through a widow-woman . . . You've got to look each week and say, what is the Senate doing in Committee this week and when will they be through, what is the House doing . . . You've got to be running into these guys in the halls, and going over and having a drink with them in the evenings . . . I want that program carried. I'll put every Cabinet officer behind you, I'll put every banker behind you, I'll put every organization that I can deliver behind you . . . I'll put the labor unions behind you.

4 All of President Johnson's recordings are available on line in both transcript and audio form at a number of locations. I found the Lyndon Baines Johnson Library to be the easiest to search, available here: http://tinyurl.com/7leetxr

Johnson's election did not just change the Democratic Congress's advantage over Republicans; it also changed Mills' political view. Seeing the writing on the wall, Mills made another speech where he announced, "I can support a payroll tax for financing health benefits just as I have supported a payroll tax for cash benefits."

With Mills' support, the measure was now destined to pass. There were still several hurdles to overcome, but, in the end, Johnson gets the legislation he wants regardless of the consequences. On March 23, 1965, Johnson's Oval Office taping system records the call he has been waiting for from Wilbur Cohen (architect of much of Social Security and Medicare), Wilbur Mills, Carl Albert (Democratic Majority Leader) and John McCormack (Speaker of the House) telling him the bill has just passed out of the Ways and Means Committee. It is the first time Johnson finds out what Cohen has just actually agreed to in Johnson's name:

> ***Mills**: We wound up, and I got instructions, we'll introduce the bill at noon tomorrow, and will report it at 12:15 . . . I think, we've got you something that we won't only run on in '66 but we'll run on from here after.*
>
> ***Johnson**: Wonderful. Thank you, Wilbur.*
>
> ***Mills**: Now here is Wilbur Cohen.*
>
> ***Johnson**: When you going to take it up?*
>
> ***Mills**: We could have it on late next week, if not, early the following week.*
>
> ***Johnson**: For God sakes, let's get it before Easter.*
>
> ***Mills**: Oh, there's no doubt about that.*
>
> ***Johnson**: . . . I sure do congratulate you on getting this one out . . . I congratulate you and thank you.*
>
> ***Cohen**: I think it's a great bill Mr. President.*
>
> ***Johnson**: Is that right?*

Cohen: *Yes sir. I think you got not only everything that you wanted, but we got a lot more . . . It's a real comprehensive bill.*

Johnson: *How much does it cost our budget over what we estimated?*

Cohen: *Well, it would be, I would say, around $450 million more than what you estimated for the net cost of this supplementary program.*

Johnson: *What do they do under that? How is that handled? Explain that to me again, over and above the King-Anderson, this supplementary that you stole from Byrnes.*

Cohen: *Well, generally speaking, it's physician's services.*

Johnson: *Physicians. All right, now my doctor that I go out and he pumps my stomach out to see if I've got any ulcers, is that physicians?*

Cohen: *That's right.*

Johnson: *Any medical services that are M.D. services?*

Cohen: *Any M.D. services.*

Johnson: *Does he charge what he wants to?*

Cohen: *No, he can't quite charge what he wants to because this has been put in a separate fund and what the Secretary of HEW would have to do is make some kind of agreement with somebody like Blue Shield, let's say, and it would be their responsibility . . . that they would regulate the fees paid to the doctor. What he tried to do was make sure the government wasn't regulating the fees directly . . . the bill provides that the doctor can only charge the reasonable charges, but this intermediary, the Blue Shield, would have to do all the policing so that the government wouldn't have its long hand . . .*

> ***Johnson**: That's good. Now what does it do for you the patient, on doctors. It says you can have doctor's bills paid up to what extent or how much? Is there any limit?*
>
> ***Cohen**: The individual patient has to pay the first $50 deductible, then he's got to pay 20 percent . . . of everything after that . . .*
>
> ***Johnson**: That keeps your hypochondriacs out?*
>
> ***Cohen**: That will keep the hypochondriacs out. At the same time, for most of the people it will provide the overwhelming portion of their physician's costs.*
>
> ***Johnson**: Yes sir, and that's something nearly everyone could endure. They could borrow that much, or their folks could get them that much to pay their part . . . I think that's wonderful. Now remember this, nine out of ten things I get in trouble on is because they lay around. Tell the Speaker, and Wilbur, to please, get a rule just the moment they can . . . That damn near killed my education bill, letting it lay around. It stinks. It's just like a dead cat on the door. When a Committee reports it, you better either bury that cat or get it some life.*

In the end, Medicare and Medicaid became the law of the land. And, as can be seen by the earlier chart, Mills was correct to have his doubts about the actuarial basis of Medicare, Medicaid and Social Security when the bill was passed in 1965. But, like the Social Security Act of 1935, the 1965 Act was not an ending but a beginning of a perpetual series of expansions of the benefits provided by the programs.

So concerned were many over the potential cost of Social Security, Medicare, and Medicaid, Ronald Reagan on behalf of the AMA said in a speech, in 1961, as part of Operation Coffee Cup, "If you don't stop Medicare, and I don't do it, one of these days you and I are going to spend our sunset years telling our children and our children's children what it once was like in America when men were free."

Operation Coffee Cup was an AMA campaign during the late 1950s and early 1960s in opposition to the Democrats' plans to extend Social Security to include health insurance for the elderly, later known as Medicare. Doctors' wives would organize meetings in order to convince more like them to write letters to Congress opposing the program. Ronald Reagan was a strong supporter, who, in 1961, produced a LP record to be played at the meetings, *"Ronald Reagan Speaks Out, Against Socialized Medicine for the AMA,"* outlining the main arguments against what he called "socialized medicine".

Since its inception in 1965, Medicare has had a series of expansions, including at least one signed by President Reagan. In 1964, the system covered 19 million at a cost of $10 Billion. In 2004 Medicare covered 244 Million people at a cost of $1.2 Trillion.

The Battle of the Sexes

The psyche of the country, in the late 1940s to early 1950s, was dealing with the lingering effects of those that had seen warfare up close; the recognition of just how fragile the world's peace and economies were, and the realization that our economic might was still very tenuous. The generation entering the 1950s was very aware of poverty, as most had suffered hunger and poverty of the Great Depression. They were also very aware of the fragility of life, and the daily cost of survival as few had any extra after shelter and food had been obtained. As they moved from the war economy, the men were focused on regaining their role as the breadwinner, and building a nest egg to help their family weather the next potential problem that they imagined lurked just around the corner.

The burgeoning prosperity of the 1950s was reflected in movies and television shows of the day. It was the age of *Leave It to Beaver, Father Knows Best,* and *Ozzie and Harriet*. The advent of television rapidly began to shape the lives and values of those who watched it. Gaining a nightly-view into the lives of the Cleavers, the Nelsons, and the Andersons provided a template for Americans to see their idyllic life. The show, *Father Knows Best,* is a good example of the changes that were occurring during the 1950s. Having originally been produced as a radio show, in the late 1940s, the original father, played by Robert Young, was cast as a Midwestern insurance agent named Jim Anderson. Life with Anderson's wife, Margaret, his daughters, Betty and Kathy, and son Bud reflected the mores of the day. What is indicative of the times, however, is that the characterizations of the family dynamic changed from the radio show of the late 40s to mid-50s, along with the other shows that wound up on television, in 1954.

For instance, on the radio show, Jim was not the kindly man, we later saw during the television period. The radio Jim was domineering and sarcastic. Routinely, he said things like "What a bunch of stupid children I have!" He called his children derogatory names. His wife Margaret was portrayed as the paragon of solid reason and patience. Betty, on the radio program, was a status-seeking, boy-crazy, teenage girl to whom, everything that happened was "the worst thing that could ever happen." On radio Bud was the all-American boy who always seemed to need just a little more money, and he worked hard to make it. And, Kathy, she was the source of family irritation as she constantly whined, cried, and complained about her station in life.

As the show segued over to television, the times were changing, and the characters evolved to reflect the new era. In 1949, just a few years after the men returned from World War I, women were seen as the stalwarts of the home life. The men had mostly been away at war and women had manned the factories, become the breadwinners, and learned the necessary skills and trades to keep the homes productive. In sum, they were the backbone of the family. Boys, like Bud, were seen as productive, willing to work, and always striving to earn more. Nevertheless, as the country moved in to the post-war years of the prosperous mid-50s, the perception of roles began to shift. By the time the show aired on television, in 1954, Jim was now both patient and wise, a fountain of common sense, and Margaret became relegated to play the dutiful wife who followed her husband's instructions, a bit ditsy, not always understanding the nuances of the world, and seemingly lost if her husband was not on hand to keep the family on track. Bud became a bit more industrious, but sometimes he was portrayed as a reckless child. His drive to earn money would as often as not be based on a get-rich-quick scheme. Betty became more the virtuous teen-age daughter, rising in the mold of her mother; remaining devoted to her father. Kathy was the one character that did not exhibit much change between the radio and television show, except to become more of a tom-boy on television.

What we noticed in this contrast of characterization is a reflection in the changing mind set of America. As men came home from the war, the strong role of women in society at first allowed for a period of decompression. The returning veterans, imbued with a strong love of country, also had to contend with the tail end of the Depression and the stress of changing the wartime production economy to a general industrial one.

As men resumed their role of father, provider, and master of the home, women were relegated to their prior role as subservient, dependent, and vacuous. The new ideal wife was becoming the "Geritol Wife." She cleaned, she cooked, she took care of the kids, and most importantly, she served the husband's every need, whim, and wish. Upon the husbands arrival home, dinner was to be waiting, the kids were to be quietly out of sight and out of mind, the wife should be dressed, made up, and gloved with drink in hand, fresh cigarettes at the ready, and clean ashtrays laid out conveniently.

The "Geritol" generation of women was portrayed as taking this modern nostrum to help them fulfill their role as dutiful wife. One long-running commercial theme, painted the ideal wife as the "Geritol Wife." This popular commercial showed a woman walking to the front door of their home dressed-up with hair and makeup perfect, holding a cocktail to present to her husband as he walked through the door. Upon his arrival, the wife was known to say that two teaspoons of Geritol helps her get through the day and be prepared to greet her husband after his long and stressful day, and to see to his every need. As she hands him his drink, he kisses her—turns to the camera and says, "My wife—I think, I'll keep her."

Another version of this advertising has the wife staring, somewhat vacantly, into the camera saying, "I take Geritol every day and my husband likes me this way." The fact that the actress was obviously intoxicated, and slurred the lines, gave rise to a famous *I Love Lucy Show* episode where Lucille Ball got a job as a spokeswoman for "Vita-meata-vegemin." By the end of the commercial, as portrayed in the show, Lucy was so looped she could not stand up. This parody was based on the very real fact that one tablespoon, *two were recommended*, of Geritol introduced, in 1950, by Pharmaceuticals, Inc., contained about 20 percent alcohol by volume—almost equal to one typical cocktail of bourbon and water.

Like the patent medicine period before, this alcoholic drink was passed off as an off-the-shelf medicine with predictably harmful results. But, the real harm of this product and others marketed in this manner was that it was used successfully for a time to reinforce the stereotype of the role of women as only happy when serving the needs of their husbands. Soon, many women felt trapped in this role: guilty at not being happy as a maid and servant. This led many into deeper and more pronounced alcohol addiction, depression, and despair.

Vietnam: the Made-for-TV War

Unknown to most of our generation, the first protests of America's involvement took place in 1945, when U.S. Merchant Marine sailors condemned the government for using their ships to transport French troops to "subjugate the native population" of Vietnam. The earliest civilian protests of the Vietnam War began in 1963, in England and Australia. American pacifists mounted them during the annual remembrance of the U.S. bombing of Hiroshima and Nagasaki.

By 1964, hundreds of students participated in anti-war demonstrations, in New York's Times Square. Another 700 marched in San Francisco with smaller groups in Seattle, and Madison, Wisconsin. The rhetoric of the protesters gained ground after the "Gulf of Tonkin" incident, in which the USS Maddox fired on three North Vietnamese torpedo boats, killing four North Vietnamese sailors and wounding six.

From its beginning, Vietnam was a TV war. Nightly images of the action in Vietnam filled the nightly news. For those with loved ones in the conflict, it heightened their fears by offering them a continued belief that they would catch a glimpse of their spouse, friend, or relative on the news and gain validation that they were all right. In many ways, this unrealistic expectation kept them engaged on a daily basis in the conflict that had not been available in any of the prior wars. As the U.S. involvement in combat escalated each night, television brought the public the vivid horror, death, and destruction in living color. To cater to the demands of the news media for progress measures, the Pentagon provided daily body counts.

The effect of the media on the Vietnam War did not just affect the well-being of the families and loved ones waiting at home. As the war moved on, the media and its daily reports also began to fuel the flame of discontent and anger at our participation. It also fostered terrible treatment of the returning veterans. Protestors, not content just to damn their government, began to take their anger out on the returning veterans. Mid-way through the war, many returning, soldiers, sailors, and airmen changed to civilian clothes en-route if possible to avoid the confrontations with protestors, who sometimes shoved, spat on, and threw things at the returning combatants.

Lastly, not only did the mediagenic nature of this war affect those at home, it affected the prosecution of the war itself. Unlike earlier conflicts, or those since, the Vietnam War was prosecuted with direct, detailed control by the President, his advisors, and Congress. Everything, from what target should be attacked, to how, when, and with what, were often decisions that were made by people in Washington, not soldiers and commanders on the battlefields.

As such, the mission of the war to the average soldier rapidly began to seem pointless. Many patrols went after targets that had long since left the area and yielded "no joy," meaning no contact. Routinely, troops were sent out to attack a position, which the soldier dutifully performed only to find out that there was nothing there of value to conquer or claim. Worse yet, they would be ordered to attack an enemy village or move through a safe zone only to find the "intel" was completely wrong resulting in significant troop casualties or the death of innocent civilians.

Anyone who lived through this period can clearly give you chapter-and-verse on this Nixon-era mind-set. Born from the anxiety, frustration, and anger with the government during the Vietnam War, it was during this period that the country's youth became concerned about being drafted and sent away to war—a war that was not very popular. Many people were asking "Why are we there?" Others, who believed we had made a grave error in entering Vietnam, were protesting in different forms.

"Make love, not war" was a common cry. "Peaceniks," and later, "Flower Children," as some were called, dressed with flowers in their hair. In some, cases these youths formed communities and called them communes. Peaceniks experimented with drugs in order to meditate. In essence, during this time period, the norm and the standard (establishment) became socially and culturally archaic.

Protests and anger of our involvement in the war escalated from 1965 to 1969. Events continued to deteriorate, culminating with the May 1970 shooting of four students, wounding of nine others on the campus of Kent State University in Ohio. This event has been recorded in history as the Kent State Massacre, or the May 4 Massacre. Photographs of the dead and wounded at Kent State that were distributed in newspapers and periodicals worldwide amplified sentiment against the United States' invasion of Cambodia and the Vietnam War in general. In particular, the camera of Kent State photojournalism student John Filo captured a fourteen-year old runaway, Mary Ann Vecchio, screaming over the body of the dead student, Jeffrey Miller, who had been shot in the mouth. The photograph, which won a Pulitzer Prize, became the most iconic image of the protest events, and one of the most enduring images of the anti-Vietnam War movement.

The shooting led to protests on college campuses throughout the United States, and a student strike, causing more than 450 campuses across the country to close with both violent and non-violent demonstrations. Students expressed a common sentiment, at New York University, with a banner that was draped out a window which read "They Can't Kill Us All." On May 8, 11 people were bayonetted at the University of New Mexico by the New Mexico National Guard during a confrontation with student protesters. Also, on May 8, an antiwar protest at New York's Federal Hall held partly in reaction to the Kent State killings was met with a counter rally of pro-Nixon construction workers organized by Peter J. Brennan, who was later appointed U.S. Labor Secretary by President Nixon, resulting in the "Hard Hat Riot".

More than any anti-war event, the Kent State Massacre shocked the nation. Unknown at the time, it sparked a series of discussions and events that eventually ended U.S. participation in Vietnam.

From a health perspective, Vietnam was like other wars, it had a significantly negative influence on America's health. Aside from the rampant drug addiction endemic in many of the returning veterans, and venereal diseases spiraling out of control and typical of most wars, the war in Vietnam also influenced the rise in drug addiction among the youth in America. Vietnam was the first war that saw veterans publicly suffering long-term mental and physical effects. Just as in prior wars, the same effects may have been apparent: the systematic approach to identify and deal with these issues simply did not exist. Long-term effects from exposure to carcinogens like Agent Orange, battle fatigue, tropical disease, and mental illness affected this generation of soldier more than any other soldiers before them or since. Vietnam, more than any other event during this period, changed the nature of who we were as a people.

Some say, we lost our innocence during this troubled historical period, but I believe we lost our faith in who we were, our belief in what we aspired to be, and our conviction that America was, is and always can be, a force for good. More than anything, we lost our ability to see and accept that there is a clear separation between the ideals that we aspire to and the failures of ourselves as humans. We lost the ability to see that we could aspire to ideals and fail as human beings at the same time. It is in our failures that we assess our progress toward the ideal, but we should not allow our failures to define our potential.

While the Korean War had been a, much more costly and forgotten war, Vietnam lives on in the scarred soul of our country. While World War II gave rise to the "greatest generation," Vietnam gave rise to an unprecedented period of protest, unrest, and rejection of our own image of us as a nation. The vapid patriotism of World War II was replaced with the violent hatred for our government and for a long period of our own military. Public displays of American Exceptionalism, common in the 1950s, became public cries of our own immorality.

Antidisestablishmentarianism began as a British word—one that was coined as a political position that originated in nineteenth century Britain. It rose as a phrase to coin the opposition to proposals disestablishing the Church of England that were an attempt to remove the Anglican Church's status as the state Church of England, Ireland, and Wales. The word was used in 1838, in *Church and State,* by William Gladstone, under whose administration the Irish Church Act 1869 was passed. Again borrowing on our overseas cousins Vietnam War protestors revitalized this word to encapsulate a policy or attitude that viewed a nation's power structure as corrupt, repressive, or exploitive.

Antiestablishmentarians, as defined by the 1960s, adhered to the doctrine of opposition to the social and political establishment. Their purpose was to subvert from within. This doctrine held that establishments lose connection with the people and have their own agendas, which frequently destroy the things they blindly don't address.

A counter-culture emerged, which adhered to the doctrine of opposition to the social and political establishment. Their purpose was to subvert from within. This doctrine held that authority figures and the established orders that support them lose connection with the people and have their own agendas, which frequently destroy the things they blindly don't address.

This rising distrust of authority helped set the stage for further changes that would come in the 1960s as first the youth rebelled, "turning on, tuning in, and dropping out" giving rise to the "sex, drug, and rock 'n roll" culture of the period. Later on, women felt too rejected by the narrow definition of their cultural role and limited opportunity. The phrase, "The Personal is Political" was coined, and the second wave of the feminist movement began to define a new, empowered and self-fulfilled societal role for women. First the youth burned their draft cards to protest the war and their lack of trust in their government, as well as in business, and society. Next, women in the early 70s burned their bras to proclaim their freedom from the binding mores and stereotypes of the 50s and to protest their puny role. They also began to force the expansion of their role into a more free and equitable position in American government, society, and business.

America's New Drug Culture

As pointed out throughout this book, America, like much of the rest of the world, has had a long history of addiction. In this era, while government regulation, social engineering, and religious activism had significantly reduced the incidence of addiction in the prior period, the 1950s began to signify resurgence in consumption and abuse of addictive drugs.

For instance, marijuana use began to rise among the youth of America. Originally an affectation of the "beatnik" subculture, while it was not socially acceptable during most of the 50s marijuana thrived as a hidden vice. Its use continued to be condemned as a degenerate act leading to many social and physical problems. The socialization of marijuana became a major part of pop culture in the 1960s. *Joints, Pot, Reefer, Ganja, Herb, Hemp, Bud, Dope, Weed, Laughing Grass, Loco Weed, M.J., Mary Jane, Love Weed, Match Box, 420, Rope, Sweet Lucy,* and many other terms of the period were often used to describe it. Its widespread use and acceptance were a clear indication of the rebelliousness of that period's counter culture. Hardly anyone came of age in the 60s who had not at least tried the drug. Most notably, President Bill Clinton became famous for saying he had tried it, but he "did not inhale!"

The 1959 biopic, *"The Gene Kruppa Story"* starring Sal Mineo, attempted to help instruct the youth of the day as to the dangers of dope. This film set the standard of this period as a means to reinforce the stigmatized view of marijuana smokers as out of control dope fiends. It is debatable, however, whether the film discouraged any youth from the evils of marijuana as the 1960s experienced not only a significant increase in its use, but also the gradual socialization of its use.

Such "cautionary tales" from cinema soon became admired in the drug culture for their ironic value. A movie, called *Reefer Madness* (originally released as *Tell Your Children*), was a 1936 American exploitation film that depicted the crazed events that could ensue when high school students were lured, by pushers, to try "marijuana"—from a hit and run accident, to manslaughter, to suicide, to attempted rape, and finally a descent into madness. In 1971, *Reefer Madness* was discovered in the Library of Congress archives by pro-marijuana activist Keith Stroup, who bought a print for $297.00. The film, with its the poor production values and grotesque overacting, became a crowd-pleasing favorite among pot smokers on college campuses around the country. For this modern audience, the film was an uproarious comedy. Its success as a cult hit helped bankroll the burgeoning film distribution company, New Line Cinema.

Another rising drug of the day was Dexedrine, also known as "speed." While used by the younger generation of the day, Speed was more an addiction among housewives than others of the period. As a result of the increasing pressures on home makers to be the perfect "Geritol" wife, a significant portion of these women graduated from Geritol or alcohol products to this methamphetamine. Speed also had another benefit—that of helping women reduce their weight. Many of the first addicts came to use this drug—often abusively—as a means of weight control. The drug's stimulant effect increased energy levels and elevated moods, both of which were necessary to get their work done and put on that happy face.

The practice of injecting drugs had waned significantly from the early part of the twentieth century, but it revived in the 1960s. While never socialized into the culture, like marijuana and alcohol, heroin addiction, and amphetamine injection skyrocketed during the 1960s and early 1970s. In 1962, a crackdown on San Francisco pharmacies known for selling injectable amphetamines drew national attention to the problem of amphetamine "mainlining." This led to the emergence of underground production facilities referred to as "speed labs." While many of these labs, located primarily on the West Coast, were small "Mom and Pop" operations, the amphetamine trade was historically dominated by outlaw motorcycle groups. Amphetamine use began to decline in the late 1970s, due to increased public awareness of its dangers, as well as FDA scheduling of the drug.

If marijuana was the poster child for the 1960s, the signature daemon seed was LSD. LSD was accidentally discovered and ingested by Dr. Albert Hofmann, a Swiss chemist, who was working for Sandoz Laboratories. He found himself embarking on the first LSD "trip" in history, in 1943. Soon after Hofmann's initial experimentation with LSD, he provided samples of the drug to psychiatrists at the University of Zurich for further testing into possible uses. In the 1950s, the U.S. military and CIA researched LSD as a possible "truth drug," which could be used for brainwashing, or inducing prisoners to talk. However, after military interest in LSD waned in favor of other drugs choices for that purpose, the psychiatric community began to research and issue reports on the drug's possible therapeutic capabilities for psychotic, epileptic, and depressed patients.

Non-therapeutic use of LSD increased throughout the late 1950s and 1960s. Among the first groups to use LSD recreationally were research study participants, physicians, psychiatrists, and other mental health professionals, all of whom later distributed the drug among their friends. Before 1962, LSD was available only on a small scale and generally used among those who had connections in the medical field, Most of the LSD was produced by Sandoz Laboratories, in Basel, Switzerland, then distributed to health professionals. However, the drug was not difficult to produce in a chemical laboratory. The formula could be purchased for fifty cents from the US patent office, and the LSD itself could be stored inside blotting paper. Soon, a black market for LSD emerged across the country.

In 1966, the Grunsky Bill was passed by the California State Senate. This piece of legislation prohibited the possession, manufacturing, sale, and importation of LSD. Illegal manufacturing of the drug, however, continued despite the new law, but soon LSD users experienced growing problems with contaminated or adulterated LSD produced by amateur chemists. The product was not of the same quality as that produced by Sandoz.

Dr. Timothy Leary, who had conducted earlier experiments with hallucinogenic psilocybin, was introduced to LSD in 1961. His personal uses of the drug lead to his dismissal from a teaching position at Harvard University in 1963. Writers such as Aldous Huxley, Allen Ginsberg, and Ken Kesey and his band of Merry Pranksters, were known for their use of LSD. In 1967, the "summer of love" attitude in San Francisco linked the drug to counterculture music and the philosophy of "sex, drugs, and rock 'n roll"

While the use of LSD declined in the 1970s and 1980s, the drug made a resurgence in the 1990s, particularly in the rave subculture. It is typically manufactured in clandestine laboratories, in Northern California, and it is believed that a limited number of chemists manufacture nearly all available LSD products, although at a potency level nearly 90 percent weaker than the typical dose used in the 1960s

If the 1950s were the alcohol and tobacco years, and the 1960s were the marijuana years, the 1970s were the cocaine years. Cocaine had been around for a long time. As shown in earlier chapters, cocaine addiction was a significant by-product of the patent medicine era. Again, even the venerable Sears & Roebuck catalog of 1890 offered an injectable cocaine kit for about $1.50. The Harrison Narcotics Act of 1914 had done a very effective job at eliminating cocaine's widespread availability, and after the 1940s, cocaine use had declined significantly. In the 1970s, cocaine regained popularity as a recreational drug and was soon glamorized in the popular media. Articles from the time proclaimed cocaine was non-addictive. In fact, the drug was viewed as harmless until the 1985 emergence of crack. Cocaine, in much the same way as marijuana in the 1960s, became a socialized part of the counter-culture. Its use became so wide spread and accepted by the mainstream that clubs, like Studio 54 in New

York, occasionally had bowls of cocaine sitting on the tables and bars of its club available for patrons to use at will.

Treatment of addiction began to change with the drug culture. Once again the country witnessed significant increases in the rate of addiction among the population. The period, from 1929 through 1959, was generally characterized by the strict enforcement of increasingly severe laws against drug possession and sales, by relentless opposition to maintenance, and by treatment that was essentially doled out in asylums. Many were given supervised probation. In 1961, California passed legislation permitting the compulsory treatment of drug addicts (including marijuana users) and established the California Civil Addict Program within the Department of Corrections. From 1962 to 1964, more than 1,000 people were committed to a seven-year period of supervision, which, at the time, typically involved an initial year of residential treatment in a facility surrounded by barbed wire in order to discourage premature departure from those facilities. In 1964, New York passed similar legislation but assigned the implementation to a special commission rather than to the Department of Corrections. As in California, New York's residential treatment facilities were also "secure." As late as 1966, the federal Narcotic Addict Rehabilitation Act (NARA), in most respects a piece of "modern" legislation, nonetheless, provided for the compulsory treatment of addicts making the hospitals at Lexington and Fort Worth into the institutional bases of the NARA program.

The tough laws and the anti-maintenance mentalities of the prior period were clearly breaking down. Both the American Bar Association and the American Medical Association issued a combined report, in 1961, that cautiously favored outpatient treatment and limited opioid maintenance as alternatives to overcrowding jails and prisons. In 1962, The U.S. Supreme Court struck down a California statute that made drug-addiction a per se crime. The court found that medical treatment, not the cruel and unusual punishment of incarceration, was the desired outcome.

The 1963 and 1964 landmark studies by Vincent Dole and Marie Nyswander, funded by Rockefeller University, showed that methadone maintenance was an effective method to block withdrawal symptoms. (Rettig and Yarmolinsky 1995) It also found that in easing these symptoms methadone could allow motivated addicts to return to sobriety. Strongly resisted by the federal Bureau of Narcotics, methadone maintenance did not become widespread rapidly. The most fundamental criticism of maintenance has always been that it presumes "incurability," encourages users to continue to rely on a narcotic medication, and thereby undermines abstinence-based approaches. During the 1960s, and especially during the 1970s, when methadone maintenance programs expanded dramatically, this criticism came mainly from two sources: (1) abstinence-based programs run by recovering addicts, more or less in the mutual-aid tradition and (2), minority poverty activists who saw in Methadone a palliative strategy to treat what they saw as a symptom of economic deprivation without addressing its causes.

Opposition from those working in the mutual-aid tradition came mainly from veterans of therapeutic communities inspired by Synanon (established in Southern California, in 1958), and Daytop Village (opened in New York City, in 1964). While most therapeutic communities saw addiction primarily as a result of 'characterological' deficits and immaturity, some drew financial support from the Office of Economic Opportunity (OEO), the short-lived, principal arm of the War on Poverty, and relied on an analysis of heroin addiction that located its social sources in adaptations to poverty.

Despite the resistance, a new age of drug treatment emerged. By 1969, a connection between drug use and crime came to the forefront as part of the necessary action in order to stem the tide of addiction. The passage of the Controlled Substances Act of 1970, signed by President Nixon, and the reorganization of federal enforcement agencies led to Nixon's declaration of the War on Drugs. It also spawned the creation of the Special Action Office for Drug Abuse and Prevention (SAODAP). SAODAP directed an unprecedented expansion of treatment facilities. In 1971, there were thirty-six federally funded treatment programs in the U.S. By January 1973, there were almost 400. During the Carter Administration, high hopes for the continuation of expanded attention to the war on drug addiction stagnated. By the 1980s, federal support for treatment was cut almost in half.

While much was gained in the treatment of drug and alcohol abuse during this period, by the beginning of the 1980s the drug culture was not slowing down. In fact, the use of illegal drugs was just getting started, and the impact to Public Health would continue to skyrocket. By 1992, the Office of National Drug Policy estimated that the national cost of drug abuse was $172 billion. By 1998, the NIH reported that a total cost of $246 billion was spent on drug abuse. By 2001, the National Institute on Drug Abuse estimated the number was more like $484 billion.

Free Love - Free Clinics

Arising out of the counter-culture, with its social mantra of "Sex, Drugs, and Rock 'n Roll" the consensus seemed to be: "if it makes you feel good—do it." Many took each of these options to the extreme. Woodstock, the "summer of love," Altamont, and other gatherings of these "peacemakers" came to epitomize the history of the time. All social interactions soon combined the social interplay of intoxication, fornication, and gratification. It was a free world, and some of us, living at the time, took spectacular advantage of it. The historical boundaries of sex crumbled. It was not just in the area of drugs that experimentation was societally encouraged: pre-marital sex was nonchalantly expected and socially promoted. Experimentation among male to female, male-to-male, female-to-female, one-on-one, threesome and "moresome," was not only highly accepted but enthusiastically encouraged!

Popular counter-culture literature that perpetuated these new ideals such as advertising, movies, and magazines began to sprout up everywhere. At first, the message was via innuendo, but by the end of the 1970s, innuendo was replaced with explicit depictions. The pornography industry, long a small and reclusive community with limited distribution exploded. First via Super 8 movies and coin-operated video machines, soon after home video tapes provided mass distribution.

Into this free and open expression of hedonism, in all its forms, came the rise of the free healthcare clinic. As drug abuse, once again, took over the population and venereal disease and mental health issues began to spread rapidly, a counter-culture solution was needed to address the problems that resulted from the free-spirit mind-set. An illustrative example was the Haight Ashbury Free Clinics, Inc. Founded as a free health clinic by Dr. David E. Smith in Haight-Ashbury, San Francisco, California on June 7, 1967, during the counter culture of the 1960s. Today, the Haight Ashbury Free Clinic is an iconic representation of the clinics that arose during the "summer of love." As thousands of youth arrived in the city, many were in need of substance abuse treatment, mental health services, contraception, treatment for sexually transmitted diseases, and other medical attention. The clinic became the model for the modern form of the free clinic. These clinics rapidly developed to cover four core programs:

- ✓ Neighborhood medical clinics
- ✓ Substance abuse treatment centers
- ✓ Jail psychiatric services
- ✓ Rock medicine: on-site medical services for public events and concerts

Free clinics quickly spread to other Californian cities and the rest of the United States. In 1972, a meeting was held at the Shoreham Hotel in Washington DC where clinic staff from around the country gathered to hear speakers, including Dr. Smith. At this meeting, the slogan "Healthcare is a Right Not a Privilege" emerged as a theme.

Quite rapidly, these free clinics became the front line on the war on drugs, mental health, and venereal disease that was destroying the state of public health in many American cities. Members of the counter-culture had an innate fear of authority and the government, and most simply refused to go to the public institutions for fear of reprisals or incarceration. Free clinics provided a culturally sensitive and effective method to address the needs of the underserved population.

During the 1970s and 1980s, free clinics continued to evolve and change to meet the needs of individual communities, though not all were able to survive. Each free clinic was unique in its development and services—each was based on the particular needs and resources of the local community. There is a saying among free clinic organizations that if you have been to one free clinic, you have been to one free clinic. The common denominator is that care is made possible through the service of volunteers, the donation of goods, and community support. Funding was generally donated on the local level, and there was little, if any, government funding. Some free clinics were established to provide medical services in the inner cities while others opened in the suburbs. Many student-run free clinics emerged to serve the under-served as well as to provide a medical training site for students in the healthcare professions.

While both free and community clinics provided many similar services, free clinics, as of this writing, were defined by the U.S. National Association of Free Clinics as "private, nonprofit, community based organizations that provide medical, dental, pharmaceutical and/or mental health services at little or no cost to low-income, uninsured, and under insured people. They accomplish this through the use of volunteer health professionals and community volunteers, along with partnerships with other health providers." Some free clinics have evolved to rival local government health departments in size and scope of service, with multi-million dollar budgets, specialized clinics, and numerous locations.

The Rise of the HMO

There were 6,000 hospitals in the U.S. in 1960. According to the American Hospital Association, there are actually fewer hospitals—approximately 5,795—in the U.S. today. By the time John F. Kennedy had taken office, the long problem of access to quality healthcare in the U.S. had been solved.

As the discontent with basic access and quality receded, the nation's concern moved to the cost issue and the breadth of services available for coverage. Through the early part of this period, most employer-based insurance plans offered general health coverage. Items like: maternity, vision, and dental were not typically part of the employer's paid plan. Other items like cosmetic reconstructive surgery, with only rare exception for some extreme disfiguring accidents or illness, were not covered at all. As consumers approached the end of the period, some would remark that insurance was great at "covering everything except what you lost." Pressure mounted for employers (always trying to remain competitive in job offerings) to continue to expand coverage under their employee plans by adding additional paid coverage like, vision, dental, maternity, etc.

Health insurance, like other forms of insurance, is a method to spread the risk of expense over time and across a large number of people. Under this collective pool of risk, the insurer makes a reasonable bet that a small amount of monthly payment by all of the insured will accumulate to a pool of funds that will be sufficient to cover the expenses of medical treatment because not all people in the pool will get the same level of illness and not all will get sick at the same time. By calculating the projected level of illness, in a population, over time, the insurer can estimate the minimum monthly payment, based on historical expense patterns, with enough accuracy that the amount of the monthly payment, required to build sufficient reserves to cover the maximum potential loss of the population in any period, is less than customers are willing to pay. Theoretically, the insurer is able to generate much more in reserves over time than the population will actually use for the services based on the projected services covered over the future time period.

The dominant form of insurance, which rose through the 1940s and into this period, was indemnity-based health insurance. Indemnity insurance compensates the beneficiaries of policies for economic losses, up to the limiting amount of the insurance policy. It generally requires the insured to prove the amount of its expense before they can recover. Recovery is typically limited to the amount of the provable expense, even if the face amount of the policy is higher. The key to the adequacy of the indemnity reserve funds is in the limits of what the policy covers and the fact that not all of the patients choose to receive care and a significant percentage die before chronic age based illnesses sap the reserve pool—the latter two items no longer hold true today.

The facts of the Massachusetts General Hospital, Insane Asylum, and Life Insurance Company aside (chartered in 1811), most scholars say that accident insurance, the earliest form of health disability insurance, was first offered in the U.S. by the Franklin Health Assurance Company of Massachusetts. This firm, founded in 1850, offered insurance against injuries arising from railroad and steamboat accidents. Sixty organizations were offering accident insurance in the U.S. by 1866, but the industry soon consolidated thereafter. While there were earlier experiments, the origins of sickness coverage in the U.S. effectively date back to about 1890. The first employer-sponsored group disability policy was issued, in 1911.

Before the development of medical expense insurance, patients were expected to pay healthcare costs out of their own pockets, under what is known as the fee-for-service business model. During the middle to late twentieth century, traditional disability insurance evolved into modern health insurance programs. Today, most comprehensive private health insurance programs cover the cost of routine, preventive, and emergency healthcare procedures and most prescription drugs, but this was not always the case.

Hospital and medical expense policies were introduced during the first half of the twentieth century. During the 1920s, individual hospitals began offering services to individuals on a pre-paid basis, eventually leading to the development of Blue Cross organizations.

In the 1950s, indemnity insurance as provided by the various companies like Blue Cross and Blue Shield plans was considered a fair and adequate method to offset the catastrophic cost of a sudden and unexpected illness. Expected illnesses were not something that was covered.

Since the basis of indemnity insurance, is to spread the cost and the risk across the widest population so that the average cost for anyone in the plan would be shared by both the equally sick and the equally well, insurers could not knowingly provide insurance to people with a known illness. Clearly, if insurers were willing to cover a person with heart disease or cancer after it was disclosed that they had heart disease or cancer most of the insured would not pay for the insurance until, after they got the disease. If mostly sick people were the only ones to purchase the plan then the average cost would rapidly become unaffordable. Insurance plans in this period soon excluded preexisting conditions from coverage. This was seen as, the only way to make sure the population would buy the insurance before they got sick, and then fairly pay into the system, supporting all of the insured in the pool fairly and equitably.

Even the venerable Massachusetts General Hospital and Insane Asylum quickly found that, without conditions and controls, the fiscal realities of treatment were vastly in excess of their ability to provide free beds. By 1826, the hospital board had determined that the policy, of housing incurable patients, was not consistent with the mission of the hospital. Within a week of the decision by the board, twenty-six of the thirty-two patient-residents were released.

As the country entered the 1960s, and despite the best efforts of insurance companies to keep costs down, a number of unanticipated issues with indemnity insurance plans emerged. As more and more people purchased insurance, it had long been felt that there would be reductions in the overall medical expenses of the population due to the widening of the actuarial risk and economies of scale. What had not been accurately predicted was the continuing rise in the sheer number of treatable conditions and the rapidly increasing cost of newer and better technological diagnostics.

During the 1950s, most of those insured paid for the services directly and received reimbursement from the insurance company for the eligible services. Insurance of the day did not cover everything or in some cases most things. Insurance was seen more than anything else as home protection in case of a catastrophic illness. Routine doctor's visits, vaccinations, and other more routine treatments were not often covered.

The average life span was extending rapidly, due to new and better treatments of what were only a few years earlier, untreatable and often fatal conditions. As people began to live longer, the cost of coverage, particularly in later life, was growing exponentially. The risk (actuarial) calculations were no longer working and what had been relatively inexpensive monthly premium payments were suddenly rising rapidly. Healthcare was getting more expensive in a number of areas. At the time of the writing of this book, statistics indicated that due to the longevity of the people in this period, and the number and cost of effective treatments and technologies for the diseases and illnesses of old age, in 1995, two-thirds of lifetime healthcare costs were spent in the last five years of life. (Lubitz, M.P.H., Beebe, B.A. and Baker, M.P.P. 1995) Recent data indicates that this percentage has increased to between 80–85%. George Halvorson reports in his recent book, *Health Care Will Not Reform Itself*, that the average annual cost of care for a twenty year old is $1,448, $2,601 for a 40 year old, $10,245 for a 65 year old, and for and eighty-five year old it is $17,071—an 1,184% increase over the 20 year old. (Halvorson 2009) Such a strong and unexpected back-end weighting of these costs is one of the significant causes of what is now contributing to the rapid rise of the actuarial costs of Medicare, and contributing to the rise of insurance premiums.

The average life expectancy in 1950 was 68.1 years of age. By 1980, it had been extended to 73.9 years. Overall, healthcare had improved, diagnostics and treatments had continued to expand, and the role of technologies had continued its progressive march. A new term began to take hold in our vernacular. Before this period, people were fundamentally concerned with extending their lives to a reasonable age. By 1979, however, people were now becoming concerned about the "quality of life." They recognized that the mere extension of years of life was bringing increased sickness pain and sufferingdue to a rise in the diseases of the aged, not seen as prevalently in prior decades.

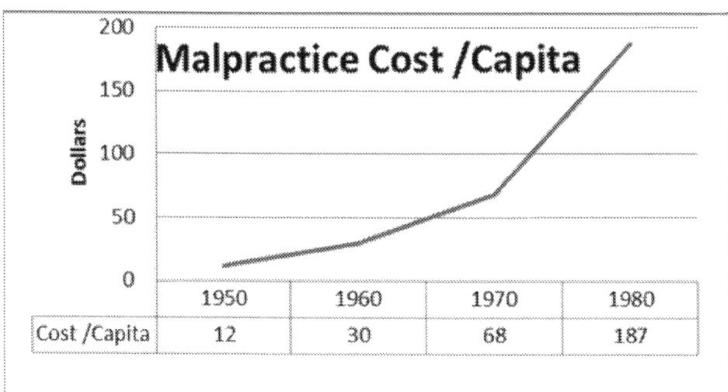

	1950	1960	1970	1980
Cost /Capita	12	30	68	187

Chart 5: Malpractice Cost

Consumers were finding that they needed to see the doctor more often. There were continually more new tests to be done, the price of the services themselves was rising, the cost for training and education for doctors was rapidly increasing due to continually rising standards and requirements, and more drugs and vaccinations to help offset or prevent disease were suddenly available. Doctors were developing new and more complicated procedures and methods to treat illness, disease and accidents—patients before then simply would have died. Now more survived, but it was not the survival that became the issue, it was those who underwent the risky procedures and did not survive that became problematic. With more doctors, more treatments, and more options to treat risky patients, malpractice insurance costs began to escalate. (Chart 5)

One other item of interest is that there was a significant, and rapid, rise in the number of lawyers being admitted to practice at the end of the 1950s. Between 1951 and 1971, the number of lawyers in the U.S. had increased 326 percent. So much so that, by the late 1960s, many lawyers were chafing at the long-standing rules of ethics by which they were bound—particularly the ones prohibiting solicitation and advertising. In 1977, however, the U.S. Supreme Court unshackled attorney commercial speech with their ruling in *Bates v. State Bar of Arizona, 433 U.S. 350* (1977). Many lawyers of the day like Judge Loker's son, Wm. Aleck, felt the new-found freedoms would significantly damage the professional nature of the occupation, and would lead to a rapid rise in frivolous cases and ever increasingly expensive judgments as lawyers competed to secure larger and larger awards. Looking back through the hindsight of history one would think this very prophetic.

Insured patients saw their cost of healthcare rise in every possible area, both in terms of what they paid out-of-pocket and what they were paying as monthly premiums. Insurers were also seeing costs rise out of control and the former sound actuarial reserves were being depleted. They reacted by raising premiums and restricting coverage.

Consumers and the nation were rapidly becoming disenchanted with the current form of coverage and cost. As the dissatisfaction grew, other methods of coverage were investigated and entities like Kaiser or Ross-Loos (now CIGNA) provided an optional alternative.

While the basic tenets of Health Maintenance Organizations (HMOs) can first be seen in a number of prepaid health plans, beginning as early as 1910, like Ross-Loos Medical Group, and Kaiser Permanente, The predecessors of today's Health Maintenance Organizations originated beginning in 1929, through the 1930s upward to World War II.

As the nation moved into the 1970s, the demand for a cheaper and better alternative to indemnity insurance was reaching its peak. One of the problems with a large scale move to HMO style care plans was that, by 1970, the number of HMOs had declined to less than forty. Paul Elwood seized the initiative. He was considered the father of the HMO. He began having discussions with what is today the Department of Health and Human Services that ultimately led to the enactment of the Health Maintenance Organization Act of 1973.

The Health Maintenance Organization Act of 1973 (Public Law 93–222), also known as the HMO Act of 1973, 42 U.S.C. § 300e, had three main provisions:

1. Grants and loans were provided to plan, start, or expand a HMO.
2. Certain state-imposed restrictions on HMOs were removed if the HMOs were federally certified.
3. Employers with twenty-five or more employees were required to offer federally certified HMO options alongside indemnity upon request.

This last provision, called the dual choice provision, was the most important, as it gave HMOs access to the critical employer-based market that had often been blocked in the past. The federal government was slow to issue regulations and certify plans until 1977, when HMOs began to grow rapidly. The dual choice provision expired in 1995.

In 1971, Gordon K. MacLeod, M.D., developed and became the director of the first federal HMO program. He was recruited by Elliot Richardson, former secretary of the U.S. Department of Health,

Education and Welfare. The act solidified the term HMO and gave HMOs greater access to the employer-based market.

The promise of the HMO model was considered to be three fold for consumers. (1) Consumers would gain additional choice in the type of coverage they could select. (2) HMOs theoretically would be able to provide the services in a much more efficient care model due to reduction in duplicated services, and better negotiation with providers, and (3) Long-term care costs would be lowered as HMOs would better focus part of their practice on the effective prevention of disease.

Although businesses pursued the HMO model for its alleged cost containment benefits, some research indicates that private HMO plans did not achieve any significant cost savings over non-HMO plans. Although out-of-pocket costs are reduced for consumers, controlling for other factors, the plans don't affect total expenditures and payments by insurers. A possible reason for this failure is that consumers may have increased utilization in response to less cost sharing, under HMOs.

At the time of this writing, we saw that while prevention may have reduced the incidence of some lifestyle-related illnesses, there are critics who argue the additional up-front expense of preventive care may not, in the long run, lead to real savings. Only time will tell if there are a true actuarial savings or if better prevention will again extend life which, in turn, will again increase the cost of care during the last five years of life. Clearly, prevention has the potential to improve the quality of life in the later years, though that is not the question. The question is: at what cost?

While this period was also characterized by a significant number of technological and medical achievements, the relative change to the general welfare of the day appears to have been less impactful, or at least less-noticed, by the average individual. While the advances continued to arrive, people became less focused on the gains they were achieving and more on the things yet to be achieved.

The effect of this period today is more characterized by this changing level of expectation as to what was wanted, than by the gains achieved. In the prior periods, any gain had a significant effect on one's life span and in such profound ways. Culturally, people were simply grateful for the benefit. Conversely, during this period, the mood of the country had shifted and each gain was countered with a demand for additional gains. The desire now was not simply to extend the years of life, but to improve the quality of those years, as well.

The period of 1950 to 1979, will likely be most remembered for the resurgence of our national addiction to tobacco, drugs, and alcohol and all the associated, human, and economic costs. The main differentiator between this period and the early 1900s, is that the addiction of this era was completely voluntary and clearly with our own knowledge and consent.

By the end of 1979, much of the core issues and systems that define our current healthcare structures and relationships had been forged and continue to build up to the dysfunctional system that we have today. A major factor facing us today is the cost and inefficiencies of Medicare and Medicaid, also a remnant of this period.

Chapter 6 Addendum
Medical Advances 1950 – 1979

1950s

- 1950, development of the first cardiac pacemaker.
- 1952, Jonas Salk develops the first practical polio vaccine.
- 1954, the first kidney transplant is performed by Dr. Joseph E. Murray.
- 1959, the first artificial heart is transplanted into a dog.

- 1951, IBM develops the Gibbon Model II heart-lung machine; delivered to Jefferson Medical College Hospital.

- 1952–53, James Watson and Francis Crick describe the structure of the DNA molecule. Maurice Wilkins and Rosalind Franklin began to study DNA. Controversially Watson and Crick announce their discovery, smoking is determined to be a health risk, and Ultrasound employed in prenatal care and heart disease, first national conference on air pollution highlights a growing health problem without sharing credit with Wilkins and Franklin, even though Wilkins shared his and Franklin's research. Watson, Crick and Wilkins share the Nobel Prize for the discovery.

- 1957, first birth control pill Enovid goes to market.

1960s

- 1960, oral vaccine for polio

- 1961, sleeping pill thalidomide taken by pregnant women in Western Europe is shown to have caused birth defects in their babies; FDA officials kept drug from being marketed in U.S.

- 1965, Ralph Nader publishes "Unsafe at Any Speed," charging that the American automobile industry is neglecting consumer safety issues.

- 1964–1980, the National Aeronautics and Space Administration (NASA) provide numerous contributions to medicine. Examples not only included the observation and documentation of metabolic and physiological stress but inventions like telemetry, Teflon, titanium, freeze-drying, microwave, fiber-optics, advances in computerization, etc.

- 1960, first coronary bypass operation.
- 1963, vaccine for measles.
- 1967, Dr. Christian Barnard performs the first human heart transplant, vaccine for Mumps invented.

1970s

- 1970, vaccine for Rubella.
- 1972, Magnetic Resonance Imaging MRI is discovered.
- 1975, British scientists George Kohler and Cesar Milstein, of Cambridge's Medical Research Council Laboratory of Molecular Biology, develop the monoclonal antibody.
- 1977, vaccine for Pneumonia, Dr. Willem Kolff, University of Utah, designs a nuclear-powered artificial heart (Westinghouse Corporation).
- 1971, introduction of Computerized Axial Tomography, the "CAT-scanner.
- 1974, vaccine for Chicken Pox.
- 1976, Robert Jarvik, Ph.D. designs the Jarvik series of artificial hearts.
- 1978, first "test-tube" baby is born in the UK, vaccine for Meningitis.

VII. (1980 – 2010) Helplessly - Hoping:

Time to Make a Change

Imagine . . .

"This is not an innocent heart murmur!" you hear the doctor say. Out of the corner of your eye, you see the mother of your newborn son begin to swoon. As you turn to reach out and hold her, you struggle to keep her upright and provide comfort at the same time—trying to make sense of what has just happened. Your mind can only think, Please, God, not again!

Just a week ago, on September 2, 1998, your son was born and all seemed happy and healthy. The only worries you felt were those of anyone becoming a parent of a newborn child. Perhaps less so, because your last child had so many things happen you just knew that lightening would not strike you like that again!

Now here you stand, holding your wife and trying to understand what the cardiologist is saying, trying to shelter your wife from the pain that you know, will soon be coming. "We need to do some additional tests right away," the doctor says.

The diagnosis is rendered within a few hours: Tetralogy of Fallot (TOF) a congenital heart defect which can involve four anatomical heart abnormalities—although only three of them are always present. It is the most common cyanotic heart defect, and the most common cause of blue baby syndrome. But, your son was not blue! His oxygen levels appeared normal during the birth and after. Christ, you are a biologist, you have been around biology and healthcare much of your life, and you were paying attention to the vitals. All was completely normal. How the hell can this be?

You want to challenge the doctor, but you don't want to right now with your wife in your arms. She is reeling and scared. So you keep quiet, and together you and your wife begin the process of learning what this journey will entail. For your wife, this is all new, but for you, this is an unpleasantly familiar story.

While today this story is unfolding near the San Francisco Bay, fifteen years ago another story in your life unfolded on the opposite coast next to another bay, the Chesapeake Bay. It began within yards of where your ancestor, Thomas Loker, first came ashore at the founding of the Maryland colony . . .

"Bobby, I need you to move that beam another two inches—the tenon isn't lining up in the mortise, and I can't get the wooden pin in to drive it tight." You yell across the room to Bobby Abell from the high rafter that you're sitting on. It is now Tuesday, December 7, 1982, in St. Mary's City, and already the cold weather is settling in. You and the guys have been building your new bookstore, and while the end-result will be stunning, the decision to build it in the seventeenth century style of the historic campus at St. Mary's College of Maryland has proven to be a whole lot more work than you expected.

When you began in April, you had hoped to have the new bookstore open before the start of the school year. The main delay had been that the original source for the large hand hewn posts and beams had fallen through, so for the past few months, the raw timbers had to be debarked, then left to dry and then hewn to shape by hand with adz and broad-ax. The summer students had a lot of fun learning to use the old tools, but not without some skinned shins and other cuts and bruises. In the end, they had gotten the timbers shaped and then they had to dry in the humid Maryland summer sun for a few months more. So here you are, up in the rafters of this new old-style post-and-beam building that will be the new campus bookstore. Your ancestor, Thomas, had come ashore and made his life in the New World right here. Now, over 200 years later, you are sitting high up mating two timbers with exactly the same type of construction, as he would have done, using the same tools. Not bad for a biologist, you think.

As Bobby drives the beam tighter into the mortise joint, you sit back and gaze out the tops of the high windows. You see one of your student assistants, Christie Engle, running across the campus in your direction. She is tall, very slender and always perky, but there is something about the way she is running that worries you. Just as the tenon seats the rest of the way in the mortise, Christie bursts through the door—she screams that there is an emergency, and you have to go to the hospital right-away.

You scramble across the rafter and down the twenty-one feet to the floor. Christie is out of breath, but explains that the hospital called, and they said you need to go there, right-away. When you ask her what is going on she gets more upset. When she heard that it was an emergency, and you needed to come right away, she neglected to find out why, and now she feels stupid and worried that she somehow has let you down. Your mother, stricken with breast cancer, has been in the hospital in a coma for the past two weeks, so you assume something has happened with her. Poor Christie now feels guilty, and is getting more, and more, flustered, so you tell her not to worry as you jump into your truck and begin the one hour ride to the hospital.

You pull into St. Mary's Hospital's parking lot and run inside. Taking the steps two at a time, up three flights to the top floor, you run down the hall and burst into the room where your mother has been for the past three weeks. Fully expecting the worst when you rush in the room, you are startled to find your mother awake and alone sitting up in the bed. As you pause to catch your breath, "What are you doing here, and in such a rush I might ask?" she says. "Well, Mom, I got a call to come to the hospital right away and frankly I thought you were passing!"

"Not yet," she says," but that will be soon I am sure. Why did they call you, I wonder?" she continues. You realize it must be because of your wife. She is twenty-five weeks pregnant with your second child, and all had been going well. You simply did not even consider something on this front.

You call down to the emergency room and speak to Ann Smart, the ER charge nurse. She tells you, they have just transferred your wife up to obstetrics in premature labor. "Mom, it's something with the pregnancy I am going downstairs, I will come back when I know something," you say as you head out the door and back down the stairs to the first floor.

When you get down to obstetrics, Dr. Bent the OB/GYN sees you in the hall and tells you your wife went into labor. "Tommy, you can't see her at the moment," he says. "We have her elevated, almost upside down, to let gravity help pull the baby and the amniotic sac, which has not yet burst, back inside. We are giving her something to try to arrest her labor. "If the baby is born now," he says, "there is nothing they will be able to do—the baby won't survive."

Unable to see your wife, and with nothing to do here, you go back upstairs and to talk to your mom . . .

You come back into yourself in 1998 from your daydream escape. The cardiologist is telling you and your wife that the prognosis for your son is uncertain. There is an open-heart surgical procedure that can be done to correct some of the defects in the heart, but you should delay the surgery till your son is three months old. Then after this surgery, he will need annual visits and monitoring as he grows. It is likely he will need additional surgery when he is around fourteen years old because, even if they can make the repairs to the affected areas, most of the time the affected valve will need to be replaced as the repaired valve will not grow proportionately to the rest of his body and will become insufficient. If that happens, then he will need to have that valve replaced with one from a pig's heart.

You look at your wife. She is holding up well under the circumstances, which makes you feel proud of her. But, you also know the heartache the next few months, or years, will bring. The continual worry, and uncertainty of a chronically sick child never goes away. Each trip to the doctor will feel like a game of Russian roulette. Will the news be good or bad? When will the next shoe drop? Why our son? Why us? Why me? Will our son have a normal life span? Will our son have a decent life?

How much will this cost? Will insurance cover it? The questions are endless and will always remain unanswered regardless of the prior results.

Days later, you take your now-very-fragile son home. For the next three months, you wait and anticipate the surgery that you know, will be horrible. You shift between wanting to learn everything you can about the disease's potential treatments and the fear that grips you as you become fully aware of all of the various worst-case scenarios.

Two weeks later, at the next office visit, you are introduced to another couple that has a son born almost the same day as yours, who also has TOF. It is a relief to be able to speak to someone else who is going through the same experience. You son's surgery has been scheduled first. Theirs will come a week later. You are now on this odyssey together. For the next three months, you will compare notes, share articles and stories, and most importantly get together with both of your sons hoping they will each survive and do well. Many times you will escape the current problem and drift back in your mind to 1982 and your last experience as you try to draw some lessons and, again, help you cope . . .

In your mind, it is 1982, and you are back in your mother's hospital room. "Mom, she is in labor, and they are trying to get it to stop," you say. "They say there is an outside chance if they can stop the contractions and get the baby and the amniotic sac to go back in her womb they can stitch her shut, and with a little luck, allow the baby to develop for a few more weeks to where he may survive. They need to get him up to at least two pounds."

"Well, son," Mom says, "you just need to believe it will all work out."

For the next two hours, you and your mom talk about everything that is going on. You speak about the good times in the past, and the recent couple of years as she has been declining from the breast cancer. Five years before, a bilateral radical mastectomy took both her breasts, followed by two separate bouts of radiation and chemotherapy. Looking at your mom as she chats while sitting up in bed, she appears frail but better than she was a few days ago while she was lying unconscious. Since the cancer metastasized a few months ago, it seemed your mom was on a downhill spiral leading to the inevitable. That is why, when you got the call, you fully expected to find her either on her last breath or passed-on. But, right now she is lucid, vibrant, apparently not suffering much pain and both at ease and at peace. She is more concerned for your unborn son than for herself. At 5-foot-1 and 85 pounds, your mom never seemed to be a strong woman. Nevertheless, here she sits awake and still alive. Her concern is focused, as always, on others.

At about 3:30 that afternoon, your sisters Peggy and Lucy, your brother Aleck, and your dad, all show up. For the next half-hour, the family simply sits together and talks about life, family, and friends in a way you have not been able to do for quite a while.

The quiet revelry is suddenly broken when Joan Wise, a friend you have known since the first grade and an OB/GYN nurse, calls you into the hall. She tells you, they have your wife stabilized and are about to transport her to Georgetown Hospital—two-and-a-half hours away. This is the only hospital in the area that can provide some potential for hope. Joan pulls some strings, and you will be allowed to ride up in the ambulance and comfort your wife during the long drive. It is going to be a long week . . .

As the memory fades, you find yourself back in 1998. Three months have passed. It is now December 7, coincidentally the same day that you were in the rafters when your second son's odyssey began sixteen years before. Tomorrow morning at 4:15, you will drive your wife and fragile son to the hospital for the surgery that will, hopefully, correct the congenital defects of his heart. Neither of you has gotten much sleep, during the past few days. When you arrive at the hospital, once again you feel that same feeling of disconnect you felt the last time, all those years ago. The fabric of time seems to tear apart and fall back on itself. Events begin to teeter-totter between long slow never ending waiting, anxious worry filled periods, and periods when time just seems to slip where you don't seem to know how you got to where you are and what was just happening.

The final X-rays and cardiac tests are done. The long nerve-wracking tedium in the waiting room suddenly comes to end. The moment you both hope for, and wish never would come is finally here. The surgical prep team enters the room. Carefully, confidently the staff says, "Its time." Your wife desperately holding your son for just that one more second seems to begin to fold in on herself, but thankfully her strength rebounds. She holds your son for that last little bit as you both give him a kiss and then reluctantly hand your precious, fragile, outwardly perfect child to the awaiting team. As they leave the waiting room and pass through the door, you and your wife hold each other and are left alone with nothing else to do but pray and comfort each other. The next five hours will be the longest of your life. Again, you seek some solace in the past, and you again drift back . . .

The second week of December of 1982, the first few days after arriving in the ambulance at Georgetown Hospital remain in memory a disconnected blur. You arrive at 6:30 in the evening after the two-and-a-half-hour drive. Your wife is subjected to tests, medications, and more tests. Much of this time you sit alone in a nondescript waiting room.

After an hour, or more, a group of doctors appears. An obstetrician, neonatologist and numerous other specialists greet you. The OB doc begins to tell you what is going on. "While things have improved," he says, "your wife is now resting in her room; there are a number of things to be aware of. First, labor has still not been arrested completely. She is still having contractions, and if we cannot get these to stop soon there will be further complications. Second, the cervical cerclage, also known as a cervical purse stitch, was correctly applied by the doctors at St. Mary's and is helping, but it is too early to know if there will be infection as a result of the presentation of the amniotic sac during the premature breach. Third, the team is working hard to determine how well-developed your son is now, and how much longer we need to keep him in vitro to give him some chance of viability. At twenty-five weeks, he likely weighs less than two pounds, which is usually too small to survive. At this stage, your son's lungs have not developed enough to breathe on their own and typically they are too delicate for mechanical ventilators."

"There is some good news, however," says the neonatologist. "While a few weeks ago a child less than two pounds would have no chance, we just received a neonatal micro ventilator for kids just like your son. If we can determine that your son is over about 1 pound, he will have a slim chance. The key is to get him over about 450 grams."

"That is where Dr. James comes in," says the OB doc. "He is one of the pioneers of using ultrasound in obstetrics, and has recently been working on a method to estimate birth weight based on ultrasound density readings."

"I will be taking a series of readings over the next few days to determine your son's weight and development and should be able within a week or so to predict when he can be born," says Dr. James. "For now, though, "concludes the OB, "We need to try to keep your son safe and sound in his mother's womb and try our best to make sure no infection or other complications develop. Do you have any questions?"

Of course you have questions, thousands of them. But, now does not seem like a good time to get into any of them. The main thing that you want now is to see your wife and sort it all out. So, you ask to see your wife.

They take you down the hall to the room you both will share for the next few weeks, and it all starts to hit you. Until now, everything has been guided by the focus of the moment, but as you approach her room it all just seems to be overwhelming. Now standing outside her door, you realize that everything in your life has changed today, all your hopes and dreams and most importantly right now you don't have the time to fret or worry about it, you have to be strong and support your wife and trust in modern medicine and technology—something that until a few hours ago was an abstract thought that had little to no consequence on your day-to-day life. In fact, self-reliance, not an expectation of help from medicine, has been something your family has traditionally valued ever since your ancestors' time.

Then next morning you find out that your mother slipped back into a coma. Your dad tells you, it happened two hours after you left St. Mary's Hospital in the ambulance. You spend the next two days and nights alternating between getting something to eat in the cafeteria and sitting or sleeping in the chair next to your wife's bed in the hospital room. By Friday, the OB doc reports that finally the contractions have completely subsided, and there is no sign of infection. Your wife appears to be stable, but she will be confined to bed rest. You and your wife agree you need to go back home for a day or so. You didn't pack anything before you left, and have been in the same clothes for four days. You didn't have much cash, but fortunately you had a credit card, and the hospital gift shop had some sundries like toothbrush, tooth paste, soap, and deodorant.

Your truck is still parked at St. Mary's Hospital, more than one hundred miles away. After work your brother, Aleck, agrees to make the long drive from Leonardtown to pick you up at the hospital. After a short visit with your wife, you reluctantly leave for home. Along the way, you stop at Billy Martin's Tavern, in Georgetown, to grab a bite to eat. By the time Aleck drops you off at your truck in the hospital parking lot, it is 11:30 at night.

Even though you are tired, something drives you to visit with your mom before you go home for the night. You make your way into the hospital, and you walk up the stairs to see her. As you enter the room, she looks at peace, as though she was merely resting and not in a coma. The prior weeks, when she was in the coma she looked in distress, but now she simply looks asleep. You've been told that it is good to talk to people in a comatose state, so you sit down and begin to give your mom an update.

You begin by telling her about the previous few days at Georgetown, but soon you are telling her about everything. The bookstore construction, sitting in the rafter making the mortise and tenon joints, driving the beams together and having them held together with wooden pins just like in the original, Thomas Loker's, time. Growing up in Leonardtown, the Fourth of July picnics, Judge Loker wading in the bay up to his calves, still wearing his suit and tie, all the kids swimming in the pond—all of these thoughts flood your mind as you talk with your mom. Somewhere deep in your mind, she is there speaking with you as you share the moments of your past hopes and dreams. For a moment, you have both forgotten your worries. At 1:15 in the morning, December 11, you finally leave the hospital to go home . . .

Another hospital, and another place; your mind reels again, back to 1998. Two hours have elapsed since the surgical team took your three-month-old son from your arms. You and your wife have alternated between sitting anxiously in the cardiology surgical waiting room and restlessly sitting in the cafeteria.

As you return to the waiting room, you see your best friend, and longtime business partner, Ken Waters, standing in the doorway to the room. He has flown in, from his home in Arizona, to help share your vigil, and lend his support to you and your wife. An open-heart patient himself, he knows first-hand the miracle of modern-day medicine and what your son is going through. And, more than most, he knows just how hard the recovery will be for everyone. The fact that he is standing here with you, is something that will separate him from all others in your family's heart, for the rest of your lives. For the next few hours, he is there at your side, much of the time in simple, quiet support, but there nonetheless to help ease the fear and anxiety and, providing an extra set of shoulders to help you carry your burden.

Three hours later, the door to the waiting room opens and Dr. Frank Hanley, the pediatric cardio-thoracic surgeon, enters the room. His life's research and clinical work have been focused on the development of interventional techniques for fetal and neonatal treatment of congenital heart disease, pulmonary, vascular physiology, and the neurologic impact of open-heart surgery. He developed and pioneered the "unifocalization" procedure, in which a single technique is used to repair this complex and life-threatening congenital heart defect rather than several staged open-heart surgeries as performed by other surgeons. The exact surgery that he has just done on your son that is now the standard for treating Tetralogy of Fallot was developed by this gifted man. There is no one better to have performed the surgery, but still as he walks across the room it makes little difference. The next words out of his mouth will tell the tale. For all three of you standing there, you both desperately want to hear them, but you fear them at the same time.

"It went very well!" he says. "Sit, sit. Let's chat about the surgery! I may write this one up—it was a textbook repair. In all the hundreds of these repairs I have done, I do not recall one ever having gone as well as this one did. We repaired the ventricular septal defect, the hole in the wall between the heart's chambers, first, and it went off

without any problem at all. Next, we corrected the overriding aorta, the thickening of the aorta that was restricting the blood flow, and again this went perfectly. Better than perfectly actually, normally we have to cut down through the aorta to free the Aortic Valve. When that happens, there are lifelong issues that happen and typically the valve has to be replaced when the patient reaches twelve to fifteen years of age; but here we did not have to cut into this area significantly. Finally, I was able to go inside the aorta and repair the valve itself without having to go in through the side of the heart. This again, is almost never the case and the benefit to your son is that we were able to preserve the valves integrity. I can say now, that your son's heart is performing better than most children born with so-called normal hearts. This is one for the books."

In just a few minutes, the shift in mood has been enormous. First, your son has survived the surgery. Second, the surgeon is telling you that the prognosis is better than good. It's excellent. Finally, your hopes for your son's future, something most parents have when children are first born but were robbed from you and your wife, is starting to return. Your wife, in tears, is hugging the surgeon. You, in tears, are shaking his hand. Kenny is in tears, too, with his arms around both you and your wife. As emotions overrun your mind, again you drift back to 1982 . . .

You are awakened Saturday with the news of your mother's death. She passed away less than half-an-hour after you left. You can't help realizing that, if not for the issue with your unborn son, you would not have had any time with your mother prior to the transport when she was awake for the short period from the coma, nor would you have seen her last night, to spend her final moments reminiscing. As you move about the quiet, lonely house, you are lost trying to figure out what you have to do.

Arrangements need to be made and since for a time you worked for Clark Mattingly at his funeral home, your dad wants you to accompany him to help with the preparations. By noon, it has been decided, both by family tradition, and an approaching blizzard, that Margaret Bell Wigginton Loker, born in 1914, will be laid to rest in

Leonardtown at Our Lady's Chapel cemetery in the family plot, on Monday December 13, 1982, at 11 in the morning. Prayers will be Sunday evening at the Mattingly Funeral Home. After speaking with your wife on the phone, you have decided that you will go back up to see her on Tuesday, the day after the funeral.

The next day is spent in taking care of family matters both surrounding your wife's hospitalization and your mother's funeral. By the time you attend the prayers Sunday evening, you are again in something of a stupor. You know there were many people at the vigil, but you don't remember seeing or speaking to anyone. It is as if you were on autopilot. By the time you arrived home at 9:30 that evening, you had barely noticed that the snow was starting to fall. Almost immediately upon walking in the house, you are in your bed asleep.

Ring! Ring! Ring! It's the old wall phone in the kitchen, the only phone in the house. You are wrenched from sleep, wondering what is happening. It is still dark outside, and you feel like you just got to bed. As you jump to your feet, and run into the kitchen, to answer the phone, you see it is 5:13AM. You answer the phone, out of breath and hear a female voice say, "Is this Mr. Thomas Loker?"

"Yes it is," you reply. "Mr. Loker my name is Mary Peterson. I am the charge nurse on your wife's ward at Georgetown Hospital Center. You need to get here right-away. The baby is coming. I am sorry to wake you this way, but it is best if you leave quickly," she says.

"What about the baby?" you ask. "Mr. Loker I don't have any information on that at this point," she replies politely. "I know the doctors are evaluating, but there is not much hope. How soon will you be able to get here?"

"Two hours!" you say. "Please take care of my wife!" You hang up and start pulling on your clothes.

Reconciled to the loss of your son, you pray that your wife will survive. Again the phone rings. Two doctors from Georgetown are on the line, the one with the ultrasound and the neonatologist. The ultrasound guy, Dr. Jones, says, "Mr. Loker, we have finished the review of the ultrasound information, and I think your son will be slightly over one pound. I think he has a fighting chance, but there are very significant risks."

"Mr. Loker, I agree with Dr. James," says the neonatologist. "Between his new measurements and the new equipment that we just received we should be able to provide good ventilation to your son, I think there is a chance he will survive. But, as Dr. James said, there will be very significant challenges . . ." As the doctor continues, the details start to get lost as you grapple with what he is saying. You were told that there was no chance for a child this small to survive. Now, he is talking as if there is some chance. You were just resolving yourself to the inevitable and now . . .

". . . but in the end this has to be your decision," the doctor is saying. "Do you want us to try this?" ask the doctors. The end of the sentence wakes you from the fog.

While you heard everything he said, you never expected there to be a choice. At least not a choice you needed to make. That is what doctors do, they make these choices so we don't have to—don't they? How can a man make such a choice? On the one hand, your son will definitely not survive a vaginal birth. On the other hand, he may survive, but the sheer extent of the laundry lists of potential problems, ranging from severe mental retardation, multiple physical defects, countless surgeries, and potentially permanent institutionalization are unimaginable. And, now they need you to make a decision about this? How does anyone make such a decision? Nowhere in your life could you ever have contemplated to have to make such a decision. These decisions should only reside in the hands of God, not Man!

As they await your reply, you realize that your last thought is your guidance. This is not your decision. It is God's decision. If you choose to withhold the miracles that they have come up with to offer your son a hope at life, then you are acting in God's stead, and that is something you simply cannot choose to do. "Do what you can for my wife, and my son, Doc," you say. "I will be there, as soon as I can."

You rush outside, and find your truck covered in two feet of drifting snow. A blizzard hit last night while you were sleeping. You try to back out your truck, but it gets hopelessly stuck. Your wife's car, smaller and lighter, gets similarly stuck. You slog across your sister's property to your father and mothers home. Your dad agrees to let you borrow his station wagon. You fill the back with bags of fertilizer to add enough weight for the wheels to gain traction, and slowly, carefully begin the long drive to Washington, D.C., and Georgetown Hospital.

The drive takes almost five hours. As you rush up to the ward, you see the nurse who called you on the phone. She has been awaiting your arrival. Before you can say anything, she greets you with, "Congratulations, you have a son. He is in the NICU, the neonatal intensive care unit. Your wife is in recovery from surgery, and she is doing fine."

As you continue to walk down the hall toward the NICU, she tells you to be prepared for what you will see. Your son is very tiny; he has tubes coming out all over his body. They will look massive in proportion to his small size. He weighs about fifteen ounces.

As you walk into the NICU, there are five patient areas. Each of areas has a team of five or six nurses in constant attendance. As you come closer to one area, you see lots of equipment but don't really see what it is connecting to. At first, you think your son is not yet in the incubator, but as you take the last step to the incubator and the nurse's part to let you see, there is a tiny doll inside the box. Your son is not much bigger than the Barbie dolls your sister Lucy once played with, but this doll has tubes and wires coming out of his chest, throat, arms, and legs and wires seemingly everywhere. Except for the fact that there is movement, you would not believe this is real. How can this be? How can something this small survive? He looks so small so fragile so helpless and hopeless, yet he clearly is alive and struggling to keep that way.

At once, you know your decision was correct and that no matter what happens, this child's chance at life has as much purpose, meaning, and hope as anyone else. While you are fearful of the future, you know this was the correct thing to do.

In a matter of moments, one of the nurses takes you to the side and shows you how to wash your hands and how to gown and glove, so you can hold your son. They place your son in the palm of your hand, and he lies across your palm as if in a small bed. His head rises only slightly above the top of your wrist and his toes stretch only slightly off the end of your fingers. One of the nurses slips off your wedding ring and places it on his arm near his bicep. My God you think it looks huge on this small child. So small, but lying on your hand you feel his heartbeat, his muscles stir. You know this kid is fighting for his life, and you know the doctors and nurses here are his best chance at survival, something that hardly anyone would have believed was possible just two weeks ago.

Your son was born at almost the exact moment that your mother was being laid to rest. His birth is a miracle of modern science and technology. Just a few weeks before, there was no path any of the doctors here would have supported to give this small infant a chance at birth, but today, here he lies, in the palm of your hand, clinging to life. A combination of research, technologies, advances in antibiotics, therapeutic practice, in both the process of birth, and the process and development of early life had culminated in the new chance afforded to your son, your wife, and your family.

On this day, there was no question of cost, or of the liability of taking risks. For all the people in this room, it was just about giving another human being the chance for life, whatever it took, whatever the risk, whatever the cost.

Your son, named Justin, has survived but with some issues. A lack of oxygen during a critical part of his birth by caesarian section damaged a part of his brain. His immature lungs, despite the benefit of the newly developed micro ventilator, kept him in the hospital for almost five months, most of which was in the NICU.

Only later would it be understood, as the result of a medical study begun just before Justin's birth, that the bright lights and loud sounds of NICUs had a very bad effect on the development of the neonatal brain, causing a lifelong series of issues. Even today at twenty-eight, your son jumps at almost any sudden noise or flash of light. For many years, he has had multiple surgeries to correct spasticity in his legs. Lifelong physical therapy has brought him good use of both of his arms, but despite the surgeries, he is now confined to a wheelchair for extended mobility. When not in his chair, he gets around his home by crawling. Initially, he had difficulty learning as he struggled with the ability to recall specific words or phrases, but he also has been blessed with a photographic memory. His problem, as observed in stroke patients, is not in the learning of information, but the ability recall facts in a timely manner.

Most importantly, he is a happy and healthy adult. He brings light and pleasure to all who know him. He is kind, patient, loving, and gifted in many ways. He has touched so many, so profoundly, how would all of your lives have been altered if you had simply not given him a chance?

The cost of delivering him into the world was astronomical. By the time he was released from the hospital, the bills had topped $500,000. Insurance paid for most of it, but not all. Hospitals, doctors, and other providers discounted some of the bills and forgave another large portion of the debt. Still, in the end you will pay for over $48,000.00 out of your own pocket during the ensuing years just for the cost of the birth.

Throughout the rest of his life, you will continue to deal with large medical bills, surgeries, complications and weekly physical therapy. If not for organizations like Easter Seals, you never would have been able to handle it all.

But, when you finally made that long drive home from Georgetown Hospital, bringing your now-five-month-old son home for the first time, you were faced with a long future full of unknowns and medical necessities. That long drive was difficult and frightening for you and your wife. The constant support of the professional staff had been there to help with all the daily therapy—they were there when the monitors went off scaring the bejesus out of you. They were there when he stopped breathing or, when tubes came out.

Now, you are both on your own. Only the two of you are left to deal with the uncertainty of not knowing what will happen next. What happens if he stops breathing? If his heart stops? Would you be able to do what they did and get his little body working again? All you really know is that, there was going to be a long, lifetime of challenges that you will all have to face to continue to provide for your son's survival . . .

As if from a deep dream, you find yourself again back in 1998. Here you are again, in the car going home alone with a small, fragile child! As you leave Children's Hospital in Oakland, driving back to your home, things look better than they have in months, but still you are plagued with the doubts and worries of what could happen.

When you and your wife first saw your son Aleck Ford after the open heart surgery, it was simply overwhelming. There are no words to describe how a parent can cope with such a small child clearly in such distress. Unlike your son Justin's traumatic birth in 1982, where he seemed like an unreal doll, today in 1998, Aleck Ford is a small baby. He is someone you have spent the last few months playing with, bonding with, and finding his personality. For you, at the beginning, Justin started the drama as a small, pitiful thing that became a person, and then your son. For Aleck, by the time of the surgery he was already your precious son, a son you handed to others, who then cut him open, dissected and re-sculpted parts of his heart and then stitched him back together with a needle and thread in order to try to give him a shot at a long and valuable life. As you sit in the recovery unit and look at your son, deathly pale, swollen, chest taped where it had been split open—hooked up to monitors and breathing tubes—again you and your wife hold each other and pray. At the time, you could not help but flash back again to that small, one pound, helpless child that became your loving son and note the difference between the two experiences and feel humbled. Now, just a few days later, you are in the car and driving home.

Within the first few minutes after arriving home, your fears begin to subside, unlike the last time. For a moment, you are sitting on the couch in your living room, your son Aleck in his travel chair on the floor, your wife lying next to him coo-ing with him and kissing his cheeks as he waves his arms and smiles. You realize that he will be OK, and no matter what happens all three of you will enjoy each and every moment from now on. Together, you are prepared to take on everything that may come . . .

It is 2010, and Aleck Ford is twelve years old. His visits to the cardiac unit of Children's Hospital have become less frequent, and he has continued to have his test results on the extremely favorable far right edge of the bell curve. While the initial prognosis included the likelihood a valve replacement operation in his teen years, today this is no longer an item routinely discussed.

In his first three years, there was a worry whether his heart could stand the rigors of sports. You were told you needed to keep a close eye on him for telltale signs of problems while playing, but none has appeared. Today he plays soccer, and basketball, and seemingly can run for days. In his first eight years, every visit to the dentist required a treatment of antibiotics for a week before the appointment, due to the potential of cardiac infection, but no longer. While the visits to the cardiologist have grown less and less frequent, each visit, once again, brings back to you that familiar gut-level displacing fear as you worry, will they find something. So far, they haven't, but the fear will always be there. As they say in finance, past results are not an indicator of future performance.

Both of your children survive today as a direct result of the advances in healthcare, in America. In both cases, it was the ever-expanding role of technology and medical science that provided timely options for the treatments that both of them received. Had either of them been born a few years earlier, these options would not have been there for them. Neither of them would be alive today.

Contrasting this experience to the life of your grandfather, Judge Loker, you can't help seeing how good you have it today. Finally, in both cases you also keenly understand the cost in agony, ecstasy, and dollars and cents of these miraculous cures. If it was not for insurance, philanthropy, non-profits, family, friends and neighbors, and your own personal ability and responsibility, either case could have left you destitute.

What did allow this to happen, was the coordination, by effort, and accident, of all of the various benefits, and sources of care that allowed for each of the myriad programs, and factors that helped you get what you needed, and allowed you to provide what you could, in order to support your two sons and deliver them an opportunity for a future. Each entity, from hospitals, to physicians, to laboratories, to insurers, to non-profits like Easter Seals, played a part in helping you get all the things that were necessary. Some provided free services, some waived all or part of the bills, others paid for part of the services, and still others just volunteered. Most importantly, you also paid as much as you could. You accepted as much of your own responsibility as possible. You came to realize, that only if every part of the equation does what it can, would everything work out the best for everyone. If you had simply not done your part, then others in the equation would have had to do more, and that would have taken resources from those other parents that could do less than you, or who needed part of what you received for their own children's survival. Both at Georgetown, with Justin, and again at Children's Oakland, with Aleck, you saw many other parents coping with the same problems as you and your family. Some had more resources than you. Others had significantly less.

You realize that anything you fail to pay for, or find a way to cover yourself, is simply going to get drawn out of the combined pot that everyone is reaching for. You know that the only way America will ever be able to afford care for everyone is if we find a way to coordinate all benefits and services from across all resources.

Years later, someone who grew up with you will ask you how you were able to cope with both your mother's death and your son's traumatic birth at the same time. A great question! Will you ever find the answer? Or, is it simply that it was everyone and everything in your life, then and now, that ultimately was there when you needed them.

Reform, Reform, and Reform Again....

The pace of technical change, both in medicine and our daily lives, skyrocketed, in the 1980s. As a result of the creations of the space program and NASA's efforts in the 1960s, a technological revolution took hold—so much so that by the 1980s, the scientific benefits were in full bloom. Corporations began to focus on healthcare, and many entered healthcare-related businesses. Some began to aggregate hospitals into holding structures. Overall, there was a shift toward privatization and consolidation of control over healthcare.

Medicare shifted its payment system from payment for treatment to payment based on diagnostic related group (DRG). Private plans quickly followed suit and reimbursement rates began a rapid and significant decline. As healthcare costs began their rise "Capitation" of payments to doctors became much more common. Under a capitation system, healthcare service providers are paid a set amount for each enrolled person assigned to that physician or group of physicians per period of time, whether or not that a person seeks care. The amount of remuneration is calculated on the average expected healthcare utilization of that patient.

Healthcare costs began to rise at double the rate of inflation in the 1990s. A major push to control costs took shape in the expansion of the concept of "managed care." Managed care is a process intended to reduce unnecessary healthcare costs through a variety of mechanisms, including economic incentives for physicians and patients in order to select less costly forms of care; programs for reviewing the medical necessity of specific services; increased beneficiary cost sharing; controls on inpatient admissions and lengths of stay; the establishment of cost-sharing incentives for outpatient surgery; selective contracting with healthcare providers; and the intensive management of high-cost healthcare cases. As managed care became the norm, Americans began to notice a significant change in the quality of interaction with their providers. Levels of dissatisfaction have grown, as a result.

Under the general category of healthcare industrial change, the 1980s proved to be a period of rapid and dramatic expansion of HMOs. Competition and regulatory pressures, combined with developing technologies, ever increasing diagnostic or treatment related options—and a significant increase in both the demand for, and the scope of requested services—contributed to an ever expanding rise in the cost and pricing of care. These factors pushed providers, payers, and consumers into new and increasingly more costly behaviors.

As costs rose out of control, Medicare and Medicaid reimbursement rates became the focus of targeted spending reductions. Consumers began to experience an increase in the cost burden disproportionately as these entitlements grew, and their costs were then shifted to non-governmental payers who were forced to make up the difference. As these costs in the public sector shifted, providers became defensive in their pricing strategies. Payers became more aggressive in driving down reimbursements to providers. As HMOs rose in utilization and popularity, the initial fee for the service model that began a decade earlier began to exhibit signs of fatigue. As we entered the 1990s, the effectiveness and efficiencies promised to public and private enrollees became at issue, and remained so throughout the end of the period. In most cases, providers became disenchanted with the model and public and private payers became less and less willing to pay for services. In the early 1980s, the main issue with the adoption of HMOs was the restrictions on the numbers and scope of physicians and hospitals invited into the HMO's network.

Employees did not flock to HMOs, to say the least. HMOs responded by developing individual practice association (IPA) HMOs. In the IPAs, the patient could select from a list of community physicians whose participation in the plans initially represented a small part of their overall practice. The resultant lower reimbursement rates that the participating physicians received were initially easily offset by transference to other private payers. Employees began to select HMO IPA plans as they felt more comfortable with the choices offered and increasingly found their physicians willing to participate.

The initial success of the wider choices available through the IPA model gave rise to other options. As such, this offered wider choices for both the consumer and the physician. These choices eventually included the development of the preferred provider organization (PPO). PPOs, in general, offered the consumer a wider range of full (HMO-like) coverage of ambulatory and inpatient care with a selected panel of providers combined with a limited (indemnity-like) range of coverage for out-of-plan use. These plans were not regulated by the Federal HMO Act or by any State HMO mandates. They also were not required to offer the broad range of services or the community premium ratings mandated for federally qualified HMOs. Consumers typically enrolled in the indemnity plan. They were able to decide whether to use providers in or out of the plan (preferred providers) at the time of service. Enrollment counts, therefore, were very difficult to estimate, yet these plans continued to grow steadily in physician, employer, and insurer participation. The rise in enrollment did not guarantee financial success for the HMO industry. In 1987, the HMO industry as a whole lost $692 million according to a report by Ellen Morrison and Harold S. Luft in *Healthcare Financing Review,* fall of 1990, titled "Health maintenance organization environments in the 1980s and beyond." They also found that nearly three quarters of the plans in existence at the time lost money.

However, as time passed the percentage of business that physicians received from these IPA and PPO plans, offering continuingly lower discounted reimbursement rates had grown to encompass most, if not all, of physicians' practices. With few other reimbursement options, physicians have found themselves once again in a declining revenue model. Compounding the issue for a physician's business models is that the reimbursement rates for Medicare and Medicaid have also dropped precipitously over the past fifteen years. Today, those patients are, in effect, being subsidized by increasing demand for higher fees on the backs of private payers. By 2010, many physicians were finding it difficult to maintain their practices due to the available reimbursement rates.

The continuing growth in the number of devices and services available to treat more and more diseases—particularly chronic conditions during this period—led to higher and higher demand for services and abundant increases in costs for healthcare on a national level. A combination of escalating Medicare and Medicaid costs, rampant health-related issues related to tobacco, drug and alcohol abuse, and epidemics of deadly and dangerous diseases like cancer, heart disease, and HIV/AIDS pushed the nation to expand the size and scope of offerings from federal and state government subsidized programs.

By the end of the century, the burden of healthcare in America was breaking the bank—though few in government seemed aware of it. Healthcare costs continued their rise unabated through the 2000s. Medicare again became viewed as unsustainable under the present structure. Direct-to-consumer advertising of pharmaceuticals and medical devices became permissible and were soon on the rise. Changing demographics, uncontrolled increases in demand and utilization of services, and continual increase in employment costs led some to question if employer-based insurance could last.

It's the Economy, Stupid

One of the main myths dispelled by reviewing our history is that recession, depression, inflation or other economically debilitating situations are not the exception for the U.S. economy. These conditions have been the norm since the country's inception.

On July 5th, 1687, Sir Isaac Newton wrote in his seminal work, Philosophiæ Naturalis Principia Mathematica, (*Natural Philosophy of Mathematical Principles*)

The above quote is Newton's third law of natural principles, and

> *Actioni contrariam semper et æqualem esse reactionem*
>
> *To every action there is always an opposed and equal reaction.*

like his observations governing the rest of the natural world, we also have seen that our nation's historical, economic problems have had a definitive impact on our national health. Our national health has an equal and opposite impact on our national economy.

It can be effectively argued that while America was successful at throwing off the shackles of British colonialism—during, both the American Revolution and the War of 1812—the battle against America has never truly abated. While we successfully defeated their military ground game, the war against America simply became an economic conflict. It is also historically naïve to believe that France and Germany were aligned with America. The European countries had less in concert with America's success than with the economic damage that the defeat of Britain by America would have and the benefit of the reduction in British power would have for Spain, France and Germany's economic interests. Despite lulls based on differing European self-interest and the need for American economic support during both world wars, by and large, it remains, to this day, an economic "battle royale." This ongoing war is now simply prosecuted by banking interests instead of troops on the ground.

As we will discuss at the end of this book, one of the prime issues that we have today related to the cost of healthcare, is simply the economy itself. As we moved through this period, several economic decisions were made that significantly changed the checks and balances, and altered the fundamental nature of our economy. In the process, this altered the relative valuations of all the tangible and intangible segments of the economy in often specious and arbitrary ways. Most importantly, with no fixed control point over the amount of currency in circulation, the money supply itself was increased so dramatically during this period that any product, good, or service that brought a new value proposition benefited disproportionately over prior long standing staples of the American economy. As a result, these industries, many of them technology based, have yielded a significantly disproportionate rise in the cost to consumers. Healthcare is a prime example.

The Breton Woods Accord established the rules for commercial and financial relations among the world's major industrial states through the mid-twentieth century. Under the accord, Franklin Roosevelt agreed with forty-four other Allied Nations to the re-institution of a modified gold standard. Under this system of monetary management, many countries fixed their exchange rates relative to the U.S. dollar. The U.S. promised to fix the price of gold at approximately $35 per ounce. Implicitly, then all currencies pegged to the dollar also had a fixed value in terms of gold.

Initially, the policies as agreed with by the various nations appeared to be in the best interests of America. The gold coffers in Fort Knox continued to fill through the duration of World War II as U.S. materials and production capacity supported the allies' efforts. As has been discussed in the prior chapters, the U.S. economy continued to boom as post-war Europe rebuilt and found a willing supplier for almost everything in America and her companies.

But as with most other things, silver linings often have dark clouds: the Breton Woods accord was no exception. Countries like Britain, France, and others continued their maneuvers against the American economy and the U.S. dollar and its limited growth against the fixed gold reserves. These countries reduced their dollar reserves by exchanging them for U.S. gold. As they made this exchange, they reduced the amount of gold in Fort Knox, diminishing, under the control formula, the relative amount of U.S. dollars in circulation. This instigated a gradual but effective reduction in U.S. influence and control abroad.

The cost to the country of the Korean War, and then the Vietnam War, were added to by the expansion of entitlements like Social Security, Medicare and Medicaid, as well as the conscious reductions and eliminations of the staple and dominant U.S. enterprises. Those included steel, oil, clothing, fisheries, and agriculture which led to the persistent and problematic balance of payments deficits. From the middle of the 1950s to the beginning of the 1960s, America was well on its way to transferring herself from the world's dominant producer, to the world's dominant consumer. By 1970, the American economy was suffering an annual inflation rate of 5.84 percent. The growing deficit became such a problem that by 1971, President Richard Nixon was forced to end direct convertibility of the dollar to gold, resulting in the system's breakdown, best known as "Nixon Shock."(Chart 6)

As the economy began to circle the drain, President Nixon imposed a ninety day wage and price freeze and a 10 percent surcharge on all imports. More importantly, he closed the gold window, ending convertibility between U.S. dollars and gold. The President—and fifteen advisors—made this decision without consulting the members of the international monetary system, so the international community informally named it the Nixon Shock. By the time Nixon made his announcement before the stock markets opened on Monday, August 15, 1971, the public at large was desperately seeking a solution. The price control plans proved very popular and began to raise the public's spirit. Despite the legacy of Nixon's failures with Vietnam and Watergate, he deserves some credit for finally rescuing the American public from foreign price-gougers, and later, a foreign-caused exchange crisis.

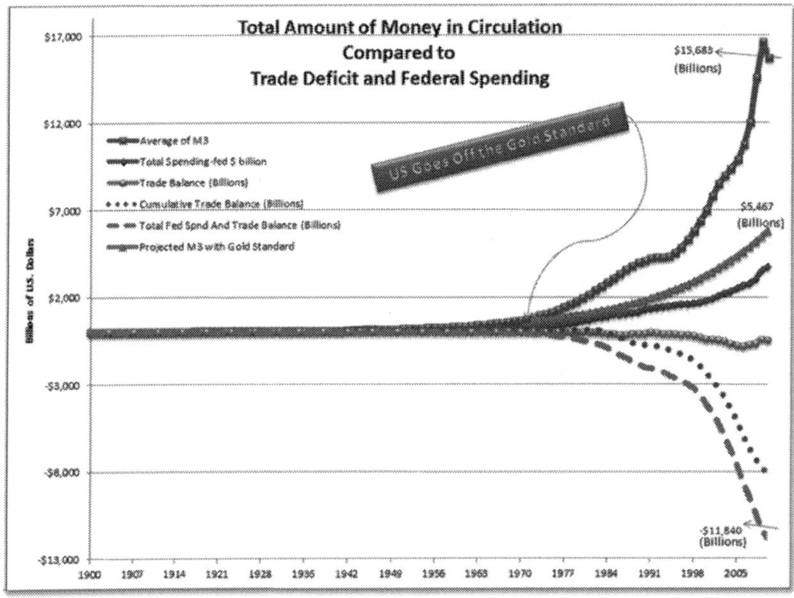

Chart 6: Total Currency in Circulation (CinC)

By March 1976, the world's major currencies were floating. In other words, the currency exchange rates were no longer the principal means of administering monetary policy. We clearly took great advantage of these new fiscal freedoms.

Economist Paul Krugman summarizes the post-Nixon Shock era as follows:

The current world monetary system assigns no special role to gold; indeed, the Federal Reserve is not obliged to tie the dollar to anything. It can print as much or as little money as it deems appropriate. There are powerful advantages to such an unconstrained system. Above all, the Fed is free to respond to actual or threatened recessions by pumping in money. To take only one example, that flexibility is the reason the stock market crash of 1987—which started out every bit as frightening as that of 1929—did not cause a slump in the real economy.

While freely floating national money has its advantages, it also has risks. Between 2005 and 2010, the dollar has been worth as much as one-hundred-twenty yen and as little as eighty. A system that leaves a country's monetary managers free to do "good" also leaves them free to be irresponsible, both within a countries fiscal policy as well as between countries.

The same song of economic warfare, which started at the end of the Revolutionary War, continues to this day. But, now the damage to our economy has not just been due to foreign governments and their maneuvers, it also has been due to the maneuvers within our own economy by governmental and industrial naiveté and avarice. Like most other things, what looked good initially has brought significant problems along the way with the then perceived benefit. Perhaps one day we will learn there is no free lunch!

By the 1990s, we again were in the grasp of a great desire of our politicians to solve our problems by giving us more. President Clinton made much of his presidential agenda predicated on a national healthcare plan. It was such a key part of his agenda that he appointed his wife and first lady, Hillary Clinton, to head the effort. (We will discuss this in more detail in a later chapter, but for now, it is significant to note that the Clinton bill did not pass.)

Given what we now know, it has been a blessing that President Clinton's effort, dubbed "Hillary Care," was not enacted. We now know that the economy was in a much more fragile state at that time than we thought it was. As the government continued the rapid expansion of the money supply in an attempt to bull our way out of the recession, our politicians enacted another series of legislative changes that altered many of the historic banking limitations that were seen as necessary by the legislators in 1933 to protect our economy.

The Glass-Steagall Act of 1933 was a law that established the Federal Deposit Insurance Corporation (FDIC) in the United States. It introduced banking reforms, some of which were designed to control speculation. As Franklin D. Roosevelt was working to finance the "New Deal" and later World War II, he was forced to make some concessions to the banks and the Federal Reserve to assure the required capital. As he negotiated the necessary deals, he also stimulated legislation that fostered the creation of Savings and Loans in conjunction with the Banking Act of 1933 (Glass-Steagall), an act that would provide checks and balances over the Federal Reserve and the banks. When they were repealed in the 1980s, and 90s, most of the controls, such as regulation "Q" which prescribed how the Federal Reserve regulated interest rates in savings accounts, and the provisions that prohibited a bank holding company from owning other financial companies, like Wall Street investment banks and depository banks, were lost. It is becoming clearer to economists and historians that the loss of these checks and balances played the pivotal part in the enablement of the financial crisis of 2007 – 2011.

One other set of changes that were implemented as a simple change to accounting rules, which were enacted on behalf of the banks during this period, was the establishment of the "Mark to Market rule of fair value accounting." This took place during Clinton's presidency. This action directly led to the death of the savings and loan industry, long a thorn in the side of the traditional fractional-reserve lending-based banks.

This simple rule change effectively killed the savings and loan institutions that were not able to lend at the 10 to 1 fractional reserve formula of the traditional banks. Their lending cushion was based on the future value of their portfolio. When the "mark to market" rule wiped out their ability to project this future value into their asset base, not only was their lending ability curtailed but their portfolios were now upside down. Traditional banks could have lent $100 for every $10 in reserves. Savings and loans had to have an equal amount of reserve to the amount lent out. Overnight the savings and loan industry collapsed. And, who was there to reap the benefit? They collapsed directly into the waiting arms of the traditional banks. I am sure that the Federal Reserve and the banking industry said a silent prayer to the gods for the providential legislative changes. (Chart 7)

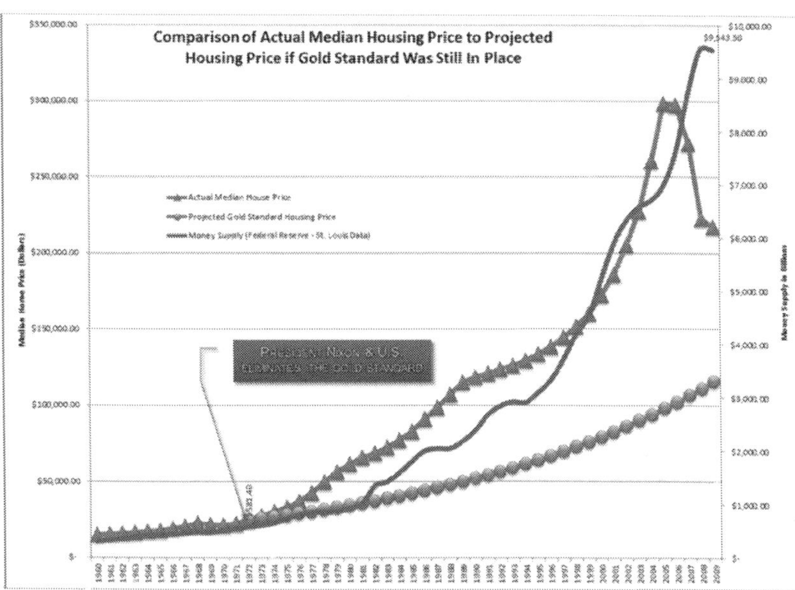

Chart 7: Median Home Price to CinC

Even with the ability effectively to create currency out of thin air, the traditional banks still needed additional legislative help legally to acquire and effectively finance the assimilation of the savings and loans portfolios. The elimination of the Glass-Steagall prohibition of banks from owning other financial companies, including investment banks, allowed the creation of what is now called the financial derivative market. Derivatives such as the mortgage backed securities that most recently collapsed Wall Street, killed the housing industry, and reduced the real equity of many Americans significantly below their debt base. Many have gone bankrupt, at least on paper, for more than 25 percent of the American population. There is no doubt that this crisis has led both America in general and most of the individual states to the edge of bankruptcy, as well. (Chart 8)

While it is not the intention of this book to provide a dialogue on the final failure of the American economy, it is clear that the uncontrolled rise of currency, starting in 1971, has become the prime cause of much of the economic problems we now face. Our federal government, as well as most of our state governmental structures, is visibly perceived as not financially sustainable. They have joined with a number of prior events including the "dot-com" stock crash, numerous recessions, inflationary periods, and depressions, to begin to show fundamental flaws in our current fiscal policy. The catastrophic collapse of the real estate market that has been seen as the driver of the current financial meltdown is really more of an effect than the cause. (Chart 7)

All of these events are actually derivatives (pun intended) of the changes in fiscal policies that have occurred as the country disconnected from a standard that limited currency production to changes in banking regulations allowing an already irresponsible fractional reserve banking system controlled at the rate of 10 to 1, to develop financial instruments that have subsequently taken our Total Currency to real GDP values to well over 10,000 to 1.

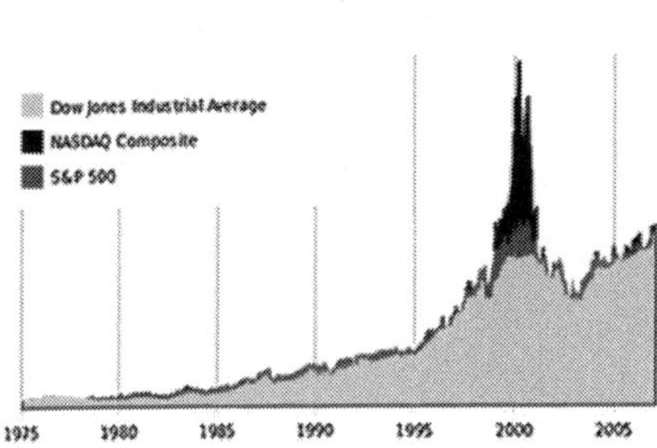

Chart 8: Stock Market Value

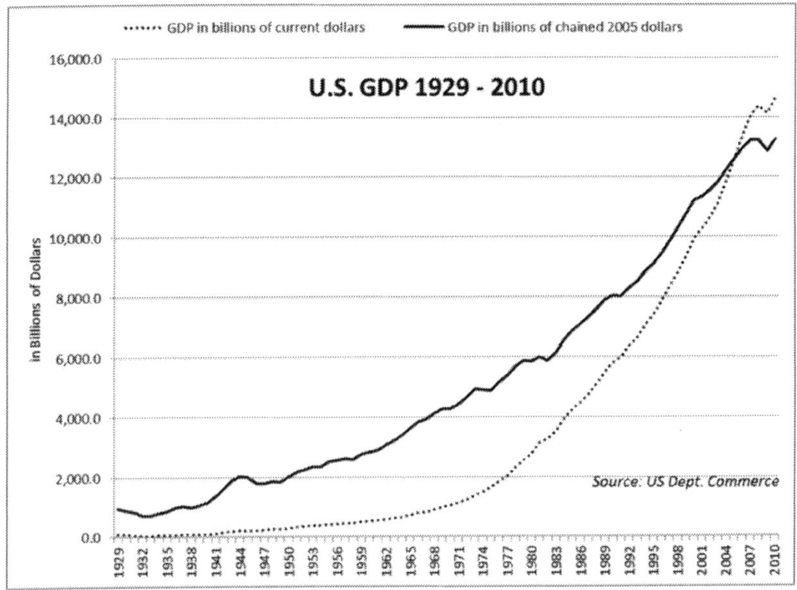

Chart 9: GDP Current $ to GDP Chained $

While the government has not reported the M3, the total amount of U.S. currency in circulation, in all its forms, since March of 2006, it is estimated that the total amount of currency circulated, including the value of derivatives like the mortgage backed securities, singled out as the crux of the current crisis, exceeds over 1.5 quadrillion dollars. A quadrillion is a million-billion! It looks like this!

$1,500,000,000,000,000.00

Many, including Objectivists, Libertarians, and other followers of the Austrian School, advocate a return to a gold standard because they object to the role of the government in issuing fiat currency through central banks. A significant number of the gold standard advocates have called for a mandated end to fractional reserve banking.

We now live within a system in which, on both the federal and

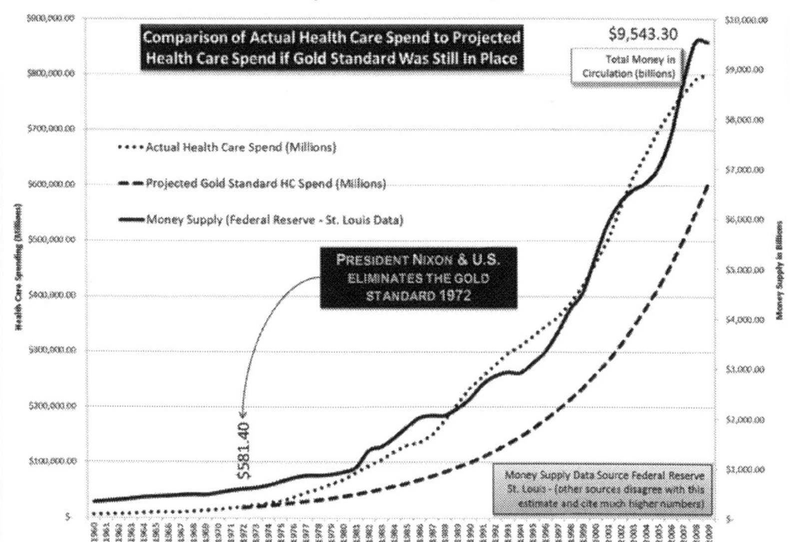

Chart 10: Healthcare to CinC

state level, programmatic entitlements can no longer be funded with new printed money. Actions that President Nixon took at the behest of the banks and the Federal Reserve have obscured the deleterious effects of the impact of the rapid and uncontrolled increase in these programs for the past forty years. The costs of these items now have tangible and dangerous effects on the individual taxpayer. Economically, it can also be argued that the rapid rise of healthcare costs has been further disproportioned to the rest of the economy because they do not truly exist in a free market system where consumers are making choices based in whole or in part, in their available buying power or willing discretionary expenses. Clearly, some health related issues, particularly those that involve life and death, are not discretionary; but as we have moved past 1971, the benefit of the constant and profligate increase in currency by both the government through borrowing, and the Federal Reserve, through back-end hidden funding to the banks, has been disproportionately available, to be applied to, government entitlement programs, like the healthcare industry. (Chart 10)

Is it possible this is one of the reasons the costs of care have risen so substantially? Was it simply because there were more dollars funding the program costs from the federal government, so more goods and services could be created to capture these free dollars? We are now keenly aware that they were not free. Without a doubt, one of the main contributors to the need to increase our currency has been both the continued trade deficit and government, deficit

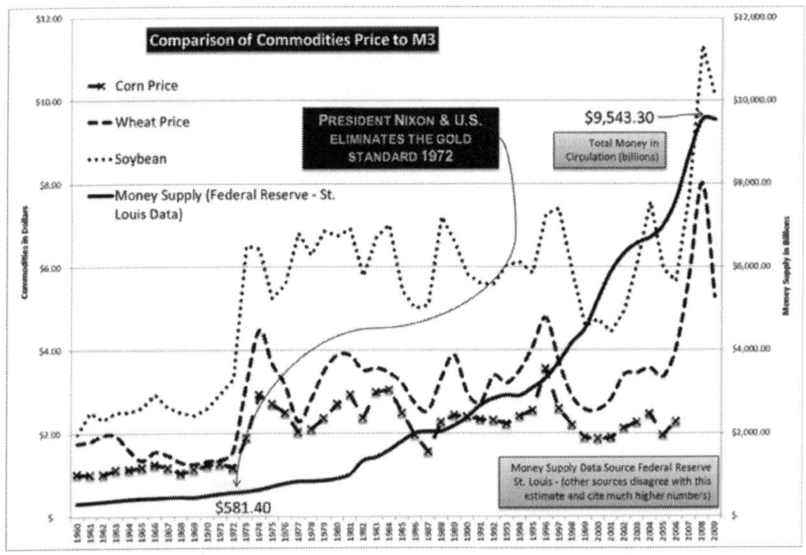

Chart 11: Commodities to CinC

spending to fund entitlements. We can now see that Wilbur Mills'' worries were justified, but the esteemed actuarial expert of Congress would never have predicted the mess we find ourselves in during these pressing times.

This period, more than almost any other, illustrate the broken economic basis of the current healthcare system. Further, it serves as a keen reminder that government intervention does not offer unbridled costless solutions. It also clearly demonstrates that healthcare and the economy in general are truly a zero sum game. There is no free ride, no free years of life, and no costless bad life choices. In the end, economic entropy will be the result. Naturally, to resist entropy takes energy and effort. In the case of healthcare, it takes energy in the form of money, and effort—work for more efficient and deliberate systems with appropriate market and individual controls—add to that personal responsibility.

Originally Medicare was meant only for people over sixty-five years of age. In 1972, President Nixon expanded coverage to people under the age of sixty-five with long-term disabilities and end-stage renal disease. In 1980, Congress expanded Home Health Services and Medi-Gap coverage under federal oversight. In 1982, hospice services for terminally ill patients were added. Under the current program requirements, no matter what the wage level, marital status, or retirement date, a man or woman will receive far more in benefits than the taxes they paid in to the programs. Costs for Medicare have doubled every four years since 1966.

Chart 12 shows the CBO's recent analysis of the cost of Medicare and Medicaid since inception in 1965, overlaid with the total tax revenue collected by the government and as projected into the year 2072.

What is clear from the chart is that the cost of Social Security, Medicare, and Medicaid alone consumes the available federal revenue by 2062, if left as is. What is further clear is that Social Security, Medicare, Medicaid and the other federal spending have outstripped our revenue line for most of the modern era.

Annual hospital admission per thousand people increased from 56.7 per thousand in the period of 1930 to 1949, to 99.4 per thousand by 1958. Science continued to improve the outcomes of treatment for the average patient, and with more cures came more and more costs. The Johnson administration's intent was to keep down

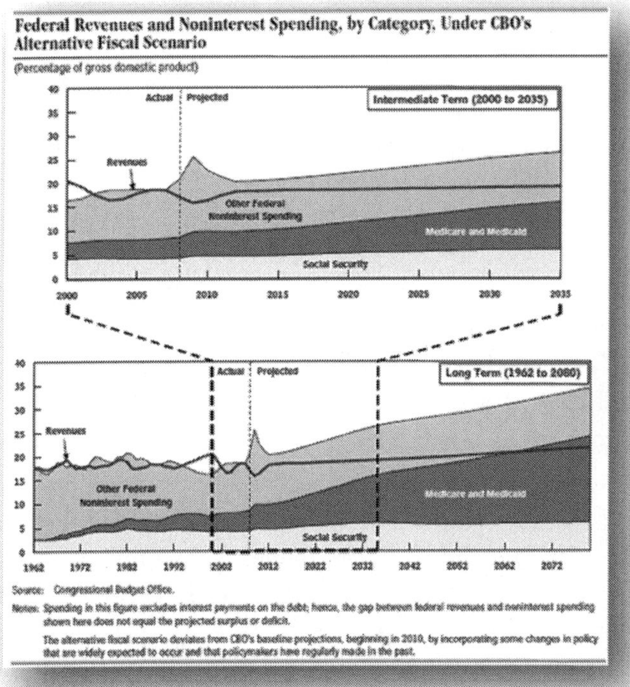

Chart 12: Medicare Medicaid Cost Chart

opposition from the AMA and hospitals by accepting a cost-based payment system that had been worked out between the hospitals and Blue Cross plans. Former Health, Education, and Welfare official Robert Ball pointed out that, "After-the-fact reimbursement for hospital costs clearly was a flawed policy." Health economist Ted French has pointed out that "this attempt to adopt the practices of the private market as they existed, in 1965, was already out-of-date even as Medicare was being implemented. The private market was beginning to move away from cost-based reimbursement, while the Medicare legislation locked the government program into a historical straitjacket." By 1983, Medicare was revised to change hospital payments to a system of fixed amounts based on 500 diagnostic codes (DRGS). With additional modifications, this is the system we have today.

The continual expansion of services available, diseases defined, and cost of services provided, now yield a staggering 14,432 diagnostic codes as of the most current Centers for Medicare and Medicaid Services (CMS) code list effective October 1, 2010—and the current administration is proposing adding thousands more. With all these various treatment options and the continual rising cost of care CMS has been forced to continue to lower reimbursement rates. We are now at the point where many physicians simply refuse to take Medicare and/or Medicaid patients because the rate of reimbursement forces the doctor or hospital to lose money. They either refuse to treat the Medicare or Medicaid patient, or raise their rates for everyone else to offset the losses.

Additionally, the actuaries of the day did not take into account the role of immigration and increasing eligibility. Over the past thirty years, we have seen not only a steady rise in immigration, but also the average age of immigrant has slowly crept up from an average age of twenty-two in 1979 to an average age of thirty-nine in 2009. Further, as a result of continual expansion of the legislation over time, the spouse of immigrants becomes eligible after their death if they have been employed and paid into the system. For the most part, middle aged immigrants have maintained more of their cultural identities and, as a result, fewer immigrant households have had both people working. As a result, the system is paying out an even larger proportion of immigrant families that they would have paid in as native born. This issue is not addressing the impact of illegal immigration. The total estimate of the fiscal burden (taxes paid minus services used) of immigration on public programs was recently estimated as $20.2 billion annually by Steven A. Camorota, in a 2006 Testimony before the House Ways and Means Committee on behalf of the Center for Immigration Studies.

After forty-eight years of experience, we now know the basic design of Medicare and Medicaid is fundamentally flawed. The relationship between Government monopoly and purchasing power does not either yield the ability to control costs, manage program expansion, or keep consumers satisfied. Continually reducing reimbursements, regulations, and paperwork for provider participation and continuing to expand the eligibility and services available to the population is a magnificent perversion of the discipline of an open marketplace. Would Wilbur Mills be surprised?

The Medicaid-Medicare Confusion

In any debate over entitlements, today Social Security and Medicare are the defined topics of discussion. To anyone who has read the Social Security Act of 1965 it is curious why Medicaid is left out of the discussion. The answer is that Medicaid is a much larger problem and one in which the nature of the program gives the federal government some political cover. While it is politically expedient to think of these programs as separate, they are, in fact, all just different parts of the Social Security Act of 1965. They are more tightly integrated than most acknowledge.

Medicaid is the United States health program for eligible individuals and families with low incomes and resources. It is a means-tested program that is jointly funded by the state and federal governments, and it is managed by the states under federal guidelines. Medicaid is supposedly voluntary for states to participate. Arizona was the last state to participate in 1982.

The biggest little secret of Medicaid is that the cost of this system to taxpayers dwarfs that of Medicare. Medicaid is funded by both federal taxes and state taxes on an approximately 50/50 formula. Federal spending figures in 2008, show Medicare costing $391 billion and Medicaid $244 billion. Medicaid appears to be less costly, but the reality is the federal expenditure is only 50 percent. The states spend about the same for programs on average plus each state has to support its own infrastructure to administer the program adding another few hundred million of program administrative costs to the equation. There is no transportability of Medicaid benefits across state lines as each program is state specific. Additionally, as the economy of the US has been depressed and the number of jobless and homeless has risen, the cost of Medicaid is skyrocketing.

At a recent conference of state governors, Medicaid was listed as the biggest threat to state solvency. While it can be argued that, in some states, Medicaid provides an effective safety net this does not hold true on a national scale. In fact, Medicaid and Medicare have been routinely cited as suffering exceedingly poor efficiencies in the delivery of benefits to the needy. In a meeting with Republicans, in 2010, at Blair House across the street from the Whitehouse, focused on the discussion of the Patient Protection and Affordable Care Act, the President himself cited a recent Congressional Budget Office study that showed only about one third of dollars make it to effective patient services. By the governments own projections, about two thirds of monies collected are lost to fraud, waste, inefficiencies, and duplications of services. Medicaid is not the government's poster child for an effective program, and it seems clear it is not a program that is being brought into the current conversation.

Recently, there has been a trend of federal legislators, including President Obama, referring to Medicaid as a state program. Many states are now looking to find out what they need to do to un-volunteer to participate. While the federal government is adopting the policy that Medicaid is a state responsibility, many states are now trying to find out how they pass back to the federal budget, the cost of a program that over which they have little legislative say. The reality is Medicaid, like Medicare, is becoming a federal program that neither the federal government nor the states can afford.

An argument can be made that, for many of its recipients, Medicare has funded vacation homes, new cars, flat panel televisions and other luxury purchases made in the years before retirement, much more than it does elder year healthcare needs. Prior to 1965, when Medicare did not exist, these purchases often would have been deferred in order to save for those elder rainy days. In the case of Medicare, the $1.00 of savings would have translated into much more than the 33¢ worth of Medicare services we receive from the current system.

The HIV-AIDS Epidemic

In the mid-1970s, physicians and other healthcare providers began noticing an unexplained increase in the death among young adult males. Often citing the cause of death as pneumonia, some health anomalies like Karposi's sarcoma were consistently showing up in disparate cases of unexplained death in other parts of the country.

Slowly, the realization set in throughout the medical community that the men who had sex with other men were dying of an otherwise rare cancer. The syndrome was often referred to by the colloquialism "gay" cancer. Medical scientists discovered that the syndrome included other manifestations, such as pneumocystis pneumonia, a rare form of fungal pneumonia. It was given the nickname "GRID," or Gay Related Immune Deficiency.

In the late-1970s, San Francisco-based providers recognized they were in the middle of an unexplained epidemic. The Haight-Ashbury Free Clinic and San Francisco General Hospital would become the front line of the next emerging healthcare crisis. While originally classified as "wasting disease," due to the rapid and then irreversible effect on the body, by 1983, HIV was identified as the virus that caused AIDS. Within a few years, it was recognized that a number of the prior, unexplained deaths in the country going back before 1970 were a result of this new virus.

From 1981 to 1987, the life expectancy for people with HIV was just eighteen months. Initially isolated in the gay community, the combination of its high infection rate and its evident death sentence sent a panic across the U.S. This had a profound effect on boosting homophobia and adding stigma to homosexuality in the general public, particularly since it seemed that unprotected anal sex was the prevalent way of spreading the disease. For a country still not at ease with the sexual liberation that was spreading across the country, this disease did little to foster acceptance of the gay or lesbian lifestyle.

The early years of the U.S. AIDS epidemic caused an unimaginable holocaust for the family members and loved ones of patients and for healthcare professionals, as well. Hundreds of young people died each week, and the healthcare system lacked the medical, ethical, technical, and spiritual resources to soften the blow of so many young people dying of such a mysterious illness. Many of the family members only found out about their loved ones "alternate" lifestyle when their infection forced them to come out of the closet.

Throughout the next few years, other forms of potential transmission were identified not specific to gay men having sex with men. Blood transfusion, intravenous drug use, heterosexual, and bisexual women, and new born babies were added to the list of those victimized by the disease. A national panic ensued. Blood Banks became suspect and more people became self-donors. The method of infection for women became a strong cause for concern. The role of infected women passing the infection on to their newborn babies again increased the national anxiety. As a result, the nation and the Centers for Disease Control mobilized and soon research funding was being appropriated, flowing into institutions like San Francisco General and others in order to understand and attack the disease.

Along with some other national figures diagnosed in the early years with HIV/AIDS, one young victim stands apart in becoming the national face of the disease, fostering an unprecedented federal funding effort that directly led to the gain we have today.

Ryan Wayne White (December 6, 1971 – April 8, 1990) was an American teenager from Kokomo, Indiana who became a national poster child for HIV/AIDS in the United States, after being expelled from middle school because of his infection. A hemophiliac, he became infected with HIV from a contaminated blood treatment and, when diagnosed in December 1984, was given six months to live.

Doctors said, he posed no risk to other students, but AIDS was poorly understood at the time. When White tried to return to school, many parents and teachers in Kokomo rallied against his attendance. A lengthy legal battle with the school system ensued, and media coverage of the case made White into a national celebrity. Soon he was named a spokesperson for AIDS research and public education. He appeared frequently in the media with celebrities such as Elton John, Michael Jackson, and Phil Donahue. Surprising his doctors,

White lived five years longer than predicted. He died in April 1990, a month prior to his high school graduation.

Before White, AIDS was a disease widely associated with the male homosexual community. That perception shifted as White and other prominent HIV-infected people, such as Magic Johnson, the Ray brothers, and Kimberly Bergalis, appeared in the media to advocate for more AIDS research and public education to address the epidemic.

The U.S. Congress passed a major piece of AIDS legislation, the Ryan White Care Act, shortly after White's death. The Act was reauthorized in 2006 and again on October 30, 2009. At the time of this writing, Ryan White Programs were the largest provider of services for people living with HIV/AIDS in the United States. These programs continue as the basis by which many can now continue to live and work productively in their communities—to exist with near normal lives. The impact of the Patient Protection and Affordable Care Act on the Ryan White Care Act is yet to be determined. There are those that believe it is destined to provide an excuse for the elimination of this, and other, disease-state based, carve-out programs. The argument will be made that, since PPACA provides insurance for all, there will be neither the need for this kind of program, nor the funding available to support such a specific populations set.

As San Francisco was desperately trying to get a handle on how to treat this rising epidemic, health officials there were confronted with another significant problem brought by fear and social stigma of the disease. As the first Antiretroviral (ARV) drugs were coming to the market to treat the disease, there were few pharmacists willing to either stock the drugs or those who would accept the patients into their pharmacy. This was due to both the high expense of the drug and the perceived risk from the infected patients or the apparent risk to their business due to a loss of clientele, who no longer wished to shop alongside infected and supposedly contagious patients. As a result of this problem, San Francisco General Hospital had to stock, and dispense, these drugs to their ever growing infected population out of one location; in a crumbling and sorely maintained hospital.

The monthly process to see the patient and to dispense the drugs could take up to two days for a patient. The system was becoming overwhelmed.

The city and county of San Francisco approached one courageous African American pharmacist with a long history of treating the mentally ill, those with drug addictions, and the underserved populations around the San Francisco Bay area. He agreed to rally his peers to stock and dispense the drugs and open their doors to these patients. Sylester Flowers, a 1958 graduate of Howard University, developed and automated an effective model. This, in conjunction with the Ryan White Care Act, set the stage for, and then later provided the outcomes based payer of last resort management model that gave rise to the current Aids Drug Assistance Program or ADAP programs offered across much of the United States.

HIV/AIDS continues to be a growing problem, imperiling our national health. Many technological and pharmacological strides have transformed the disease from a short-term condition with assuredly fatal results, to a long-term treatable chronic condition. The upside is the significant reduction in the human cost of the disease but the converse is a steadily increasing fiscal burden for all to shoulder since, we as a society feel we must do something to help support those who have acquired this debilitating disease. We continue to incur the treatment costs and the very expensive and damaging co-morbidities that result from both the damage the disease does to the body and the damage these powerful medications inflict on the infected patient, as well.

It is not just in the area of HIV/AIDS that we have such a mixed blessing. In almost every area where we have a complicated and deadly health-related issue, we have made tremendous strides and have converted what would have, just a few years ago, been a death sentence into a treatable and livable condition. Moreover, cancer in numerous forms, hepatitis, diabetes, neurological disorders, kidney diseases, congenital defects, neonatal disorders, and genetic disorders have benefited from improved technological and procedural gains, allowing for effective treatments, and conversion from deadly to chronic conditions—the list goes on, and on. But, in every case, the cost has continuously spiraled up and up and the demand for new technologies and treatments to cover the maladies that would not have shown up if the patient had not survived the initial problem in the first place, continue to grow.

Compounds have continued to get much more potent, manufacturers of these highly reactive and dangerous products tend to push the limits of containment in modern factories. Simply put, soon it will be required that prior to a drug being prescribed, the person's genotype (genetic code), and phenotype (body chemistry), will need to be assessed. The pharmacologicals coming to market, will be effective in one person with few to perhaps no side effects, but then again, in another person, they could be potentially very harmful, even fatal.

Biotechnology still has several promising years to go in the discovery of the so-called large molecular drugs and treatments. The underlying process is much better suited to a personalized medicine production approach, but this industry suffers from a different problem. While Big Pharma can produce blockbuster drugs in the billions of doses capacity, in numbers of factories around the world, Biotech (due to the process of how their molecules are synthesized) cannot produce at such capacity. They currently are, and likely will continue to be limited in their production for a long time.

Therefore, both sciences are pushing us ever closer to a need for personalized medicines, tailored to be effective based on the specific variant of the disease, an individual's unique body chemistry, and their personal genetic makeup. This is an even more expensive treatment system and one that is simply not supported by the current healthcare systems and underlying supply chain practice that we have today.

So then, we have not fared very well in our battle against the environment and other species in the past thirty years, despite many unprecedented technological and biological discoveries and achievements. Also, we have not trended well in the battle with ourselves. As a nation, we have continued to foster bad habits and, most importantly, bad diets. Obesity is at an all-time high and continues to spike. In general, health of the population is not improving. It is instead, portending of a long-term decline. This is not simply because we are living longer and suffering more and more chronic diseases related to old age. Nor is it just because we have simply found ways to convert what, in years past, would have been fatal conditions, which today are now simply chronic problems. There is one other fly in the ointment.

We have done a great job as a species of taking ourselves out of our environment and extracting ourselves from the Darwinian equation. Simply put, we are no longer subjected to the rules of natural selection the same way that we were just fifty or so years ago. All of the advances from electricity to central heating, to penicillin, to anti-retrovirals, and many other societal and scientific marvels have effectively removed us from the food chain and environmental influences.

In the not so distant past, those that got ill or injured did not reproduce as effectively or as often as they do today. Diseases, conditions, and behaviors that would have virtually ensured the elimination of a genetic trait, currently do not impede our reproductive success in the least. As a result, are we getting sicker? Are we subject to more maladies and conditions than we were before? Is the rise in obesity an early indicator? I do not think that we know yet, and those who may have theories are likely hesitant to say. Even if we did know the answer, and it was in the affirmative: what would we do about it? What could we do?

The DOCs Split With the DOCtrine

As we entered the 1980s, doctors, in high numbers, began to leave the healthcare industry. The continual rise in the cost of malpractice insurance as a result of larger and more costly punitive damage awards against doctors quickly outpaced the ability for some to maintain their practice. It appears now that the initial effect was seen in the areas of cosmetic surgeries and obstetrics. All of the factors that have been discussed before began to meld, discouraging many physicians from continuing to practice medicine.

As this period continued, other factors arose that would impinge a physician's ability to manage the cost of his/her practice. The rising role of regulations and requirements for technological tools, and the continued decline in reimbursement rates have collided to push many doctors out of sole practice, and more recently, out of the practice of medicine altogether. For physicians, today there are few options for a successful practice model. The office-based sole practitioner business model requires a huge up-front investment in equipment, real estate, high, ongoing monthly costs for staff, systems, and supplies, and the rising, uncontrollable costs of liability insurance. Now there is no predictability on what reimbursements will be due in terms of reductions in reimbursement rates. There is also the complete ineffectiveness and unprofitability of Medicare and Medicaid reimbursements, and significant difficulty in processing claims due to constant demands in documentation requirements and purposeful delays by payers. Most physicians just say it's a mess.

As the country became embroiled in political debate over healthcare reform, the AMA, historically the dominant voice of the practicing physician, found itself at odds with its base of support. Nowhere was this more evident than the AMA's public support of Obamacare. Once the arbiter and choke point for what was good for physicians, the AMA has found itself in a position where a significant portion of its members, if not a large majority, disagree with AMA positions. As one of the three historical main drivers of the form and substance of the current healthcare system, the AMA has found itself in the position of losing its constituency.

On March 15, 2010, the *New England Journal of Medicine* reported that nearly one third of practicing physicians might leave the practice of medicine if the healthcare bill were to be signed into law by President Obama. The survey illustrated there was a disconnect between the AMA (who proactively supported the legislation) and its members. The survey also underlined and punctuated the problem that physicians have as they attempted to operate profitable medical practices. Some other interesting statistics from another survey published by the Physicians' Foundation in October, 2008 include the following:

- ✓ 60 percent of doctors would not recommend the medical profession as a career to young people.
- ✓ 78 percent of physicians believe there is a shortage of primary care doctors.
- ✓ 49 percent of physicians, more than 150,000 doctors, said they plan to reduce the number of patients they see or stop practicing entirely.
- ✓ 94 percent said the time they devote to non-clinical paperwork in the last three years has increased, and 63 percent of the respondents said this paperwork has caused them to spend less time with their patients.
- ✓ 82 percent of physicians said their practices were unsustainable.
- ✓ 33 percent said they had closed their practice to Medicaid patients, and 12 percent have closed their practice to Medicare patients.
- ✓ 65 percent said Medicaid reimbursement was less than their cost of providing care and 36 percent responded similarly to Medicare reimbursement rates.

Presently, individual doctors are seeking alternative methods to continue to practice their art. Individual physicians are returning to the practice methods of their forefathers in the 1800s. Some are eschewing the private office model and returning to a general practice with "house call" care. Coupled with this practice method, is the reduction, by these practitioners, on the reliance for reimbursement from plans and other commercial payers. Some physicians are once again on a "fee for service" basis. But, this is *not* the fee for service model as practiced in the past thirty years. Oh no, this is becoming a "you pay me a fee, and I provide you the service you want model . . . Reimbursement to you by someone else is entirely your problem . . ."

Concierge medicine is now being investigated in many forms. The main tie that is binding all of these new systems together is a pragmatic decoupling of the physicians prices, from arbitrary reimbursements, that is further reconnected to the consumer's choices at purchase. Even those models that continue to offer basic services that will fit in many plan cost structures are simply offering the enhanced services as separate expenses from the base plan coverage.

We have continued to expect more and more from providers. At the same time that our expectations have grown, we have continued to drive a system, incentivizing providers to do less and less—all justified in the name of lowering the cost. In the past thirty years, we, as consumers, became fully decoupled from the "purchase" of care. Still, we have come to expect that the least cost providers should give us the most personalized services.

Try walking into any high-end fashion shop ask for a pair of "Seven for all Mankind" jeans ($249.95 retail) and demand they sell them to you for $39.95, the price of a pair of jeans at J. C. Penney. Then try complaining to the store manager because the sales clerk laughed at your request. We know not to try this stunt because the free and open market has taught us that you get what you pay for. As educated consumers, we know better than to expect designer clothes at discount prices. The level of service you should expect is always tied to the value point and profit you are willing to pay.

This is a lesson that the current supply system and politicians have spent a lot of time and money telling us is not necessary, and something we should not expect for healthcare. They have effectively convinced us that when it comes to healthcare it should be someone else's responsibility to pay for what we want and need. So we sign up for Kaiser Permanente's low cost, but very efficient and effective, industrialized medicine model. Then we expect to have one-on-one, personalized services as if we were still going to the same family doctor our parents, or grandparents, did back in 1955.

We need to make a choice as to how we can develop a system that will offer both basic services and value services and stop trying to demand that everyone get the same treatment, regardless of means. If we want more services that effectively get equally provided to everyone, we will need to pay more than an equal access price to get it. If the goal is for everyone to get everything for no cost or at least to have no concern over cost, then everyone will use all the services they can. Then, all must receive exactly the same options. Margin entropy predicts that the profit in such a system will sink to the lowest possible point because the system prohibits anyone to pay any more for perceived value. Do you really want to receive your care from the lowest bidder? The lowest performing student? The cheapest hospital?

Unfortunately, we can see from history that as we attempt to move to this increasingly government-controlled utopian dream, several negative outcomes will likely be the result.

- ✓ Good doctors will quit or will be driven out of business! This trend has already emerged in the past thirty years.
- ✓ Doctors will be amalgamated into an industrial-type practice in which they will continue to operate their practices with less revenue and profit, ultimately forcing them by their employer to provide the least common denominator services. Again, this looks really familiar!
- ✓ Healthcare will be rationed based on remaining quality of life estimates or rationed based on remaining societal value estimates. Does this ring any bells?
- ✓ Large numbers of practice areas, more and more likely in quality-of-life areas, will cease to be readily available.
- ✓ Fewer dollars will be available for research and development of new devices, technologies, drugs or treatments.
- ✓ Fewer and fewer students will take on the rigors and the cost of training in any of the healthcare professions because the financial burden will outweigh the benefit.

As the current system collapses, we will be left with only a government subsidized model where all healthcare professionals work for the government and all medical and health related research are tax-funded. Innovation and excellence will likely be replaced with a less costly extension of existing technology, and a focus on cheaper, and marginally effective, solutions.

As Jim Morrison said, "The future is uncertain, but the end is always near!"

Hillary Care: It Took a Village

During the presidential election of 1992, candidate Bill Clinton campaigned heavily on healthcare for America. As can be seen in any of the economic charts at the start of this section, the period between 1992 and 1996 represented a period of economic recession. While the government was pumping huge amounts of currency into the economy relatively unseen by the world at large, the economy continued to grow sour. As any of us today can attest, when there is an economic downturn and personal discretionary buying power reduces, the cost of healthcare becomes a significant issue.

Couple this trend with the politician's perpetual need to find something to grant, as appeasement to the masses to show how they "feel your pain," and you have what, at the time, looks like a match made in heaven. As President Johnson discussed almost thirty years before during his phone call with Wilbur Mills and Carl Albert, if we give this (Medicare) to the people we will be able to run on it for years to come. Even without the 2,000-plus page Patient Protection and Affordable Care Act, there has been more healthcare-related legislation during this period than throughout almost all of our prior history combined. The sheer number, scope, and breadth of the law during this period illustrate the amazing depth of penetration and control over many aspects of our day-to-day lives that the government has legislated since 1980. Most of these have passed by way of serial increments without our even being terribly aware.

Over the past thirty years, all these additions and amendments have been inexorably intertwined into Social Security, Medicare, and Medicaid making a matted and dysfunctional mess of conflicting regulations and compounding fiscal problems at both the federal and state levels.

After President Clinton's election, he appointed a "Task Force on National Healthcare Reform," headed by First Lady Hillary Rodham Clinton, to come up with a comprehensive plan to provide universal healthcare for all Americans. Clinton delivered his first major healthcare speech to a joint session of Congress on September 22, 1993. In that speech, the President explained the problem:

> *Millions of Americans are just a pink slip away from losing their health insurance, and one serious illness away from losing all their savings. Millions more are locked into the jobs they have now just because they, or someone in their family, has once been sick, and they have what is called the preexisting condition. And, on any given day, over 37 million Americans—most of them working people and their little children—have no health insurance at all. And, in spite of all this, our medical bills are growing at over twice the rate of inflation, and the United States spends over a third more of its income on healthcare than any other nation on Earth.*

Blazing new ground, and much of that not overly welcome by the people of the U.S., Hillary Rodham Clinton used the charter for healthcare reform as the vehicle to redefine the role of a presidential spouse. However, President Clinton's unconventional decision to put his wife in charge of the project only helped focus the ire of those opposed to the bill.

The first lady's role in secret proceedings of the Healthcare Task Force sparked litigation that led to the Federal Advisory Committee Act, which set new requirements for openness in government decision making. Soon the Association of American Physicians and Surgeons, the AMA, a number of powerful lobbies from the insurance industry, Big Pharma, the American Pharmacists Association, big business, and many others had lined up against the plan.

The main components of Clinton's plan included:

- ✓ Universal coverage and comprehensive benefits.
- ✓ A mandate that all employers pays 80 percent of the average health insurance premium for their workers, with caps on total employer costs and subsidies for small businesses
- ✓ Cost controls through competition among private health plans, and federally determined caps on insurance-premium growth (Artificial cap on spending without market control on demand and costs are doomed to fail)
- ✓ Establishment of regional purchasing pools (health alliances) through which people would enroll in insurance plans
- ✓ Financing through employer mandate, savings from cuts in projected Medicare and Medicaid spending, and increase in federal tobacco taxes.

By April 1994, the tide had definitively turned. Democratic Senator Daniel Patrick Moynihan qualified his prior statement that "there is no healthcare crisis" by stating "there is an insurance crisis." He also indicated that "anyone who thinks the Clinton healthcare plan can work in the real world as presently written isn't living in it."

Meanwhile, other Democrats, instead of uniting behind the president's original proposal, offered several competing plans of their own. Some criticized the plan from the left, preferring a single-payer system. By August of 1994, Democratic Senate Majority Leader George J. Mitchell announced that the healthcare plan was dead and would have to wait for its re-introduction in the next Congress. In the end, America was not ready for such a governmental takeover of any system, let alone one as personal and pivotal as healthcare.

The 1994 mid-term election became, in the opinion of one media observer, a "referendum on big government because Hillary Clinton had launched a massive healthcare reform plan that wound up strangled by its own red tape." In the 1994 mid-term elections, the

Republican revolution led by Newt Gingrich gave the GOP control of both the Senate and House of Representatives for the first time since 1952, ending prospects for a Clinton-sponsored healthcare overhaul. Congress did not revisit the issue of comprehensive healthcare reform until, after Barack Obama's inauguration in 2009.

Chapter 7 Addendum: Key Governmental Actions 1980 – 2009

Department of Health, Education, and Welfare was renamed the Department of Health and Human Services (DHHS).

- 1981, federal budget reconciliation requires states to make additional Medicaid payments to hospitals that serve a disproportionate share of Medicaid and low-income patients.

- 1981, states are permitted to mandate managed care enrollment of certain Medicaid groups and to cover home and community-based long-term care for those at risk of being institutionalized.

- 1987, states are permitted to expand Medicaid to children with disabilities who can be cared for at home and had previously been ineligible if not institutionalized.

- 1980, Medicare introduces Diagnosis Related Groups (DRGs) as a system for controlling hospital payments.

- The Food and Drug Administration expands the provision of patient package inserts for prescription drugs.

- The American Medical Association lifted the ban on physician advertising.

- The FDA and the Department of Health and Human Services revised regulations for human subject protections, based on the 1979 Belmont Report.

- The Federal Anti-Tampering Act passed in 1983 making it a crime to tamper with packaged consumer products.

- FDA published the first Red Book (successor to 1949 "black book"), officially known as Toxicological Principles for the Safety Assessment of Direct Food Additives and Color Additives Used in Food.

- The Orphan Drug Act passed.

- Emergency Medical Treatment and Active Labor Act require hospitals receiving Medicare payments to screen and stabilize all persons who entering their emergency rooms, regardless of ability to pay.

- COBRA (Consolidated Omnibus Budget Reconciliation Act) contained specific regulations to allow employees who lose their jobs to continue with their healthcare plan for 18 months.

- 1986, states permitted to the Medicaid option to cover infants, young children and pregnant women up to 100 percent of the poverty level.

- 1987, eligibility was raised to 185 percent of the poverty level in legislation for infants and pregnant women the following year.

- The Medicare Catastrophic Coverage Act (MCCA) expands Medicare coverage to include prescription drugs and places a cap on beneficiaries' out-of-pocket expenses.

- The Family Support Act required states to extend twelve months of transitional Medicaid coverage to families.

- 1989, the states are mandated, by Medicaid, to cover pregnant women and children under age 6 at 133 percent of the federal poverty level.

- The Drug Price Competition and Patent Term Restoration Act expand the availability of less-costly generic drugs by permitting the FDA to approve generic versions of brand-name drugs without repeating original research on safety and effectiveness.

- AIDS test for blood approved by FDA.

- The Food and Drug Administration Act of 1988 officially established the FDA as an agency of the Department of Health and Human Services, with a Commissioner of Food and Drugs appointed by the President.

- The Prescription Drug Marketing Act banned the diversion of prescription drugs from legitimate commercial channels.

- 1990, the states are mandated expand Medicaid coverage to all children age 6 – 18 whose families are below poverty-level income.

- The Health Insurance Portability and Accountability Act (HIPAA) restrict the use of pre-existing conditions in health insurance coverage determinations. It also sets standards for medical records privacy, and establishes tax-favored treatment of long-term care insurance.

- The Personal Responsibility and Work Opportunity Act delinks Medicaid and cash assistance eligibility to allow states to cover parents and children at current Aid to Families with Dependent Children (AFDC) levels and higher.

- The Mental Health Parity Act prohibits group health plans from having lower annual or lifetime dollar limits for mental health benefits

- 2003, the Balanced Budget Act includes many changes in provider payments to slow the growth of Medicare spending. It established the Medicare+ Choice program, later re-named Medicare Advantage.

- Also, part of the Balanced Budget Act (BBA), the State Children's Health Insurance Program (S-CHIP) is enacted.

- Ticket to Work and the Work Incentives Improvement Act of 1999 allowed states to cover working disabled with incomes above 250 percent of poverty and the Act also imposed income-related premiums.

- The Infant Formula Act established special FDA controls to ensure necessary nutritional content and safety

- The Anabolic Steroid Act of 1990 identified anabolic steroids as a class of drugs and classified over two dozen items as controlled substances.

- The Nutrition Labeling and Education Act requires all packaged foods to bear nutrition labeling, and all health claims for foods to be consistent with terms defined by the government. Restrictions on direct-to-consumer advertising of prescription drugs are loosened.

- The Safe Medical Devices Act requires nursing homes, hospitals, and other facilities to report incidents that implicate medical devices in patient injuries and deaths.

- The Generic Drug Enforcement Act imposes debarment and other penalties for illegal acts involving abbreviated drug applications.

- The Prescription Drug User Fee Act requires drug and biologics manufacturers to pay fees for product applications and supplements, as well as other services significantly increasing the cost to consumers.

- The Mammography Quality Standards Act requires U.S. mammography facilities to be accredited and federally certified.
- The Dietary Supplement Health and Education Act establish labeling requirements and a regulatory framework for dietary supplements.
- The Uruguay Round Agreements Act extended the patent terms of U.S. drugs from 17 to 20 years.
- The FDA declares cigarettes to be "drug delivery devices and proposes restrictions on marketing and sales to discourage smoking by young people.
- The Food and Drug Administration Modernization Act mandates the most wide-ranging reforms to FDA practices since 1938 in yet another attempt to reign in false claims and speed the approval process.
- The FDA Pediatric Rule requires manufacturers of selected, new and extant drugs, and other products, to conduct studies to assess their safety and efficacy in children.
- The Best Pharmaceuticals for Children Act improved safety and efficacy of patented and off-patent medicines for children.
- In the wake of the events of September 11, 2001, the Public Health Security and Bioterrorism Preparedness and Response Act of 2002 was designed to improve the country's ability to prevent and respond to public health emergencies.
- Under the Medical Device User Fee and Modernization Act, fees were assessed on sponsors of medical device applications for evaluation.

- The Office of Combination Products was formed within the Office of the Commissioner, as mandated under the Medical Device User Fee and Modernization Act.

- The Medicare Prescription Drug Improvement and Modernization Act required that a study be made of how current and emerging technologies can be utilized to make essential information about prescription drugs available to the blind and visually impaired.

- The Department of Health and Human Services announces that the FDA would require food labels to include trans-fat content.

- An obesity working group is established by the Commissioner of Food and Drugs, charged to develop an action plan to deal with the nation's obesity epidemic from the perspective of the FDA.

- The National Academy of Sciences released its "Scientific Criteria to Ensure Safe Food," a report commissioned by the FDA and the Department of Agriculture.

- The Animal Drug User Fee Act permitted the FDA to collect subsidies for the review of certain animal drug applications from sponsors.

- The FDA is given clear authority under the Pediatric Research Equity Act to require that sponsors conduct clinical research into pediatric applications for new drugs and biological products.

- The Project BioShield Act of 2004 authorized the FDA to expedite its review procedures to enable rapid distribution of treatments as countermeasures to chemical, biological, and nuclear agents.

- The passage of the Food Allergy Labeling and Consumer Protection Act requiring the labeling of any food that contains a protein derived from any one of the following foods that, as a group, account for the vast majority of food allergies: peanuts, soybeans, cow's milk, eggs, fish, crustacean shellfish, tree nuts, and wheat.

- The Anabolic Steroid Control Act of 2004 passed.
- To provide for the treatment of animal species other than cattle, horses, swine, chickens, turkeys, dogs, and cats, as well as other species that may be added at a later time, the Minor Use and Minor Species Animal Health Act was passed to encourage the development of treatments for species that would otherwise attract little interest in the development of veterinary therapies.
- The FDA bans dietary supplements containing ephedrine alkaloids based on an increasing number of adverse events linked to these products and the known pharmacology of these alkaloids.
- The formation of the Drug Safety Board is announced.
- President Obama signs the Family Smoking Prevention and Tobacco Control Act into law.
- The FDA Center for Tobacco Products was established.
- The FDA announced a ban on cigarettes with flavors characterizing fruit, candy, or clove.
- The Breast and Cervical Cancer Treatment and Prevention Act of 2000 allowed states to provide Medicaid coverage to uninsured women for treatment of breast or cervical cancer.
- President Bush launched the Health Center Growth Initiative, significantly expanding the number of community health centers serving the medically underserved.

- Maine passed the Dirigo Health Reform Act, a comprehensive healthcare reform plan that expanded Maine Medicaid, and created the Maine Quality Forum.

- The Medicare Drug, Improvement, and Modernization Act (MMA) passed, creating a voluntary, subsidized prescription drug benefit under Medicare.

- Medicare legislation creates Health Savings Accounts which allow individuals to set aside pre-tax dollars to pay for current and future medical expenses.

- The Deficit Reduction Act of 2005 made significant changes to Medicaid related to premiums and cost sharing, benefits, and asset transfers.

- Medicare Part D Drug benefit went into effect.

- Massachusetts passed and implemented legislation to provide healthcare coverage to nearly all state residents.

- One month following Massachusetts, Vermont passed comprehensive healthcare reform and also aimed for near-universal coverage.

- The city of San Francisco created the Healthy San Francisco program, providing universal access to health services for residents of the city.

- The Census Bureau estimated there were 45.6 million uninsured (15.3 percent of the population) in 2007.

- Congress passed two versions of a bill to reauthorize the State Children's Health Insurance Program with bipartisan support, but President Bush vetoed both bills. Congress could not override the veto. A temporary extension of the program was passed in December 2007.

- The Mental Health Parity Act was amended to require full parity.
- The Children's Health Insurance Program (CHIP) is reauthorized, providing states with additional funding.

VIII. Where We Are Now

Where Are We Now?

For those of you that have stuck with me on this journey, you know that we have undoubtedly come a long way in the past few hundred years. Comparatively, the past forty years have dwarfed, in sheer numbers, the achievements of the previous two hundred. We have had more technological innovation, more medical innovation, more legislation, and more advancement in pharmacology during the past four decades, but what we did not gain was a corresponding increase in life span, the quality of our health, or in the efficiency of the delivery of the new cures.

In fact, if you did nothing but compare the current advertising for our modern medical miracles with the advertising of the cures from the 1890s, you would see striking similarities in the quantity and the areas of focus. In the 1890s, for example, papers were full of cures for women's monthly conditions, male enhancement, and restoratives for virility in men, cures for the common cold and flu, and for the restoration of energy and the elimination of depression. The media today is filled with the same messages. Would Judge Loker think we have accomplished anything at all? One thing that is different is that, in those days, no one knew what they were taking or that most of the nostrums were narcotics that today are restricted or downright illegal—today most of the magic cures offered have a larger list of potential side effects than actual benefits!

Knowing the Judge the way I did, I can tell you what he might say about our healthcare system, "Boy, what the hell are you complaining about? You don't know how good you truly have it!" Remember what I pointed out earlier in this book: consider the context.

In a paper, for the National Center for Policy Analysis, Scott Atlas, senior fellow at the Hoover Institution (Atlas, 2009), identified ten facts you probably don't know about American healthcare. I can almost guarantee the Judge would have agreed with each and every one of the points that follow.

Fact No. 1: Americans have better survival rates than Europeans for common cancers. Breast cancer mortality is 52 percent higher in Germany than in the United States, and it is 88 percent higher in the United Kingdom. Prostate cancer mortality is 604 percent higher in the U.K. and 457 percent higher in Norway. The mortality rates for colorectal cancer, among British men and women, are about 40 percent higher.

Fact No. 2: Americans have lower cancer mortality rates than Canadians. Breast cancer mortality is 9 percent higher, prostate cancer is 184 percent higher and colon cancer mortality among men is about 10 percent higher than in the United States.

Fact No. 3: Americans have better access to treatment for chronic diseases than patients in other developed countries. Some 56 percent of Americans who could benefit are taking statins, which reduce cholesterol and protect against heart disease. By comparison, of those patients who could benefit from these drugs, only 36 percent of the Dutch, 29 percent of the Swiss, 26 percent of Germans, 23 percent of Britons and 17 percent of Italians receive them.

Fact No. 4: Americans have better access to preventive cancer screening than Canadians. Take the proportion of the appropriate-age population groups who have received recommended tests for breast, cervical, prostate, and colon cancer:

- ✓ Nine of 10 middle-aged American women (89 percent) have had a mammogram, compared to less than three-fourths of Canadians (72 percent).

- ✓ Nearly all American women (96 percent) have had a pap smear, compared to less than 90 percent of Canadians.

- ✓ More than half of American men (54 percent) have had a PSA test, compared to less than 1 in 6 Canadians (16 percent).

- ✓ Nearly one-third of Americans (30 percent) have had a colonoscopy, compared with less than 1 in 20 Canadians (5 percent).

Fact No. 5: Lower income Americans are in better health than comparable Canadians. Twice as many American seniors with below-median incomes self-report "excellent" health compared to Canadian seniors (11.7 percent versus 5.8 percent). Conversely, white Canadian young adults with below-median incomes are 20 percent more likely than lower income Americans to describe their health as "fair or poor."

Fact No. 6: Americans spend less time waiting for care than patients in Canada and the U.K., Canadian, and British patients wait about twice as long–sometimes more than a year–to see a specialist, to have elective surgery like hip replacements or to get radiation treatment for cancer. All told, 827,429 people are waiting for some type of procedure in Canada. In England, nearly 1.8 million people are waiting for a hospital admission or outpatient treatment.

Fact No. 7: People in countries with more government control of healthcare are highly dissatisfied and believe reform is needed. More than 70 percent of German, Canadian, Australian, New Zealand, and British adults say their health system needs either "fundamental change" or "complete rebuilding."

Fact No. 8: Americans are more satisfied with the care they receive than Canadians. When asked about their own healthcare instead of the "healthcare system," more than half of Americans (51.3 percent) are very satisfied with their healthcare services, compared to only 41.5 percent of Canadians; a lower proportion of Americans are dissatisfied (6.8 percent) than Canadians (8.5 percent).

Fact No. 9: Americans have much better access to important new technologies like medical imaging than patients in Canada or the U.K. Maligned as a waste by economists and policy makers naïve to actual medical practice, an overwhelming majority of leading American physicians identified computerized tomography (CT) and magnetic resonance imaging (MRI) as the most important medical innovations for improving patient care during the previous decade. The United States has thirty-four CT scanners per million Americans, compared to twelve in Canada and eight in Britain. The United States has nearly twenty-seven MRI machines per million compared to about six per million in Canada and Britain.

Fact No. 10: Americans are responsible for the vast majority of all healthcare innovations. The top five U.S. hospitals conduct more clinical trials than all the hospitals in any other single developed country. Since the mid-1970s, the Nobel Prize in medicine or physiology has gone to American residents more often than recipients from all other countries combined. In only five of the past thirty-four years did a scientist living in America not win or share in the prize. Most important recent medical innovations were developed in the United States. (Atlas, 2009)

Even without Judge Loker's historical perspective, we simply do not grasp how good we have it today, do we? We have accomplished most of what we experience now, because, over the past forty years, we reaped the benefits of many spectacular advances, both technologically and legislatively.

Recent Legislation

Despite all the wonderful progress that we have made we still cannot seem to find a workable solution to the healthcare crisis, making insurance affordable, providing care for those who can't afford it at all, and a supply chain where those who provide the services can make a reasonable living. All things considered, it is amazing—nearly breathtaking—to see how far we have come since our forefathers landed in Virginia, Plymouth Rock, and St. Mary's City in Maryland.

The listing of technological and medical advancements and the listing of legislation driven by the rapid and deep integration of governmental control into all aspects of our lives is something that most people can only see now in retrospect—and then, only if they actually look. Further, since many of those alive today do not have a historical frame of reference that precedes this forty-year period, they are, for the most part, blissfully unaware of just how far, as a culture, we have come, both for the better and for the worse.

Fundamentally, despite all the advances, the rapid rise in the average age of the population slowed quite a bit during this period. In 1980, the average life expectancy at birth was 73.9 years; by 2010 it only has advanced to 78.11 years. More importantly, the average age of the U.S. population began a rapid rise. Having slowed during the 1990s, as a result of the relatively small number of babies born or who survived the Great Depression, the percentage of the population over the age of sixty-five in 1990, 12 percent is expected to increase to 15.5 percent by 2015 and over 20 percent by 2030. Healthcare costs attributable to the diseases of the aged and chronically infirm have risen significantly during this period and are expected to increase significantly in the next decade alone.

The chickens have finally come home to roost! As I will discuss in the remainder of this section, if we do not address the fundamental economic issues of our healthcare system and the underlying hopelessly broken supply chain mechanics surrounding it, we will likely bankrupt our states, the federal government, and ultimately ourselves and our children.

WE Are a Huge Part of What Is Wrong

During a recent discussion with a friend, I commented that the only thing that we tolerate today is intolerance. This problem underlies much of what we are dealing with as a society today. And, nowhere is the problem more evident than trying to find a solution to the healthcare dilemma.

One thing I am sure of: Everyone discussing solutions to the current healthcare crisis will need to be tolerant because in every case views and ideas will emerge that Republicans will not like, that Democrats will not like, progressives and conservatives won't like, and vested special interests most definitely will not like. Throughout this section, I will attempt to address potential solutions pragmatically, not ideologically. I can only promise this, if you will read on you will find much with which to agree. You will also find much to think about, which I find important since each of us is ultimately responsible for finding an answer for this enduring problem.

We need to address the fundamental and the hard, gut-wrenching issues that are underlying as they relate to this problem. If we do not, then we will bequeath future generations much more debt with which to deal—the healthcare system itself will be much worse.

Time and again, we Americans forget what has made us great. It is somewhat ironic that our newest immigrants are the ones that remind us the most of what it means to be American. Throughout our history, adversity and injustice have been the catalysts to unite us and allow us to rise to our potential. Following these peaks, we have become complacent, reverting to our more banal, self-centered pursuits and then we begin to expect, rather than earn, the benefits that being an American brings.

During these periods of expectation, we embrace the doctrine that the government is responsible for our life, liberty, and our pursuit of happiness. At these times, we, as a people, expect the government to provide us with "things" and politicians are more than happy to fulfill our requests. The problem lies therein! We ask for the wrong "things." We ask for housing, and the government provides us subsidies, loan guarantees, and tax breaks. We ask for healthcare, and the government provides more entitlements and mandated insurance and subsidies. Where do the "things" the government gives us, as a people, actually come from? Why, from us of course!

While sounding simple enough, there are a few problems. First, government is not efficient at redistribution. If you look across any government program whether it is Medicare, Medicaid, Food Stamps, Housing Assistance, you find that after accounting for waste, fraud, and abuse, only about 30 percent of the funds collected from us, as a people, come back to us, as a people in benefits. Numerous large, non-profits have been investigated by state attorneys general in the past decade and sued for delivering less than thirty cents on the dollar to beneficiaries. Second, politicians then feel the need to either act paternalistic or to assume a superior, "smarter-than-thou" approach to governing. Third, the temptation to monetize our wants and needs into political capital becomes overwhelming, and they buy our votes by providing more and more supposedly "free stuff."

Nothing in recent history exhibits this behavior more than "The Patient Protection and Affordable Care Act" enacted by Congress in March, 2010.

The 'Let's Make a Deal' Mind-set

Having closely followed, and attempted to affect, the process of delivery, of this legislation, it became clear to me, early on, that we simply ask the Government to give us more than they could ever hope to dispense. Also, it became clear that we are not of one group asking for the same thing. In fact, we have spent the last fifty years dividing ourselves further and further, into smaller and smaller groups. More and more, typically, we have brought our groups down to our basic family unit. *US*, ME AND MY FAMILY, want you, THE GOVERNMENT, to give us what *US*, ME AND MY FAMILY, wants. Get what you need from *THEM*, EVERYONE ELSE. While this sounds ludicrous, it is almost exactly what has happened in the path to the delivery of the current legislation.

The core ideals were never anything with which conservatives, progressives, moderates, Republicans, Independents or Democrats disagreed. Most of the basic ideals that started with Senator Kennedy's HELP legislation were lost as the various legislators made their deals with *THEM* to get the votes to give *US* what we asked for, or at least what the legislators felt we should have. In the end, the law, as delivered, provided not one of the ideals, and has garnered almost total derision from all sides. Why? Is there nothing good in the bill? Of course not! There are many good pieces in the legislation that we can be proud of. Simplistically, we cannot ask our government to provide us things, stuff, "tchotchkes," with no participation or responsibility assumed by us. History shows that the government simply can't do it.

It is no accident that the sections of the bill we most agree on, are relatively small, discrete and pointed pieces of legislation that change current practice and delivery systems or provide some reasonable bridge for the underserved. Government is very good at making such changes in a free market system. The problems emerge when the government attempts to replace these systems with governmental-controlled bureaucracies. We can never get cost-effective programmatic solutions given to us through inefficient delivery systems. Shouldn't we take the responsibility ourselves, and participate in the acquisition of the services in a free and open market?

In the end, one of the biggest drivers we have in our poor opinion of our own healthcare system is our own attitudes and behaviors.

There is a Way—If WE Want to Take It!

Sometimes we all need a "do-over"! Fortunately, *WE* can learn from our mistakes. *WE* is all of the people in America, not just some. The opportunity to benefit from the debate—both during the legislative process and after the signing by the President—gives us the opportunity to learn, revise/repeal and generate a much better approach focused less on having the government "give" *US* healthcare and more on passing legislation so that *WE* can secure the goods and services we need to manage our health in a fair, open market with simplified, transparent pricing systems—so that *WE* can determine what we need and obtain it cost-effectively and efficiently. *WE* can provide for one another as well if *WE* can develop a system that facilitates coordination of the care and benefits regardless of where they are available and who they are available from so *WE* can reduce duplication of effort, minimize fraud and abuse, and stimulate behaviors where *WE* unite actually to help one another!

Should we or shouldn't we? The decision really is up to us!

ONLY WE CAN DO IT!
FRANKLY, WE MUST DO IT!

Chapter 8 Addendum Medical And Technological Advances 1980 – 2010

The following includes other noteworthy advancements that are within this 30-year period:

- 1980, W.H.O. (World Health Organization) announced that smallpox was eradicated.
- 1981, first vaccine for hepatitis B was introduced.
- 1982, Dr. William DeVries implanted the Jarvik-7 artificial heart into patient Barney Clark. Clark lived 112 days.
- 1983, HIV, the virus that causes AIDS, is identified.
- 1987, DNA identification of individuals found wide application in criminal law. Protease inhibitors were introduced allowing HAART therapy against HIV; drastically reducing AIDS mortality.
- 1990, Human Genome Project began.
- 1992, first vaccine for hepatitis A is made available.
- 1996, Dolly the sheep is cloned.
- 1998, first vaccine for Lyme disease was offered.
- 1999, The Human Genome Project was completed.
- 2005, National Geographic and IBM fund The Genographic Project, which traces every living human down to a single male ancestor.
- 2006, emerging use of robotics, especially tele-robotics in medicine, particularly for surgery came along.

- 2007, scientists discovered how to use human skin cells to create embryonic stem cells.

- 1980 – 2010, corrective eye surgery became popular as costs and potential risk decreased, and results further improved.

IX. A Road Map to Sanity

A Rational Argument for Repealing, Revising, Readjusting, or Reinventing the Affordable Care Act

The Fundamental Issues

In June 2009, Senator Ted Kennedy, the acknowledged healthcare expert in Congress, introduced what he called the Affordable Health Choices Act. Kennedy had spent years pursuing a dream for a tightly integrated, well-reasoned, and carefully crafted series of reforms to solve what he had come to learn were some of the fundamental issues in the current system. Having read this bill along with most other healthcare reform legislation, I can say that Senator Kennedy's bill, while it clearly would not have won a popularity contest from the right side of the aisle due to its pragmatic and progressive approach, seemingly provided a well thought out and tightly integrated set of actions that would have been a good basis for future change.

In the end, however, Kennedy's bill never moved forward. It was drowned in the legislative process that ensued. In an atmosphere of hyper-partisanship, numerous bills from multiple committees were put on the table. The efforts to combine them in a series of negotiations, back-room deals, trade-offs, grants, exceptions, and reductions in control yielded the disintegrated, unintelligible, convoluted, often conflicting 2,000-plus-page abomination, known as Obamacare or the Patient Protection and Affordable Care Act (PPACA).

Obamacare is another instance in which we have taken on the task of creating some artificial means to grant services to everyone, without adequate thought and debate as to the consequences suffered by the taxpayer, and, ultimately by the consumers of the services. The actual goal of the people who passed this legislation was not to provide an effective safety net for uninsured Americans. It was, in fact, to redistribute income among Americans. Such philosophical statements were publicly declared by members of the Democratic majority in Congress, during the debate over the passage of the law. Also, stated by several congressional leaders was the secondary desire to drive all profit from the provision of healthcare. While a humanitarian case may be made concerning the propriety of profiting from the sickness of others, the idea that a quality health system can be run, without the virtue of profit, to drive excellence and innovation belies and ignores historical fact.

Obamacare is almost universally disliked, for widely different reasons. The legislation was passed in a fractious and partisan manner, with the Democrat-controlled Congress approving the bill with neither support nor amendment from Republicans. Those who did not agree with the concept of reforming healthcare at the federal level hate this reform merely because it passed. Many who worked hard and diligently to pass something they felt was for the good of the American people now hate the resulting law because they see it as ineffective and likely to fail. Those who were unconcerned in the first place now hate it because they are sick to death of hearing about it. Despite promises from then Speaker Nancy Pelosi that we would all like it once we had a chance to read it, a majority of Americans now want Obamacare repealed or significantly altered.

Legal and political challenges have been brought to every aspect of Obamacare, from its constitutionality (brought by 26 states attorneys general), to the fiscal responsibility of the law—brought by numerous business groups, think-tanks, and both the Congressional Budget Office (CBO) and the actuary for Medicare and Medicaid (CMS). Continual revelations by the CBO suggest that the fiscal projections for the law continue to fall ever farther from the realm of feasibility.

Supporters of the law claim the focus of the legislation was to reform the private health insurance market, to provide better coverage for those with pre-existing conditions, to improve prescription drug coverage in Medicare, and to extend the life of the Medicare Trust Fund by at least twelve years. Detractors of the legislation claim the focus of the law was a power grab by the government to wrest fiscal control over one-sixth of the American economy in order to hide and obfuscate the problems the country has suffered from as a result of massive entitlements in the wake of the New Deal, Social Security, Medicare and Medicaid, and almost one-half a century of additional legislation.

Many components of Obamacare look good on their face but fall apart on the implementation. One such example is the promise that you can keep your "Grandfathered Insurance" plan if you prefer it. Yes, it is true. It does say that in the legislation. The issue is that if you do choose to keep your grandfathered policy, the insurer cannot ever add anyone else to the policy. Since all premium prices are derived from the actuarial base of the policy holders, as people quit the policy or die and the pool of insured gets smaller and smaller, the cost of the coverage gets spread over a smaller and smaller group and, therefore, the risk goes up significantly. Very soon, the cost of the policy will become prohibitive—and most won't want the policy. If the Secretary for Health and Human Services refuses to let the insurer raise the policy rates, then they will simply cancel the policy—so much for "grandfathered!"

Another example of the pragmatic shortfall of the legislation is the negotiated language that allows everyone to purchase health insurance regardless of pre-existing conditions. Originally, anyone was able to purchase insurance from the same policies in the same actuarial pool. In order to garner support, this provision was changed. Even though anyone can still purchase, regardless of preexisting condition, the government agreed to let insurers place those with preexisting conditions into so-called "High Risk Pools." These policies again will be priced based on their actuarial risk. If everyone in the high-risk pool is "high-risk," then you can be assured the cost of those plans will not be the same as those in the "everyone else who is not as sick" pool. And, if, as some have interpreted, the Secretary will suppress the higher high risk pool actuarial rates and thereby artificially suppress these premium costs. Where will the additional expenses be covered? By us of course!

Now, if you consider additionally the negative effect that this legislation will have on the historic excellence and innovation brought to the healthcare system by investors, physician associations, and consumer groups, you can see that we face a clear and present danger.

While you can read every page of the legislation, as I have, and you will continue to find numerous examples of provisions that either do not pragmatically work as designed or yield numerous unintended consequences, in reality it is a waste of time. While there are likely an equal number of provisions that bring some value as they also bring unintended consequences, they are mostly irrelevant because this legislation does not address the fundamental deficiencies that exist in our current healthcare system.

In this chapter, I will discuss the details of this legislation and its shortcomings. For now, it appears that the biggest issue is that this legislation simply does not address the underlying problems in our current healthcare system, including the supply chain, the underlying economic system, a pragmatic application of existing resources, or, most importantly, personal responsibility.

And yet, although I am very critical of the deficiencies in the legislation, I believe that, despite its shortcomings, the law should not be repealed. Instead, I believe Obamacare presents us with an opportunity to use what we have as a start, even if it stands only as a blueprint for what not to do. Still, we should use what we have and move forward to a better solution for ourselves, for healthcare providers, and for our nation as a whole.

In the end, I hope we can make the certain sacrifices in the system in order to design, finally, a comprehensive well-integrated healthcare supply chain. In doing so, I hope we can determine, appropriate roles for each provider coupled with a transparent, free, and open-market pricing system. In defining this system, I sense we can incorporate all the existing participants including; for-profits, non-profits, community clinics, governmental and non-governmental organizations; faith based, secular, philanthropic and volunteer organizations; physicians, hospitals, nurses, pharmacists, social workers, and others so that we can deliver the proper care. We need to assure that care is provided at the most efficient and available points of the supply chain and in a manner that eliminates duplication of services costs—the cost of defensive medicine, as well as, that of fraud and abuse—while at the same time freeing additional capacity. And, along the way, I have faith that the end system will also have the added benefit of helping us improve patient outcomes.

My intention is to address each problem pragmatically, non-aligned with any ideology and with no sacred cows, in order to open a discussion among many that drive us all to solutions that are arrived at more by tolerance than compromise.

Cost Matters

Any attempt to reform our healthcare system immediately faces a harsh reality: the high and rapidly rising cost of care. Earlier chapters discussed the historical decisions that created our current, disconnected system with its lack of functional integration. The one thing everyone in the system agrees upon is how difficult it is to control or even assess costs. If one speaks with hospital administrators, physicians, or others providing these vital services, even they will say that they are unable to determine what their own services actually cost to deliver. Why? Because, a large portion of their revenues are now based on sliding discounted reimbursements.

The California Hospital Association said:

- "There is no relationship between what is charged, the actual cost of care and what hospitals get reimbursed". (Stanley Feld M.D., 2007)

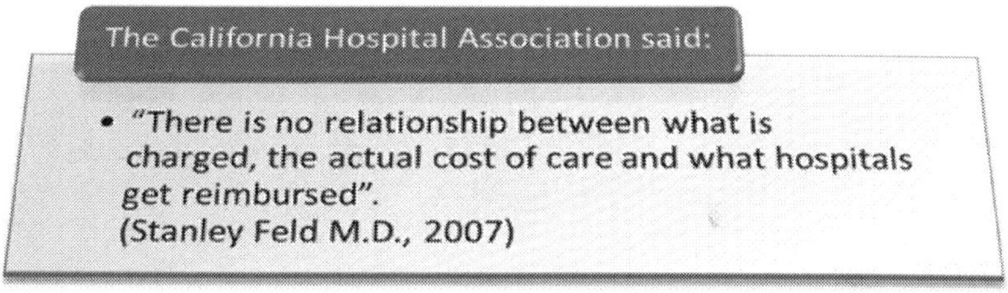

Figure 10: California Hospital Association Quote

If they are treating the truly-underserved, many dedicated providers and institutions will readily discount their services. Why? Because they never actually expect to be paid the invoice rate! The invoiced rate is merely a fiction used to arrive at the expected payment averaging 20 – 25 percent of that amount.

Herein lies the problem. Much of healthcare pricing is based upon a more, or less, arbitrary, discounted reimbursement structure. Some providers of care today are quitting their practices because they can no longer determine whether they will make money. In recent years, they have begun steadily to accumulate losses. This is unsustainable of course. It simply makes no sense to work long hours just to pay the high cost of malpractice insurance and other overhead, with no ability to predict a profit. See the following table for some examples that illustrate this disturbing phenomenon.

Table 6: Procedure Reimbursement Comparison Chart

Item Description	Invoice Price	Managed Care Reimbursement	Medicare Reimbursement
Typical 3-day Appendectomy	$28,089.62 (King, 2008)	$8,324.25 (King, 2008)	$5,322.93 (Federal Register, 2007)
Heart Failure and Shock 5-Day	$24, 875 (US Freedom Foundation, 2003)	$2,500.00 (US Freedom Foundation, 2003)	$2,217.00 (US Freedom Foundation, 2003)
Repair Complex Laceration (Scalp)	$7,702.00 (Association, 2007)	(no comparable data)	$316.00
Diagnostic Bilateral Mammogram	$460.00 (Lagnado, 2003)	$242.00 (Lagnado, 2003)	$90.00 (Lagnado, 2003)

The basic theme, illustrated above in Table 6, is that the actual amount paid to the provider of services is substantially less than the invoice to the consumer of the services. A look at the expected reimbursement rate for hospitals in the U.S. shows they expect to be paid by insurers or government programs, on average, less than twenty-five cents on the dollar for the goods and services reflected on the bill. This average reimbursement has been in steady decline over the past twenty years—ever since the managed care model became dominant. As a result, the system that providers use to establish a profit is not based on a logical formula as found in almost all other industries, but is instead based on setting the billing rate progressively higher to offset

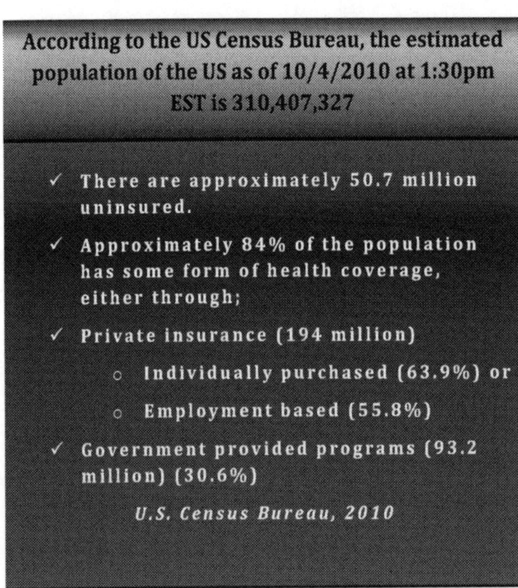

According to the US Census Bureau, the estimated population of the US as of 10/4/2010 at 1:30pm EST is 310,407,327
✓ There are approximately 50.7 million uninsured.
✓ Approximately 84% of the population has some form of health coverage, either through;
✓ Private insurance (194 million)
o Individually purchased (63.9%) or
o Employment based (55.8%)
✓ Government provided programs (93.2 million) (30.6%)
U.S. Census Bureau, 2010

Figure 11: Estimated U.S. Population 10/4/2010

the continual downward pressure from the declining percentage reimbursement rate they are paid.

For example, if one were to examine the invoice from an appendectomy procedure performed in 1990, it would be apparent that $10,000 in total charges yields an actual reimbursement from a health plan of only $2,500. Two years later, an invoice of $11,500 for an appendectomy yielded the same average reimbursed amount of $2,500. All that changed was a continued decline in the percentage rate of reimbursement.

This is problematic for patients, providers, hospitals and sponsors simply because no one can determine what is really being paid in this system. Doctors cannot predict if their practice will lose money, break even, or make a profit. Patients cannot determine if they are paying a fair price, and none of the statistics, on cost, give us any useful information.

The extent of the overall problems with a false economic structure of this magnitude is staggering. Approximately 84 percent of the U.S. population is covered with some form of health insurance, through their employers, through private purchase or through government programs. The remaining 16 percent are without insurance because they don't need it, don't want it, make too much to qualify for government coverage, or are unable to provide necessary documentation to obtain government coverage. The total amount

RECOMMENDATION

- MANDATE THE ELIMINATION OF THE CURRENT PRICING SYSTEM AND REPLACE WITH THREE MARKET BASED PRICING STRUCTURES, AND A TWO-STEP SALES OPTION.
- ALL PRICING TO BE OPENLY PUBLISHED AND EASILY AVAILABLE TO CONSUMERS VIA THE NATIONAL EXCHANGE.

spent for healthcare, in the U.S. in 2009, was projected to be over $2.5 trillion.[5] But, this number of $2.5 trillion is really still an unknown as it represents a mix of invoiced and reimbursement rate data. The true cost of care is anyone's guess and could be significantly less. If our true out-of-pocket costs are 10 percent, 20 percent, or even 30 percent less in some cases, the numbers we quote for a total cost of care become very problematic. If the numbers are off by this much, are other countries healthcare systems truly better? Cheaper? We really don't know. Simply put: until we address this underlying faulty pricing system and replace it with a common sense market price approach, no reform can yield significant results.

5 Kaiser Family Foundation, 2009

Pricing Options for Healthcare

Outside the healthcare industry, the sales of goods and services in our free market economy fall into one of three types of pricing systems: markup-on-cost (also called, cost-plus), margin-based (also called MSRP, Manufacturer Suggested Retail Pricing), and market-rate pricing. Each of these systems has evolved over several hundred years. They provide familiar and efficient methods for providers to set prices and for consumers to determine whether those prices are competitive and fair. It may be well for us to consider adopting one of these market-driven systems in the healthcare supply chain, because healthcare does not function in this manner today.

Cost-Plus: Providers set prices in this system by establishing their cost basis for goods and services and then adding to that cost a markup as a percentage "up charge" on that cost. (The markup is that percentage of the cost one adds on to arrive at the selling price.) These are different: a selling price with a margin of 25 percent results in more profit than a selling price with a markup of 25 percent. Most people find it better to work with margins. This means you can know what percentage of your gross income is profit. However, some still prefer simple markup on cost. In the formula that follows, Mu = Markup desired and C = Cost:

$$Mu = C(1 + Mu)$$

Margin-based: The provider of goods or services also may derive their pricing based on an industry-standard suggested selling price calculation derived by establishing their cost for the good or service and dividing that cost by the reciprocal of the amount of margin they expect to retain. The percentage margin is the percentage of the final selling price that is profit. In the formula that follows, Mg=Margin required, C=Cost of product:

$$Mg = \frac{C}{(1 - Mg)}$$

Market rate: The provider of goods or services can derive their pricing by relying on the competitive going market rate for similar goods or services in their area.

Two-step sales option: As can be seen in Figure 12 this option recognizes that a significant percentage of providers of healthcare services as they work in conjunction with other organizations that provide housing and care of patients during the provision of services. This approach includes pre and post-care services (Service Hubs). It is necessary to allow for the resale of the providers' services to the consumer or their payer/sponsors by these Service Hubs.

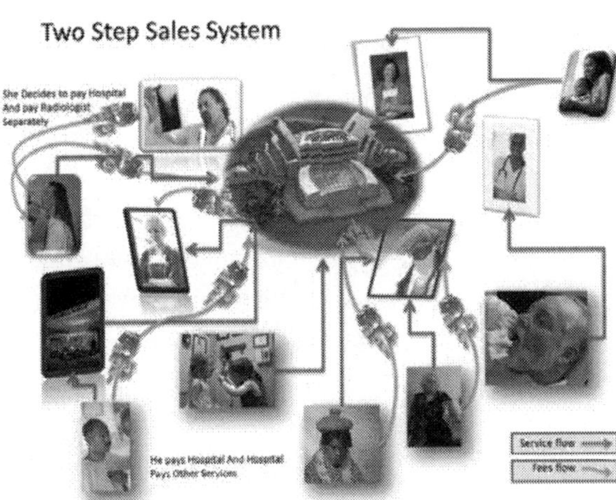

Figure 12 : Two Step System

This system provides not only convenience for the consumer, but also can bring economies of scale to providers and patients. Therefore, it is necessary to establish guidelines that will allow for the ability of these institutions, acting as hubs or aggregators of services, to bill the consumer and reimburse the providers. The efficiencies of central billing, debt carry, and central processing provided by the Hub to the providers become the basis for the discounts they offer. Consumers will be able to retain the choice to pay the provider directly or the Hub. This will help keep the costs in line and provide protection for each party in the process. If Hub fees for processing are too high, consumers will pay the provider directly. While this system will still allow discount rates to be established between providers and the Service Hubs, consumers will have the option of paying the Service Hub or the provider directly at the Providers' Suggested Price for services. Any discounts negotiated between

Service Hubs and providers will be transparent, and market forces will establish effective and value-based prices. Simply mandating transparent pricing without fixing the underlying economic structure will not work! Providers and hospitals will continue to be squeezed out of business, and service availability, already a huge concern under the current legislation, will suffer.

Rebates: Rebates exist in many industries so that manufacturers can skirt fair pricing regulations and give higher margins to various classes or channels of business partners, like distributors and resellers. All rebate programs are not created equal. Anyone who has recently purchased a piece of technology has seen some form of rebate. Some are called instant rebates and are taken at the time of purchase. Instant rebates are merely systems, so the manufacturer can reward a reseller by allowing that reseller to be able to offer a lower cost to the customer than other resellers for some period of time. Other rebate programs are "Manufacturer Rebates." In these programs the consumer often has to send the original copy of the sales receipt, the serial number, the model number cut from the box, and sometimes other information to the manufacturer's processing location. They get their rebate sent to them if they follow the instructions exactly. Manufacturers bank on the notion that most consumers will neglect to send in the rebate form or will fail to perform all of the steps correctly. Only about 40 percent of eligible rebate claims is ever paid out.

Rebate programs proliferate in the healthcare industry. Supposedly, rebates help lower costs to government. The truth is that rebates, in conjunction with other pricing mechanisms like Average Wholesale Price (AWP) or Wholesale Acquisition Cost (WAC) only serve to obscure actual costs.

In most industries, whether it's clothing, shoes, groceries, books, funerals, or other goods, rebates don't obscure costs. It is easy for people to deduce the cost, and realized profit margin, of a good or service as it passes through each step of the chain from the raw goods, to the manufacturer, to the distributor, to the reseller. In most other industries, the margins for resellers and manufacturers are consistent and similar across industries. While tough economic times will always impact the established resellers and distributors, the flux in the margin and pricing is relatively narrow.

In 2002, the National Health Policy Forum published a report that stated unequivocally that:

- ***"The 'true' cost of prescription drugs has grown increasingly elusive. Drug prices are subject to various types of discounts and rebates, seen and unseen, on both the public and private side. Each drug sold by a manufacturer, therefore, is subject to multiple prices, and little is known publicly about this pricing information."***
(Dawn M. Gencarelli, 2002)

Figure 13: National Health Policy Forum Quote - 2002

In this case, however, healthcare is an anomaly. Rebates in conjunction with arbitrary price bases like Average Wholesale Price (AWP) or Wholesale Acquisition Cost (WAC) effectively obscure actual pricing in every segment of the industry. Maintaining these confusing price schemes forces major providers and government entities to spend huge sums just to manage the process of not getting real answers! And, where did the current drug rebates come from? Why the government mandates them of course!

Across all phases of healthcare, manufacturing, and delivery, margins swing widely and often unpredictably. Rebates are a part of the problem. In order to get to rational Suggested Retail Pricing so that consumers can have transparency, we need to get to the point where manufacturers can establish real prices in the first place. The above-cited 2002 paper (Figure 13) on prescription drug costs shows how rebates are a major problem and economic drain, yet the various stakeholders have a vested interest in one form or another to preserve this flawed system.

True reform would cause pain, but the only thing that we would really lose is the camera obscura through which we see this beast. Ultimately, the consumers will win. Part of the reason that drug prices are so high is due to the issues of the false economic structure we previously discussed. The primary reason is that the use of rebates artificially inflates the price, so the rebate can bring the cost to where the manufacturer, distributor, reseller, and payer need it to be, and the hidden cash flow can continue. And, where do most of the rebates go? They go back to the government, both federal and state, supposedly to pay for more goods and services for the underserved. Some also flow back to distributors and very large pharmacy companies, and pharmacy benefits managers. The dirty little secret is that much of these funds are redirected to: (1) offset government grants to programs (thereby inflating what the government is actually saying they are spending); (2) pay for the ever expanding bureaucracies that depend on these programs for their livelihood and career advancement; or (3) to make up for the unsustainable squeeze of margin to the pharmacies and distributors. They are nothing other than another hidden tax, often disproportionately affecting the middle-class. Why not eliminate the rebates completely, save the bureaucratic cost of administration, have real pricing transparency, and cover more people with the savings?

RECOMMENDATION

- MANDATE THE ELIMINATION OF REBATES AND REQUIRE MANUFACTURERS TO SET SUGGESTED RETAIL PRICES (MSRP). ALL OTHER PRICES INCLUDING DISTRIBUTOR PRICES, MAJOR PURCHASERS PRICES, AND GOVERNMENT PRICES DERIVE FROM THIS PRICE.

Transparency in Pricing

While the word "transparency" reflects the "spin de jour" in healthcare, few, if any, in this industry truly desire to provide transparency. There is every conceivable disincentive for providers, distributors, and manufacturers to obscure the true flow of funds as they play out today. As such, each player is more than a bit reluctant to eliminate the rebates, market development funds (MDF), special performance incentive funds (spiffs), etc., so all can play fairly. I am a strong open-market advocate. In fact, much of what I am proposing is based on open-market principles. However, in this case, *there is little likelihood of change unless the whole economic structure of healthcare is addressed.* Today, pharmacies, hospitals, healthcare practices, HMOs, etc. are so bound to profit derived through rebates and other frangible and hidden sources of revenue that they simply cannot find a visible path to a more rational and transparent model. Each market segment is reliant on these false priced systems to keep their doors open. Clearly, this system is not working. Moreover, it is just as clear that the system is not working for anyone in the chain, including; providers, insurers, manufacturers, and most of all, consumers. It was not planned this way—like virulent weeds, it simply evolved opportunistically.

Let's take a brief look at how the lack of price transparency, impacts the healthcare industry.

From the program sponsor standpoint—even program sponsors, like the federal government and the various states and territories, now rely on things like rebates to find the funding to provide ser-

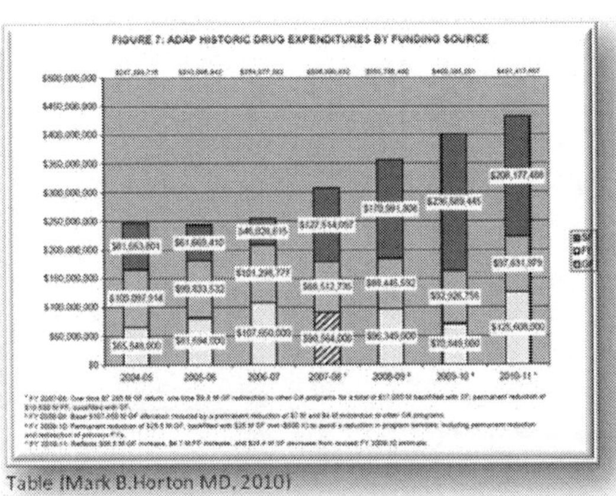

Table (Mark B.Horton MD, 2010)

Chart 13: CA ADAP Historic Drug Expenses

vices for the distressed population. For example, states receive rebates from drug companies on the dollar amount of prescriptions dispensed to users of programs like AIDS Drug Assistance Programs (ADAP), as well as mental health programs as provided by states and in some cases counties and municipalities. Even a cursory look at most states budgets for these programs will show you that the real viability of the program relies on these dollars. It takes significant resources for states to track the claims, the eligibility of the rebate claim, the price that the rebate is based on and then the processing of the claim up to the receipt of the rebate. This is neither a quick nor cheap system. Like so many other things in the government, redistribution schemes represent a significant portion of the "savings" which are lost in processing fees and interest on the funds borrowed by the states and federal government to front the expense in the first place[6]. Rebate funds account for over 48 percent of the funds applied to support the California AIDS Drug Assistance Program (ADAP). (Chart 13) It is not the fact that the funding is applied to the program that is at issue. This is a good thing for patients who need the care to have California gain additional sources to help pay for the program. The question is, "where is the money actually spent?" How much is going for the care of patients? How much is going for taking care of the bureaucracy? How much is simply a replacement of the general fund?

In California, there is no indication whatsoever that any funds get redirected to other Non-AIDS/HIV programs. That may not be the case in other states. So, how much does get diverted? How many states take the funds into the state's general fund and just spend them elsewhere? How much is spent on medications? Is that the true cost of the medication provided? Is the profit that the providers get discernible? Acceptable? Is the cost of the program justified? Is the overall program efficient? The questions driven by this lack of clarity are seemingly endless.

---

6 The included chart is reproduced from the California Governor's 2010-2011 Department of Public Health Office of AIDS - AIDS Drug Assistance Program (ADAP) budget (May Revision) (GF=General Funds, SF=Special Funds (e.g., rebates), FF=Federal Funding).

From the provider's standpoint: For those who participate in the dispensing, distribution, facilitation, and provision of services, it has become impossible to plan or predict if they will generate positive cash flow or not. What is worse is they cannot predict what they need, in a contract or business model, to control their business. They cannot project what they should charge of their own services because what they will actually derive from their effort is subject to so many other variables. In this environment, even with the strong desire to provide it, transparency is impossible.

The Physicians' Foundation commissioned a survey by the consulting firm Merritt Hawkins in 2008. One physician's response illustrates the problem from the provider's perspective.

The Physician's Foundation in a survey found:

- "I have been in practice for ten years now, the last five years as a private solo practice owner. I'm very disheartened, disappointed over the state of the practice of medicine! The combination of; low reimbursements, managed care issues and patient attitudes over the last three years have made the practice of medicine almost unbearable. If not for a son who I'm working to put through college, and a house mortgage, I would quit medicine in a heartbeat! I'm beat, tired, and under-appreciated. Sometimes I cry myself to sleep—wondering why I got into all this. Am I paying myself this month? Do I have enough to pay this month's debt and lease? (Merritt Hawkins & Associates, 2008)

Figure 14: Physicians Foundation Survey Quote - 2008

From the consumer's standpoint: So, now ask yourself this simple question: If the providers of service and the sponsors of programs, like the states and the federal government can't figure out how much they are being charged or how much they should charge, how then can the consumer figure out how to control costs or, save money? The constant evolution of these systems over the last fifty years has caused this problem. It's not a purposeful conspiracy to defraud anyone, because, in the end, while some have had sporadic periods of profitability, no one has truly received any benefit from this mess.

Transportability of Insurance

Preserved in the existing legislation is the current system of regional or state-based insurance offerings. The fact that a person who relocates from Philadelphia to Omaha can't keep his or her health insurance plan is a big problem. A bigger problem is that the insurance available to the individual, who relocates, may not have the same standards of care tied to the policy they purchase. While some of this is corrected by the minimum policy coverage standards in the current legislation, each state can mandate additions to these requirements, and many already do. So, an individual moving from state to state will still have to change policies, and each of these policies will have different terms.

Due to the significant difference in coverage and mandates state to state, the providers do not typically belong to a national network model. Under the current economic model, it is impossible for an insurer to offer a national network price, and it would be impossible for a provider to accept one. There are two problems with this state of affairs. First, most already do participate in a national network if they accept Medicare or Medicaid patients. Second, almost all other industries have a national model. These national models may or may not have a national consumer price. What they all typically do have is a suggested retail price. Local economic variances in cost and market velocity often do affect the price to consumers, and interestingly, they all seem to work themselves out, based on the free market influences. Small business owners in rural markets usually have lower economic costs. Synergistically, the market size and available capital often drive lower prices and lower margins. It is a consistent phenomenon that the relative retained earnings of like businesses in different markets often yield the same relative standard of living for the business owners. Look at most franchisees in a network and you will see that while the dollars flowing through the business vary significantly between major markets like an L. A. and New York, for instance, and smaller markets like Huntsville and Winnemucca, the standard of living of the owners relative to that of the local economy does not vary as much. While the New York owner may live in a multi-million dollar apartment off Central Park, and the Winnemucca owner may live in a $350,000 home, in the only gated community near the town, they both may live in one of the top 10 percent of homes in their respective areas. With changes in the fundamental economic system, healthcare costs will be proportional in scale to the local economy.

This problem of transportability and equality in healthcare coverage is actually much worse because there is even more variation in policy and coverage when a person is part of an employer-based health plan. Each company, in effect, becomes like a state. When an employee changes their job, that employee must often change his or her policy. These groups then carry a modified actuarial and make the system, in fact, much more complicated than it needs to be. From the employer perspective, there is a big problem in negotiating coverage with insurers every year and coming up with the policy bundles to attract new employees. The cost of the employee premium is not the only cost of maintaining these complicated option plans. Further, there is a wide disparity in insurance options from company to company.

Obamacare will restrict the ability of insurers to deny coverage to individuals for pre-existing conditions and to cancel their coverage if they get sick. The child-focused part of this provision is already in effect. The reason I say "restricts" insurance companies' ability in both cases instead of "eliminates" is because insurers still have the ability to eliminate the policies providing the bulk of the coverage in the first place. For example, within hours of the first part of this law taking effect, some insurers announced they were eliminating child-only policies in certain states. Great deal, huh?

RECOMMENDATION

- ELIMINATE THE IMPEDIMENTS TO A NATIONAL INSURANCE MARKET.
- LET CONSUMERS PURCHASE POLICIES ON AN OPEN NATIONAL MARKET.
- MANDATE THAT THESE POLICIES BE TRANSPORTABLE FROM STATE TO STATE AND JOB TO JOB.
- MANDATE MINIMUM POLICY STANDARDS.
- MANDATE NATIONAL SOLVENCY STANDARDS FOR INSURERS.
- PROVIDE EMPLOYEES FULL CHOICE IN SELECTING THE INSURER AND POLICY THEY DESIRE BY ELIMINATING EMPLOYER BASED GROUP POLICY OFFERINGS—HAVING SMALLER ACTUARIES.
- ALLOW EMPLOYERS TO OFFER TAX EXEMPT SPECIFIC BENEFIT PAYMENT AMOUNTS TO THE EMPLOYEE AS PART OF COMPETITIVE HIRING PRACTICE WITH EXEMPTIONS NOT TO EXCEED $1,000 PER MONTH.
- MANDATE THAT THE ACTUARIAL THAT INSURERS USE BE ACROSS THE FULL BREATH OF AN INSURER'S POLICY GROUP.
- ELIMINATE HIGH-RISK POOLS—ALL POLICY HOLDERS OF A SPECIFIC POLICY OFFERING IN THE SAME POOL.

Reducing the Cost of Practice

Many healthcare businesses and providers today cannot maintain a consistent, positive cash flow. They cannot predict what they will generate in revenue, nor can they identify many of the items that they can control in their business, so they can properly balance costs with the unpredictable vagaries of their reimbursements. The "payer mix" of consumers that come through their doors, significantly compounds this problem. Generally, the more Medicare or Medicaid patients a provider has the bigger that this issue is. Currently, we see a larger and larger trend line towards the elimination of services to patients, in these categories. While not a large part of the market, increasingly we see, practices where self-pay are the only acceptable form of payment. These practitioners have simply come to the point where they will no longer deal with vagaries and unknowns. The consumers all suffer. The poor have reduced access, moderate-income consumers experience higher costs, and the affluent encounter the additional burden of dealing directly with insurers.

So why is it that these providers can't make any money or figure out how to control costs? Price uncertainty is the issue, both in terms of what they pay for the services they need and in what they need to charge for their services. On the cost side are the cost of interconnection to all the others in the economic chain, including records maintenance, transmission and coordination, and duplication of services, and the large cost of a few items required for practice, such as malpractice insurance and errors and omissions (E&O) insurance.

Therefore, the lack of clarity in the costs and prices across the healthcare industry is one of the largest obstacles to true reform of the system, as well as coverage for the uninsured and under-insured. For any reform to succeed, first, the reform has to insure pricing certainty. Transparency of this kind cannot simply be legislated. For every smart person writing a law or regulation, there are thousands of smart people figuring out how to circumvent it. As we have seen historically, the disparate providers in the healthcare industry evolved self-protective practices for survival as our nation was developing its own laws and governance. It was often, not abject greed; it was simply survival.

In any other industry, what I will call "price transparity" (transparency and certainty) is achieved by natural market forces. Consumers do not spend much time, in general, researching prices. They shop and quickly determine whether, or not, prices are fair. Items that are basic and necessary are typically priced fairly and have a reasonable degree of price transparity. As services and items become less necessary, and more discretionary, they usually have more variety in the products and services offered. In other words, the more discretionary the item the higher the relative price will be and the resulting margin for the purveyor of the good or service will generally be higher.

Consider, again, the example of the $250 jeans and the $39.95 jeans. Functionally they are the same. The difference is in the desire of the consumer of the product and the area they choose to place their value when making the purchase. The person paying $250 for blue jeans is not the same customer demographically. The person who is paying effectively eighteen times the price for functionally the same pair of pants, is not buying for the function (effective value) of the service of the item, but for style and fit (intangible value). Efficacy aside, why should healthcare be any different? All people should be able to purchase affordable healthcare solutions that bring effective value, but, that said, this should not restrict those who choose to pay more for intangible value.

The other major drag on efficiency in the practice of healthcare today is the communication practices among the entities throughout the chain. Its paperwork: records creation, storage, retrieval and retention; orders and prescription transmission and processing, enrollment, benefits eligibility, tracking, and processing are some of the major cost factors. Constant, incremental, and inconsistent legislated and mandated rules and standards of practice continually and exponentially increase the cost of these communications. One of the problems addressed rationally in both the Healthcare Act and the Health Information Technology (HIT) section of the American

Reinvestment and Recovery Act (ARRA), was the need for effective standards and investment in infrastructure to develop the efficiencies to help lower the cost of care. Great care needs to be taken in application of these regulations, because history has shown that while technology always promises to reduce costs, it rarely does.

It is a mistake, in particular, simply to apply technology to an existing workflow. Instead, we need to rethink workflow based on the efficiencies technology can bring. The direct application of technology without a fundamental redesign of workflow typically yields any of three negative outcomes: decreased efficiency, broken processes, and a loss of checks and balances.

Direct administrative costs in healthcare are but one part of the much bigger problem. Duplication of services is another of the prime wasteful costs in healthcare today. Patients often undergo the same tests several times, ordered by different physicians. A man in his 60s might routinely have his PSA tested to determine his prostate health. If the same man has had some reason for concern in the past, he likely has been referred to a urologist by his primary physician. In that case, he sees his primary doctor for an annual physical, and he also sees his urologist every six months for a check-up. It is almost a given that both doctors will order the same PSA blood test, even though each is copied on the other's test results.

It has been estimated that duplication of services can account for as much as 40 percent of national healthcare spending (Kelly, 2009). If one looks across the broader healthcare arena, it is easy to see that a large portion of the tests are duplicative due to lack of coordination. This phenomenon is even more apparent in underserved communities. Along with significant administrative inefficiencies, this same lack of simple coordination leads to a high rate of fraud because some providers find they can easily game the system. Inefficiencies in the system account for as much as 12 percent of total national healthcare spending, while fraud and abuse add another 19 percent (Kelly, 2009). Thomson Reuters estimates that the total waste in this $2.2 trillion annual industry is over one-third of the total, or about $760 billion (Kelly, 2009)—of course as we discussed before, this assumes the initial numbers are even accurate.

While Obamacare represents a new attempt to address administrative inefficiencies, there are many areas that demand further review—and a few that are simply not covered in the legislation. (Some of these will be discussed below.) Overall, much of the funding we pour into healthcare is simply wasted. There are several simple things that can be done quickly to begin to address the problem and will bring significant savings, free much-needed resources, and help us cover more people for less money.

One commonly expressed panacea for this mess is the idea of going to a single-payer system. Consumer groups, healthcare unions, some physician associations, and liberal politicians all clamor to some degree for the single-payer myth. Despite strong evidence to the contrary, "single payer" has been seen as a cure-all for what is wrong with healthcare.

The problem is that the term "single-payer" is not reflective of what most of these groups and individuals really want or what taxpayers can afford. In numerous discussions with politicians pontificating on the benefits of national single payer, one question often derails the conversation: "Do you really want the federal government to be the only source of payment for all health services provided to the entire U.S. population of 350 million people?" Most of the time, the conversation stops right there, because the answer is no. On the rare occasion that the person answers "yes," a second question usually ends the inquiry, "So you expect all people that work in healthcare in any capacity to become federal employees and receive a government salary?"

What most people are talking about when they mention single payer, is really not having a single payer. Rather, they are referring to a single point of administration. To have just that one entity become responsible for the provision of healthcare services to all Americans is neither what most people want nor can we afford it.

There is a great benefit to having a system with many payers, with many sponsors to pay for the services we need. Insurance companies are sponsors; federal, state, and municipal governments are sponsors; non-profits are sponsors; faith based groups are sponsors; individual providers who provide their services pro bono are sponsors; and volunteers in effect also are sponsors. Looking across the economy of healthcare, particularly in servicing the need of the underserved, all of these entities are required to provide access and equity to deliver what is needed to the entire population. It is simply unworkable to think we can rely on one single entity, (by necessity the federal government) to provide all that we need. The inefficient 30 percent return on collected funds as goods and services alone renders this option as impossible.

Instead, we need a system to help coordinate the activities of all of these providers and sponsors in order to reduce duplication, fraud, and abuse. A single-payer system would eliminate the Glide Memorial Church's programs, the Haight Ashbury Free Clinic Programs, the other CBOs, NGOs, and state programs, and the volunteer equity from the system, which would put too much burden on the tax base. It would remove so many resources and care access points that the underserved and the vast majority of Americans will find their access to care limited and flexibility in the provision of care reduced.

In order to begin to get significant savings and increase the ability to serve more with less, we need to provide the ability for consumers of services and providers to be able to communicate, securely, with full privacy and efficiently, and work together as virtual patient-centered teams. A system that functions to address consumers' needs across the full spectrum of services available will go a long way to addressing the duplication of the services problem. Simple communication alone could solve a large portion of this costly problem. The standards and technology that will arise from the Health Information Technology (HIT) legislation will continue to bring more efficiency and lower cost. But, even a minor implementation of a basic form of communication and the ability to create virtual care teams can result in major benefits very quickly.

For example, suppose we could put those who are willing to provide healthcare services—those who will help pay for the services—and the various "middlemen"—in the stands at Candlestick Park in San Francisco. Further, suppose we could bring all the people who were in need (let us just address the underserved for a minute) into the field area. Now we bring each person to a center field microphone, one at a time, and they state what their needs are. As their needs are stated, the people who can solve the need are identified, and the person in need selects from those available who can provide the solutions conveniently. The various people providing the solution are all introduced to one another, and a care team is formed. They organize their care plan to coordinate what they will be doing and who will pay for what. As they provide the person with assistance, they continue to coordinate their actions with each other and the person in need. The person in need then begins to follow the plan, and work with each member of this team to gain the care he, or she, needs. As this care is provided, the people providing the care, those facilitating the provision of care, and the person receiving the care itself, all stay connected and in communication and coordinated. How much can we save? How much better would the outcome be for the person? How much better would the adherence be? How many more people could be covered with the available resources? Do we need Electronic Medical Records to do this? No! Do we need Electronic Prescriptions? No! They are helpful, and will increase savings and efficiencies, but are not required. We simply need a method to identify resources, make linkages to those in need, coordinate care, and communicate among the members of the needy persons virtual care group! This can be done, and, in fact, it is already being done today!

Full Coordination of Care and Benefits Across All Sources & Virtual Teams

This Coordination of Care and Benefits system can go much further in reducing duplication, waste, and fraud. Offering the ability for providers, sponsors and facilitators to work in virtual teams, as they care for the individual healthcare consumer not only reduces waste but improves the quality of care the consumer receives. Reducing the duplication of services further increases the capacity of the system to handle more consumers. Increasing capacity has been repeatedly cited as a critical need. Mandating Coordination of

Care and Benefits across all sources brings significant savings and reductions in several key areas.

Mandating the coordination of care, across all available sources, in conjunction with, permitting consumers to establish virtual care groups with the people providing the services—helping them access the services and those paying for the services—can all but eliminate duplication of services. Mandating the Coordination of Benefits spreads the cost of care across all sources lowering the burden on any one program, and reducing fraud and gaming of the system. With widespread participation in such a system, various approaches can be used for equitable sharing of the cost of care provided. No longer, would payer-of-last resort be the only solution available to sponsors to ensure efficacy and efficiency of the dollars spent.

While the work of the HIT sub-committees in the development and adoption of the standards to ensure enhanced tools like Electronic Medical Records, Electronic Prescriptions, and Electronic Lab Reporting, etc., they will provide the framework for even more systemic efficiencies and controls. Initially, a simple, free set of communication, grouping, and scheduling tools, implemented presently will provide significant savings. Much of the duplication of services is a result of the right hand not knowing what the left hand is doing.

Much of the current fraud and abuse is derived from the monetizing of the current system inefficiencies. For example, HIV/AIDS medications are among the most expensive medications for treatment of any disease, except for some cancer drugs. It is not uncommon for the annual cost to exceed $15,000 per year per patient. It has been documented that some participants in these programs also seek and become eligible for the same drugs in similar programs in other states with similar formularies and/or pharmaceutical patient assistance programs. Sometimes, these drugs are obtained over, and over, again by the same patient in the same month. So the patient is receiving two to three times the volume of medications they need at two to three times the cost to the taxpayer. Occasionally, there is a moral justification for this behavior by the patient. Some of the patients have undisclosed partners in need of the drugs. More often, however, the motive is simple monetary gain, and the excess drugs are sold on the street to other users or abusers.

Coordinating benefits across all available patient sources can ferret out these abuses, and significantly lower costs. Not long ago, an audit of AIDS Drug Assistance Program (ADAP) patients

RECOMMENDATION

- IN ADDITION TO THE NATIONAL EXCHANGE MARKETPLACE, STATES SHOULD PROVIDE A SIMPLE FRAMEWORK FOR PARTICIPANTS (CONSUMERS), FACILITATORS (ENROLLMENT WORKERS, VOLUNTEERS, AND OTHERS HELPING CONSUMERS FIND SERVICES), PROVIDERS (PEOPLE WHO PROVIDE THE GOODS AND SERVICES) AND SPONSORS (PEOPLE WHO PAY FOR GOODS AND SERVICES) TO COMMUNICATE WITH ONE ANOTHER AND THEN FORM VIRTUAL CARE TEAMS.

- THIS SYSTEM SHOULD BE PROVIDED BY THE STATE, FOR USE BY ALL, FOR FREE.

- UTILIZATIONS SHOULD BE INCENTIVIZED BY TYING REIMBURSEMENT RATES AND PROGRAM DOLLARS TO USE OF THE SYSTEM. IF THEY USE THIS SYSTEM, THE STATES' COSTS ARE LOWERED; THEREFORE THE RATES PAID CAN INCREASE.

in California and Washington State showed seventy-five patients obtaining the same prescriptions in each state in the same month. A similar review of California ADAP and the San Bernardino County mental health recipients yielded similar findings. In specific drugs where the formularies overlapped, patients were found who drew, benefits in both programs for the same prescriptions in the same month.

Each program in any given system, whether it is a state or federal program, has some form of an administrative system. In most cases, each system is composed of several legacy systems that do not integrate well, if at all. Each county, for instance, may have separate eligibility criteria and separate drug formularies. Even within a county, various programs also often have overlapping infrastructures with differing criteria. These silos do not interface with any of the others. As such, consumers, and their information, get into the system and movement between the systems is non-existent. For a person to move between counties, or programs, is often mostly a manual process. Information is lost, entry errors are compounded, and consumers have to manage multiple accounts. Sponsors that bridge multiple jurisdictions have the same problems. Reporting to sponsors of utilization and efficacy, are difficult, and benchmarking is almost impossible. The 16% administrative inefficiencies cited, in the Thomson Reuters report (Kelly, 2009), and are considered, by many, to be an underestimate.

Simply knowing where a patient is connected and receiving care goes a long way to reducing problems. Having one system for consumers or their facilitators to determine total eligibility, across all needs and program availability, will significantly reduce the administrative inefficiency.

Patient-centered team-based care has been shown to improve patient adherence and effectiveness of treatment. Ultimately, increased capacity and better outcomes would result. As previously stated, part of the problem with the current system capacity is that providers are often running the same diagnostics and tests as other providers on the same patients. For the underserved, it is compounded in that they often seek Community Based Organizations (CBOs) for care and services. It is not atypical for a patient to present at one of the CBOs as homeless, drug-addicted, HIV-positive, malnourished, Hepatitis C-positive and mentally disabled. The provider that sees the patient, and then makes a preliminary diagnosis, usually orders a series of tests, reviews the tests, develops a treatment plan, meets again with the patient, initiates treatment and sometimes meets again as a follow-up. That provider may also schedule more tests to assess the efficacy. Now suppose the typical patient shows up a few weeks or months later at the CBO across town. What does that attending provider do? Of course, they do the same thing. Time and money are wasted. The provider—rather than treating another underserved person—is treating the same person needlessly.

Now suppose this provider is at least aware that the patient was at the other clinic not long before. Even without EMR, and other enhanced tools, simply knowing allows the provider to seek patient permission for a consult. With a simple phone call, later multiple visits and tests might be avoided. Here is how it breaks down:

- ✓ Less waste with one patient, means more patients are seen.
- ✓ Less duplication frees more of existing funds to fund more treatments for others.
- ✓ Coordination of treatment and reinforcement of existing protocols increases outcomes.
- ✓ "Virtual Teaming" lowers the burden on each of the individual facilitators and providers—they are no longer alone in caring for the person in need.
- ✓ Patient-centered team-based care has been shown to improve patient adherence and treatment outcome.

RECOMMENDATION

- MANDATE COORDINATION OF CARE AND BENEFITS ACROSS ALL AVAILABLE SOURCES

Tort Reform

It seems, just like with death and taxes, no one disagrees there is a problem with the amount, scope, and justification for much of the litigation in the United States. Most people are disgusted with both the legal system and the "sue anyone for anything and get rich" mentality to problem solving. The reality is that our overly litigious society has driven up costs in almost every segment of the economy and made it all but impossible to undertake once-simple transactions. And, like death and taxes, it seems there is little we can do to overcome this problem. We simply accept it as inevitable. Americans spend proportionately far more per person on the costs of litigation than any other country in the world.

One place we are seeing a direct and significantly adverse effect from overt uncontrolled litigation is in the area of healthcare costs. We are losing providers at an alarming rate. Many are simply quitting their practice as the rising cost of insurance outstrips the declining marginal reimbursement rates.

The excesses of the litigation system are an important contributor to *defensive medicine*—the costly use of medical treatments by a doctor for the purpose of avoiding litigation. In 2001, surgeons at the University of Nevada Medical Center trauma walked off the job because they could no longer afford malpractice insurance. Their premiums increased sharply, in some cases rising from $40,000 to more than $200,000 annually. The trauma center closed for ten days until some of the surgeons agreed to become county government employees for a limited time, which capped their liability for non-economic damages. If the Las Vegas trauma center were to close again, the most severely injured patients would have to be transported to the next nearest Level 1 trauma center—five hours away.

Access to trauma care was only one problem Nevada faced during its insurance crisis. Access to obstetrics and many other types of care were also threatened (Office of the Assistant Secretary for Planning and Evaluation, 2002). This is not simply a Nevada problem. More, and more, doctors are starting to sound like Dr. Frank Jordan, a vascular surgeon in Las Vegas, who left his practice. "I did the math. If I were to stay in business for three years, it would cost me $1.2 million for insurance. I obviously can't afford that. I'd be bankrupt after the first year, and I'd just be working for the insurance company. What's the point?"

RECOMMENDATIONS

- ENACT SWEEPING AND SIGNIFICANT TORT REFORM.
- IMPROVE THE ABILITY OF ALL PATIENTS WHO ARE INJURED BY NEGLIGENCE TO GET QUICKER, APPROPRIATE COMPENSATION FOR THEIR "ECONOMIC LOSSES," INCLUDING THE LOSS OF THE ABILITY TO PROVIDE VALUABLE UNPAID SERVICES LIKE CARE FOR CHILDREN OR A PARENT.
- ENSURE THAT RECOVERIES FOR NON-ECONOMIC DAMAGES COULD NOT EXCEED A REASONABLE AMOUNT ($250,000).
- RESERVE PUNITIVE DAMAGES FOR CASES THAT JUSTIFY THEM—WHERE THERE IS CLEAR AND CONVINCING PROOF THAT THE DEFENDANT ACTED WITH MALICIOUS INTENT OR DELIBERATELY FAILED TO AVOID UNNECESSARY INJURY TO THE PATIENT, AND AVOID UNREASONABLE AWARDS (ANYTHING IN EXCESS OF THE GREATER OF TWO TIMES ECONOMIC DAMAGES OR $250,000).

RECOMMENDATIONS (CON'T)

- PROVIDE FOR PAYMENT OF A JUDGMENT OVER TIME RATHER THAN IN ONE LUMP SUM AND THUS ENSURE THAT THE MONEY IS THERE FOR THE INJURED PATIENT WHEN NEEDED.
- ENSURE THAT OLD CASES CANNOT BE BROUGHT YEARS AFTER AN EVENT WHEN MEDICAL STANDARDS MAY HAVE CHANGED OR WITNESSES' MEMORIES HAVE FADED, BY PROVIDING THAT A CASE MAY NOT BE BROUGHT MORE THAN THREE YEARS FOLLOWING THE DATE OR INJURY OR ONE YEAR AFTER THE CLAIMANT DISCOVERS OR, WITH REASONABLE DILIGENCE, SHOULD HAVE DISCOVERED THE INJURY.
- INFORMING THE JURY IF A PLAINTIFF ALSO HAS ANOTHER SOURCE OF PAYMENT FOR THE INJURY, SUCH AS HEALTH INSURANCE.
- PROVIDE THAT DEFENDANTS PAY ANY JUDGMENT IN PROPORTION TO THEIR FAULT, NOT ON THE BASIS OF HOW DEEP THEIR POCKETS ARE.

What Role for Government?

> "We the People of the United States, in Order to form a more perfect Union, establish Justice, insure Domestic Tranquility, provide for the common defense, promote the General Welfare, and secure the Blessings of Liberty to ourselves and our Posterity, do ordain and establish this Constitution for the United States of America."
>
> *Preamble to the US Constitution, 1787*

Right or wrong, the government today is the major provider of healthcare to a large portion of Americans. Over 30 percent (92 million people) of the U.S. population receives most of their care from government programs, principally Medicare and Medicaid. Even though these two programs are primarily federally funded, this is where their similarity ends. While Medicare is a national program, Medicaid is implemented in a state-by-state-based model. Providers will tell you that Medicare reimbursement rates are horrible, and the Medicaid rates are much worse. Neither typically covers the actual cost of care delivered by the provider.

> "Governments are instituted among Men, deriving their just powers from the consent of the governed, — That whenever any Form of Government becomes destructive of these ends, it is the Right of the People to alter or to abolish it, and to institute new Government."
>
> *Declaration of Independence, 1776*

Consider the case of Ms. Rebekah Nix, an uninsured twenty-five year-old Brooklyn woman who learned first-hand how bad the current billing system is. Following an appendectomy and a two-day stay in the hospital, she was billed for more than $19,000. The hospital where Ms. Nix was treated, New York Methodist Hospital in Brooklyn, typically bills HMOs about $2,500 for the same procedure and two-day stay, but it would typically receive a reimbursement of about $5,000 from Medicaid, the state and federal health program for the poor, and about $7,800 from Medicare, the federal program for the elderly (Lagnado 2003).

While some Medicaid reimbursement rates are higher than Medicare rates state by state, most providers agree that treating these Medicaid patients is bankrupting their practices and many have ceased to treat Medicaid patients. There are over fifty different programs requiring over fifty different state departments, and each state has to have administrative systems, support personnel, eligibility workers, auditors, etc. Further, many other programs, at the state and federal level, are now tightly interwoven, so the costs are actually much higher. The state of California's Medicaid program (called Medi-Cal) had a budget projected to be more than $14 billion for 2010–2011 FY, and it projected it would exceed $19.2 billion by 2015.[7] This does not include the cost of the city and county employees, and others who facilitate this program, law suits, judgments paid and many other items.

The total tax cost for Medicaid to the taxpayer in 2009 was approximately $380 billion, not including state funding. The federal share of Medicaid expenditures is 50 percent to 80 percent of the total cost.[8] Given that estimate, the total cost to the population for Medicaid could be between $760 billion and $1.9 trillion, including all the state expenditures that are duplicated in these separate programs. How many more people could we possibly cover, if we eliminated just 30 percent of the extraneous costs? At an average cost of care of $7,927 per covered person, this would equate to a cost of between 28 and 72 million more people. Since there are approximately 50.7 million uninsured in the United States, according to the federal government's vastly inflated figure, we could conceivably cover most, if not all of them, and potentially even have money left over.

The U.S. government was not established to manage industries, nor has it ever been equipped to control large sections of our economy. We need to get back to the basics of government and

7 CA Legislative Analyst's Office, 2009

8 Stateline.Org Staff, 2005.

disentangle the fog that we have in our current system. We need to create clear and distinct guidelines and limits. Government should get back to establishing the type of limited regulations and controls as were prescribed and advocated by the founding fathers. Regulations need to be in language simple enough that anyone can understand them.

One of the chief concerns of the Framers was that, in the early years of the new nation, the federal government proved unable to quell rebellion or quarrels amongst the states, either by force or persuasion. Some states had very nearly gone to war with each other over disputed territorial claims, as with the conflict between Pennsylvania and Connecticut over Wilkes-Barre. The government watched in horror as Shay's Rebellion transpired just before the Constitutional Convention. One of the main goals of the Convention, then, was to ensure that the federal government had the power to quash rebellion and to smooth tensions between states.

Welfare

welfare n. 1. Health, happiness, or prosperity; well-being. [<ME wel faren, to fare well][9]

Welfare in today's context also means organized efforts on the part of public or private organizations to benefit the poor, or simply public assistance. This is not the meaning of the word as used in the Constitution.

Posterity

posterity n. 1. Future generations.

2. All of a person's descendants. [<Lat. posteritas.] [10]

There is a role for the government to play in healthcare reform. Before we can determine what role government *should* play, perhaps we should establish what role government should *NOT* play.

9 *U.S. Constitution Online, 1997*
10 ibid

The US Constitution: Section 8—Powers of Congre
The Congress shall have Power to lay and collect Taxes, Duties, Imposts and Excises, to pay the Debts and provide for the common Defense and General Welfare of the United States; but all Duties, Imposts and Excises shall be uniform throughout the United States;
To borrow money on the credit of the United States;
To regulate Commerce with foreign Nations, and among the several States, and with the Indian Tribes;
To establish an uniform Rule of Naturalization, and uniform Laws on the subject of Bankruptcies throughout the United States;
To coin Money, regulate the Value thereof, and of foreign Coin, and fix the Standard of Weights and Measures;
To provide for the Punishment of counterfeiting the Securities and current Coin of the United States;
To establish Post Offices and Post Roads;
To promote the Progress of Science and useful Arts, by securing for limited Times to Authors and Inventors the exclusive Right to their respective Writings and Discoveries;
To constitute Tribunals inferior to the Supreme Court;
To define and punish Piracies and Felonies committed on the high Seas, and Offenses against the Law of Nations;
To declare War, grant Letters of Marque and Reprisal, and make Rules concerning Captures on Land and Water;
To raise and support Armies, but no Appropriation of Money to that Use shall be for a longer Term than two Years;
To provide and maintain a Navy;
To make Rules for the Government and Regulation of the land and naval Forces;
To provide for calling forth the Militia to execute the Laws of the Union, suppress Insurrections and repel Invasions;
To provide for organizing, arming, and disciplining, the Militia, and for governing such Part of them as may be employed in the Service of the United States, reserving to the States respectively, the Appointment of the Officers, and the Authority of training the Militia according to the discipline prescribed by Congress;
To exercise exclusive Legislation in all Cases whatsoever, over such District (not exceeding ten Miles square) as may, by Cession of particular States, and the acceptance of Congress, become the Seat of the Government of the United States, and to exercise like Authority over all Places purchased by the Consent of the Legislature of the State in which the Same shall be, for the Erection of Forts, Magazines, Arsenals, dock-Yards, and other needful Buildings; And
To make all Laws which shall be necessary and proper for carrying into Execution the foregoing Powers, and all other Powers vested by this Constitution in the Government of the United States, or in any Department or Officer thereof.
The US Constitution: Section 9—Limits on Congres

The Migration or Importation of such Persons as any of the States now existing shall think proper to admit, shall not be prohibited by the Congress prior to the Year one thousand eight hundred and eight, but a tax or duty may be imposed on such Importation, not exceeding ten dollars for each Person.
The privilege of the Writ of Habeas Corpus shall not be suspended, unless when in Cases of Rebellion or Invasion the public Safety may require it.
No Bill of Attainder or ex post facto Law shall be passed.
(No capitation, or other direct, Tax shall be laid, unless in Proportion to the Census or Enumeration herein before directed to be taken.) (Section in parentheses clarified by the 16th Amendment.)
No Tax or Duty shall be laid on Articles exported from any State.
No Preference shall be given by any Regulation of Commerce or Revenue to the Ports of one State over those of another: nor shall Vessels bound to, or from, one State, be obliged to enter, clear, or pay Duties in another.
No Money shall be drawn from the Treasury, but in Consequence of Appropriations made by Law; and a regular Statement and Account of the Receipts and Expenditures of all public Money shall be published from time to time.
No Title of Nobility shall be granted by the United States: And no Person holding any Office of Profit or Trust under them, shall, without the Consent of the Congress, accept of any present, Emolument, Office, or Title, of any kind whatever, from any King, Prince or foreign State.

Nowhere is it explicit, or implicit, in the Constitution that government should be in the business of providing healthcare. In fact, it is expressly stated that the government is to promote the "General Welfare."

It can be loosely argued by some that the term, "domestic tranquility," would also support the provision of these kinds of services. Even, if, you agree with those interpretations, nowhere is it deemed that the federal government that should provide such services! Based on the framing of the constitution, it is clear that this responsibility would fall on the states to make such a determination. The federal government's role has historically been more defined by its limitations than by its grants of power and authority. Of the seventeen specific "Powers of Congress," recognized in Section 8, nine of them deal with the provision of security. The government was chartered to provide for security, and the infrastructure necessary to support the people's provision of the necessary goods and services to and for each other in a free and open market.

Government should NOT be the *provider* of healthcare to its people. While people possess a desire for healthcare—that it be a "right" not a "privilege," and assuming we agree this is a "right," it is not the government that can provide us this right. "The Unanimous Declaration of the Thirteen Colonies of the United States of America" signed July 4, 1776, declared, among other things,

> *Governments are instituted among Men, deriving their just powers from the consent of the governed, —That whenever any Form of Government becomes destructive of these ends, it is the Right of the People to alter or to abolish it, and to institute new Government.*

PROMOTE –verb

1. To help or encourage to exist or flourish; further: to promote world peace.
2. To advance in rank, dignity, position, etc. (opposed to demote).
3. Education. To put ahead to the next higher stage or grade of a course or series of classes.
4. To aid in organizing (business undertakings).
5. To encourage the sales, acceptance, etc., of (a product), esp. through advertising or other publicity.
6. Informal. To obtain (something) by cunning or trickery; wangle.

Origin: 1350–1400; ME promoten < L prōmōtus, ptp. of prōmovēre to move forward, advance. (Dictionary.Com, 2010)

It is clear then, that from inception; it was, *and should still be*, not the government that has unalienable rights. It is *WE* the people!

But, why can't government provide us this kind of thing? Well, first it is due to the fact that the government and its powers flow from us. Second, the source of funds (money) comes from us. They simply cannot create real money out of thin air (even though the Federal Reserve has historically been, and recently busied itself with making currency out of thin air, the cost of the new currency rests squarely in our pocket books). Third, there is the little problem of the innate inefficiency of government at providing us anything.

Looking historically at various programs the government runs, or has attempted to run, government simply does not return anywhere near the kind of percentage of benefit to the people that it costs the people in taxes. Receiving one-third in benefits for each dollar the government collects is just not efficient enough. It is cheaper for us just to give directly to the people in need of help. At least, in that way, they will get one-hundred cents on every dollar and we can cover the same number with only one-third the tax burden.

Finally, and most importantly, the government will never give us what *WE* want! It is structured specifically *not* to give us what we want. While this may seem counter-intuitive, each of us has very specific things we want in healthcare. Each of us wants something different from what the other person wants. Sometimes the differences are subtle, but more often than not, these differences are drastic. And, this is in the wants area alone! If you move to how I should get it, who is it that should pay for it, and put my responsibility in the mix; then you find the differences are startling and sometimes violent. Elected officials are in the business of trading our stuff to *THEM* to get us what *WE* want. Since the *US* and *THEM*, in this case are arbitrary and capricious groupings we have adopted for convenience or to find differentiation in, or to increase the volume of, our voice. The elected officials always trade off some of what the collective *WE* wants to get the votes they need to get re-elected. *WE* simply never get what we want; never have and never will!

So then, even if healthcare is a right, then it is something we need to provide among ourselves for ourselves. In many communities, security and safety are actually provided in this manner. Through volunteer rescue squads, fire departments and sheriffs' posse—there are those who help provide these vital services, because many communities could not afford these services without all or part being provided by these volunteers.

If people need to provide the goods and services among themselves, what role should government play? Clearly government is good at creating laws for the governed. In that regard, the role for government is to create the laws that are required to ensure that the services provided among the people through the efficiencies of the free market, are fair and equitable. If there are systematic procedures that need to change, and the entrenched bureaucracy and special interests cannot address them, then Congress could, and should, create laws to force a balance.

How much legislation should be created? Only as much as is needed to balance the free market forces against the fair and equitable requirements of the people. This is clearly, easy to say yet oh so hard to do.

Recommendation

- **Preserve the laws that prohibit denial of coverage based on disease state.**
- **Preserve subsidies for the purchase of coverage for the economically disadvantaged.**
- **Require all policies to be in large national pools to spread the risk.**
- **Ban the use of high risk pools that consolidate the risk and create higher premiums to those who are sick and who are at the most risk— spread the risk across the widest population.**
- **Continue the elimination of annual and lifetime caps on coverage.**
- **Eliminate state-by-state-based Medicaid and fold this service into the Medicare system—that would provide a single safety net for the entire eligible population (saving both the federal government and the individual states, cities and counties huge amounts of money), with eligibility based on three primary criteria, age (70 years old), economic status, (under $50,000/year for an individual) and/or disability (specific disease states).**
- **Enact legislation to stimulate the states to provide a free basic single point of administration for the registration of programs, match offerings to those in need, and the simple coordination of the care and benefits for the connection of those facilitating, providing, and paying for the services, in order to reduce waste fraud and abuse.**

What Role for WE the People?

WE need to become responsible for helping one another, *not* the government. As we have seen, time and time again, we cannot rely on the government to give things to us. *WE* must each assume responsibility for our own needs and survival. The Declaration of Independence and the Preamble of the Constitution of the United States clearly sets out the role of government—what it should be.

"We hold these truths to be self-evident, that all men are created equal, that they are endowed by their Creator with certain unalienable rights, that among these are life, liberty and the pursuit of happiness. That to secure these rights, governments are instituted among men, deriving their just powers from the consent of the governed."

The authority and responsibility for goods and services, from the creation, through the distribution, sales, and use are our responsibility. *WE* are charged with first helping ourselves, then the family, and then our neighbors and our country.

"We the People of the United States, in Order to form a more perfect Union, establish Justice, insure Domestic Tranquility, provide for the common defense, promote the General Welfare, and secure the Blessings of Liberty to ourselves and our Posterity, do ordain and establish this "We the People of the United States, in Order to form a more perfect Union, establish Justice, insure Domestic Tranquility, provide for the common defense, promote the General Welfare, and secure the Blessings of Liberty to ourselves and our Posterity, do ordain and establish this Constitution for the United States of America."

Our correct role in the acquisition of the healthcare we need is first to have active participation in the process. *WE* are the check and balance on the open market costs, but only if we take responsibility for the acquisition and utilization of the goods and services. In the words of Michael E. Porter, a Harvard Business School professor, "Healthcare is a service in which physicians and patients are co-producers. Consumers need to participate actively in managing their health through lifestyle choices, obtaining routine care, and testing; seeking excellent providers, complying with treatments, and active participation in disease management and prevention. Consumers need to be the front-line participants in their health and healthcare. Even in today's flawed system, studies show that informed and involved patients tend to choose less invasive (and thus less expensive) treatments, have better results, and enjoy better compliance with medical instructions. These observations underscore the potential for all participants to benefit from a value-based positive sum competition." (Porter & Teisberg, 2006)

Time and again it has been shown that if people receive items for free, they tend to undervalue them unless there is significant and apparent intrinsic value. If people receive "free" healthcare, then they take no responsibility for consumption of the services. If there is no difference in cost for me between the most expensive procedure or the cheapest, then I will choose the most expensive, likely because I will believe it is intrinsically better. For me to give a "damn" about cost, there must be a penalty for not caring. So, on a personal, and narrow societal, level it is clear, there are benefits to my direct involvement in what I'm getting when it comes to anything, especially healthcare.

The "sticky wicket," as the British are so fond of saying, is that we also need to help those who cannot help themselves. Historically, societies took care of their own through community-based or faith-based programs and organizations. Again, historically, society has not done much for those who chose not to help themselves. Whether consciously, or unconsciously, people of prior generations let those who chose not to help themselves, pass-on. And, by the way, I am not talking about hundreds of years ago. Modern societies have been very good at letting the people that chose not to help themselves "fade away," so to speak. If you have traveled in the past fifteen years to Japan, for instance, and rode the subway, you would have seen people that do not exist in that society. I am not advocating this position in any way! I believe, we absolutely, absolutely, are obligated—we must provide a safety net for our fellow citizens. I am simply making the point that historically, people realized that those in need could be helped by their neighbors, and those who decided not to help themselves were left to the wolves, literally, in some cases. While Congress can, and should, make laws to help establish a fair pricing system, rules for transportability, interstate commerce, minimum standards of care, and a mandate for the coordination of care and benefits, should be in place to spread the burden and responsibility across a wide net. Yes, it is up to us actually to help our neighbor. *WE* are the ones who must solve our neighbor's problems. *WE* need to solve them, not "find" solutions. Finding solutions infers that others do the solving. If each of us simply (once a week) solved an issue or problem that an underserved person was facing, soon we would have little to solve except the truly large problems. Appropriately, these large problems are the ones our community groups and faith groups can unite to confront.

WE need to revisit the values we have adopted as a society, the ones we instill in our children. *WE* need to go back to the philosophy that *WE* are best in the responsibility business, and the government is best in the accountability department.

WE need to provide a safety net! *WE* need to augment what the government can provide in the combined Medicaid/Medicare program and assist those who remain underserved, because there will always be people that fall out of the sides of the bell curves.

Looking at Obamacare, it can be argued that if you ignore the relative cost, we have done more to help the truly poor with their healthcare needs than we have helped the working poor and other underserved populations. The law has increased the amount that the people can earn and still be eligible for Medicaid, provided insurance premium subsidies for families with incomes up to $87,000 per year, and we have eliminated the caps that caused middle income people to go out-of-pocket for large healthcare bills, and we have done so early in a disease state. The unintended consequences are, there is still no transparity, premiums continue to rise by the thousands of dollars, taxes, and fees are increasing dramatically to cover program costs, and, as of this writing, families with incomes over $87,000 per year will be the new underserved.

WE need to stimulate philanthropy—not stifle it, as has been the recent trend. *WE* need to expand the role of community clinics and do a much better job at connecting them to all funding sources, and do so for any patient they see. While we do that, we also need to help them with systems that make them more efficient. We need to tie their resources together with all the other resources as part of a patient-centered virtual care team for each person they treat.

WE, the people, and the commercial businesses, have to rethink what our roles and duties really are. I have argued that the government cannot do this and that *WE* must do this. How do *WE* do it? *WE* all need to begin to incorporate the needs of others into our daily lives, into our businesses. *WE* need to think about how we can pursue our own happiness and help others along the way. If you see people struggling—help! If your business has something to sell to others, it would be a good idea to find a way to give some to those in need! *WE* can develop an infrastructure to coordinate these gifts (benefits) with the work of others to eliminate duplication, waste, and fraud in this philanthropy effort, as well.

WE should develop our own philosophies of how to help our neighbors, create personal and business commitments, register our programs in a place where those in need can find them and then work with one another to team up and solve the problems of our friends and neighbors, not simply find solutions and then rely on others to do them.

I recommend giving to charities, but you shouldn't stop there to assuage your guilt. In a direct way, help others. Inculcate the concern for your neighbor in your family, your friends, and your children. Revise the values of your ancestors. Recognize that we cannot survive as simply a consumer society (*look at roman history*). We need also to produce. Production is not simply putting out commodities, like textiles, food stuffs, oil, steel, and other items from our successful history, production means offering goods and services that each of us need. I have made the argument that government is inefficient and ought to be limited.

One thing should stand out brightly: For *every dollar* of value you provide to another American, you are saving *three dollars* in taxes to accomplish the same thing.

Ask Your Own Questions

Remember what President John F. Kennedy said, but let's modify the message just a bit.

> ***Ask not what your country can do for you! Ask what you can do for one another!***

In the end, the onus is on us finally to take the time and effort to design a comprehensive healthcare supply chain. We need to start with the brightest and the best—all in one place—with the single goal of describing how we can establish a free market system that will get people the health services they need in the most efficient and cost effective manner, while, at the same time, preserving the ability for them to exercise choice and personal responsibility for the level of services they desire.

We need this team to describe a safety net that will help those that need it without obfuscating personal responsibility or completely absolving individuals of their responsibility for bad choices.

We need this group to recast the role of each provider so services by doctors, nurses, therapists, and pharmacists are delivered at the most cost effective, available, and appropriate level.

WE should bring these people together from every part of the system; put them in a bunch of rooms and not let them out until those in the room have the system fully described and documented. And, it must be documented in a manner that is simple for all to understand. Once they have this task accomplished, a small team of legislative analysts should be brought in to write up the required legislation that empowers the new system; one that contains a draft that repeals all legislation that no longer is needed.

In the end, the choice is ours to make and ours to effect! Given what you now know, will you choose to get on board? If everyone got involved, we may very well find the right answers to this draining healthcare legislative crisis.

Imagine that!

<u>Chapter 9 Addendum:</u>

Provisions of the Patient Protection and Affordable Care Act of 2010

Provisions of Obamacare take effect over a four-year period that began in 2010. The main provisions are presented here in order of their date of effect:

Effective upon Passage:

- ✓ Guaranteed issue and community rating will be implemented nationally so that insurers must offer the same premium to all applicants of the same age, sex, and geographical location regardless of pre-existing conditions.
- ✓ Medicaid eligibility is expanded to include all individuals and families with incomes up to 133 percent of the poverty level.
- ✓ Health insurance exchanges will commence operation in each state, offering a marketplace where individuals and small businesses can compare policies and premiums, and buy insurance (with a government subsidy if eligible).
- ✓ Firms employing fifty or more people, but not offering health insurance, will pay a "shared responsibility payment" (a fine) if the government has had to subsidize an employee's healthcare.
- ✓ Non-exempt persons, not securing minimum essential health insurance coverage, are also to be fined under the shared responsibility rules. This requirement to maintain insurance or pay a fine is often referred to as the individual mandate, though being insured is not actually mandated by law. Not being insured will not be a crime, and no criminal penalty can attach to non-payment of the fine. The fine serves to

encourage most people into an insurance pool and to deter the "free rider" problem of healthy individuals choosing to go without insurance until they are injured or become ill.

- ✓ Improved benefits for Medicare prescription drug coverage are to be implemented.
- ✓ Changes are enacted which allow a restructuring of Medicare reimbursement from "fee-for-service" to "bundled payments".
- ✓ A national voluntary insurance program is established for purchasing community living assistance services and support.
- ✓ Low income persons and families above the Medicaid level and up to 400 percent of the poverty level will receive subsidies on a sliding scale if they choose to purchase insurance via an exchange. (Persons at 150 percent of the poverty level are to be subsidized such that their premium cost would be 2 percent of income or $50 a month for a family of 4).
- ✓ Very small businesses will be able to get subsidies if they purchase insurance through an exchange.
- ✓ Additional support is provided for medical research and the National Institutes of Health.
- ✓ Enrollment into CHIP and Medicaid is simplified with improvements to both programs.
- ✓ Minimum standards for health insurance policies will be established, and all annual and lifetime coverage caps will be removed.
- ✓ Certain healthcare insurance benefits will be considered "essential" coverage for which there will be no co-pays.

- ✓ Policies issued before the law came into effect are "grandfathered" and are mostly not affected by the new rules.

Provisions Already in Effect

- ✓ By 2010, The Food and Drug Administration will approve generic versions of biologic drugs and grant biologics manufacturers twelve years of exclusive use before generics could be developed.
- ✓ The Medicaid drug rebate for brand name drugs is increased to 23.1 percent (except the rebate for clotting factors and drugs approved exclusively for pediatric use increased to 17.1 percent), and the rebate is extended to Medicaid managed care plans; the Medicaid rebate for non-innovator, multiple source drugs is increased to 13 percent of average manufacturer price.
- ✓ A nonprofit Patient-Centered Outcomes Research Institute will be charged with examining the "relative health outcomes, clinical effectiveness, and appropriateness" of different medical treatments by evaluating existing studies and conducting its own. Its 19-member board, independent of government, is to include patients, doctors, hospitals, drug makers, device manufacturers, insurers, payers, government officials and health experts. It will not have the power to mandate or even endorse coverage rules or reimbursement for any particular treatment. Medicare may take the Institute's research into account when deciding what procedures it will cover, so long as the new research is not the sole justification and the agency allows for public input. The Institute is forbidden to develop or employ "a dollars per quality adjusted life year" (or similar measure that discounts the value of a life because of an individual's disability) as a threshold to establish what type of healthcare

is cost effective or recommended. This distinguishes the Institute from the UK's National Institute for Health and Clinical Excellence.

- ✓ Creation of task forces on Preventive Services and Community Preventive Services are to develop, update, and disseminate evidenced-based recommendations on the use of clinical and community prevention services.

- ✓ The Indian Healthcare Improvement Act will have been reauthorized and amended.

- ✓ Adults with pre-existing conditions are to become eligible to join a temporary high-risk pool, which will be superseded by the healthcare exchanges in 2014. To qualify for coverage, applicants must have a pre-existing health condition and have been uninsured for at least the past six months. There is no age requirement. The new program is to set premiums as if for a standard population and not for a population with a higher health risk. Premiums may vary by age, geographic area, and family composition. Out-of-pocket spending is limited to $5,950 for individuals and $11,900 for families, excluding premiums.

> Just like is seen with the mandatory reimbursement required of the pharmaceutical manufacturers this cost does not simply disappear it will flow into the rest of the economic structure and we will still pay for it in the end.

- ✓ The President has established, within the department of Health and Human Services, a council to be known as the National Prevention, Health Promotion and Public Health Council to help begin to develop a national prevention and health promotion strategy. The Surgeon General shall serve as the chairperson of the new council.

- ✓ A 10 percent tax on indoor tanning services took effect.

- ✓ Insurers are prohibited from imposing lifetime dollar limits on essential benefits, like hospital stays, in new policies issued.
- ✓ Dependents (children) are permitted to remain on their parents' insurance plan until their 26th birthday, and regulations implemented under the Act include dependents, that no longer live with their parents, are not a dependent on a parent's tax return, are no longer students, or are married.
- ✓ Insurers will be prohibited from excluding pre-existing medical conditions (except in grandfathered individual health insurance plans) for children under the age of 19.
- ✓ Insurers are prohibited from charging co-payments or deductibles for Level A or Level B preventive care and medical screenings on all new insurance plans.
- ✓ Individuals affected by the Medicare Part D coverage gap receive a $250 rebate, and 50 percent of the gap is eliminated in 2011. The gap will be eliminated by 2020.
- ✓ Insurers' abilities to enforce annual spending caps will be restricted, and completely prohibited by 2014.
- ✓ Insurers will be prohibited from dropping policyholders when they get sick.
- ✓ Insurers will be required to reveal details about administrative and executive expenditures.
- ✓ Insurers are required to implement an appeals process for coverage determination and claims on all new plans.
- ✓ Enhanced methods of fraud detection are implemented.
- ✓ Medicare is expanded to small, rural hospitals and facilities.

- ✓ Medicare patients with chronic illnesses must be monitored and evaluated on a quarterly basis for coverage of the medications for treatment of such illnesses.
- ✓ Non-profit Blue Cross insurers are required to maintain a loss ratio (money spent on procedures over money incoming) of 85 percent or higher to take advantage of IRS tax benefits.
- ✓ Companies providing early retiree benefits for individuals aged 55–64 are eligible to participate, in a temporary program, to reduce premium costs.
- ✓ A new website offered by the department of Health and Human Services provides consumer insurance information for individuals and small businesses in all states.
- ✓ A temporary credit program encourages private investment in new therapies for disease treatment and prevention.
- ✓ Insurers are required to spend 85 percent of large-group and 80 percent of small-group and individual plan premiums (with certain adjustments) on healthcare or to improve healthcare quality, or return the difference to the customer as a rebate.
- ✓ The Centers for Medicare and Medicaid Services are charged with developing the Center for Medicare and Medicaid Innovation and overseeing the testing of innovative payment and delivery models.
- ✓ Flexible spending accounts, health reimbursement accounts and health savings accounts cannot be used to pay for over the counter drugs, purchased without a prescription, except insulin.

Effective by early 2012

✓ Employers must disclose the value of the benefits they provide beginning in 2012 for each employee's health insurance coverage on the employees' annual Form W-2's. This requirement was originally to be effective January 1, 2011, but was postponed by IRS Notice 2010-69 on October 23, 2010.

At the time of this writing this section of the law has already been repealed

✓ New tax reporting changes will come into effect which aims to prevent tax evasion by corporations and individuals. The provision is expected to raise $17 billion over 10 years. Under existing law, businesses have to notify the IRS on 1099 form of certain payments to individuals for certain services or property over a reporting threshold of $600. After December 31, 2011, payments to corporations and individuals must also be reported. Exceptions include: personal payments, payments for merchandise, telephone, freight, storage, and payments of rent to real estate agents are exempt from reporting. The amendments made by this section of the Act (section 9006) shall apply to payments made by businesses after December 31, 2011.

Effective by January 1, 2013

✓ Self-employment and wages of individuals above $200,000 annually (or of families above $250,000 annually) will be subject to an additional tax of 0.5 percent.

Effective by January 1, 2014

- ✓ Insurers will be prohibited from discriminating against or charging higher rates for any individuals based on pre-existing medical conditions.

- ✓ An annual penalty of $95, or 1 percent of income, whichever is greater, will be assessed on individuals who do not secure insurance. This individual assessment will rise to $695, or 2.5 percent of income, by 2016. Families have a limit of $2,085. Exemptions are permitted in cases of financial hardship or religious beliefs

- ✓ Insurers will be prohibited from establishing annual spending caps.

- ✓ Medicaid eligibility expands to individuals with income up to 133 percent of the poverty line, including adults without dependent children.

- ✓ Two years of tax credits will be offered to qualified small businesses. In order to receive the full benefit of a 50 percent premium subsidy, the small business must have an average payroll per full time equivalent ("FTE") employee, excluding the owner of the business, of less than $25,000 and have fewer than 11 FTEs. The subsidy is reduced by 6.7 percent per additional employee and 4 percent per additional $1,000 of average compensation. For example, a firm with sixteen FTE and a $35,000 average salary would be entitled to a 10 percent premium subsidy.

- ✓ Impose a $2,000 per employee tax penalty on employers with more than fifty employees who do not offer health insurance to their full-time workers (as amended by the reconciliation bill).

- ✓ Set a maximum of $2,000 annual deductible for a plan

covering a single individual or $4,000 annual deductible for any other. These limits can be increased under rules set in section 1302.

✓ Under the CLASS Act provision, a new voluntary long-term care insurance program is established. Enrollees who have paid premiums into the program and become eligible (due to disability or chronic illnesses) would receive benefits that help pay for assistance in the home or in a facility.

The CLASS provision was determined unaffordable by the Secretary of Health and Human Services in 2011 and suspended.

✓ Employed individuals who pay more than 9.5 percent of their incomes on health insurance premiums will be permitted to purchase subsidized private insurance through the exchanges. If an employer provides an employer-sponsored plan, but the individual earns less than 400 percent of the Federal Poverty Level and could qualify for a government subsidy, the employee is entitled to obtain a "free choice voucher" from the employer of equivalent value to the employer's offering, which can be spent, in the exchange, to buy a subsidized policy of his own choosing.

✓ Government savings in healthcare are realized by coverage cuts in Medicare Advantage, slowed growth of Medicare provider payments (in part through the creation of a new Independent Payment Advisory Board), reduced Medicare and Medicaid drug reimbursement rates, and cuts to other Medicare and Medicaid spending.

✓ Revenue is raised from a new $2,500 limit on tax-free contributions to flexible spending accounts (FSAs), which allow for payment of health costs.

✓ Chain restaurants and food vendors with 20 or more locations are required to display the caloric content of their foods on menus, drive-through menus, and vending machines. Additional information, such as saturated fat, carbohydrate, and sodium content, must also be made available upon request.

- ✓ Health insurance exchanges are established, and subsidies begin for insurance premiums for individuals with income up to 400 percent of the poverty line, as well as single adults. Section 1401(36B) of PPACA explains that the subsidy will be provided as an advance able, refundable tax credit and gives a formula for its calculation. Refundable tax credit is a way to provide government benefit to people with no tax liability.

- ✓ Members of Congress and their staff will only be offered healthcare plans through the exchange or plans otherwise established by the bill (instead of the Federal Employees Health Benefits Program that they currently use).

- ✓ A new excise tax goes into effect that is applicable to pharmaceutical companies and is based on the market share of the company; it is expected to raise $2.5 billion in annual revenue.

- ✓ Most medical devices will become subject to a 2.3 percent excise tax collected at the time of purchase. (Reduced by the reconciliation act from 2.6 percent)

- ✓ Health insurance companies will become subject to a new excise tax based on market share. The rate gradually rises between 2014 and 2018, and thereafter increases at the rate of inflation. The tax is expected to yield up to $14.3 billion in annual revenue.

- ✓ The qualifying medical expenses deduction for Schedule A tax filings increases from 7.5 percent to 10 percent of earned income.

Effective by January 1, 2017

- ✓ States may apply to the secretary of Health and Human Services for waivers of certain sections in the law. A state must develop a detailed alternative that "will provide coverage that is at least as comprehensive" and "at least as affordable" for "at least a comparable number of its residents" as the waived provisions. Waiver grants are at the discretion of the secretary of HHS after a public comment period. HHS must make an annual report to Congress on the waiver process.

Effective by 2018

- ✓ All existing health insurance plans must cover approved preventive care and checkups without co-payment.

- ✓ A new 40 percent excise tax on high-cost insurance plans ("Cadillac plans") will be introduced. The tax (as amended by the reconciliation bill) will be on the cost of coverage in excess of $27,500 (family coverage) and $10,200 (individual coverage), and it will be increased to $30,950 (family) and $11,850 (individual) for retirees and employees in high risk professions. The dollar thresholds will be indexed with inflation; employers with higher costs on account of the age or gender demographics of their employees may value their coverage using the age and gender demographics of a national risk pool.

X. Recommendations:

Do not just engage in a blanket repeal of the Affordable Care Act. Some of the concessions won in this legislation were hard fought and should not be reopened. Instead, read the bill carefully, all of it. Target every section, word, or phrase that is not related to the provision of care, and then place these on the top of the repeal list.

Revise the language, related to basic coverage, to require that all policies provide specific basic coverage areas with options for other at higher risk or gender specific riders like maternity, smoking, occupational, and geographic areas. Mandate that all basic policies be available in all fifty states and all territories. Mandate transportability between a state or territory, and any employer. Require that all consumers be part of the same national pool, for the policy class they have purchased. Prohibit high-risk pooling. Prohibit employer or other designated groupings for coverage. Specifically, allow employers to negotiate discounted rates based on activities the employer provides that lower the insurers costs (less marketing cost, less sales cost, and lower administrative cost if centrally managed by company HR).

Modify the language, covering the creation of the exchanges, from a state-by-state approach to a national exchange. Exchange should be for the registration and listing of all health related insurance policies. All policies offered should be required to be registered and listed in the national exchange. Information should include: the policy offerings by the insurance provider; the scope of coverage of the policies; mandate standard form of policy benefits (for easy comparison between policies and companies); mandate that all companies offer at least one policy that is specific to the base policy offering; insurance providers can have any number of other policies, but all need to provide at least the basic coverage. Optional coverage riders need to be listed, for each policy, to which they can apply with specific pricing. All exclusions that could be applied to any optional coverage item needs to be listed in the standard policy benefits format required. This service should be provided by a private sector contractor, and awarded though a competitive, public bidding process, one that is consistent with current FARS and FIRMRS.

Repeal the "navigators" section of the legislation. There is no benefit to the consumers as all individual consumers will be part of the same actuarial pool based on the policy purchased.

Recommendation: Mandate the elimination of the current pricing system and replace with three market-based pricing structures and a two-step SALES OPTION so that all pricing will be openly published and easily available to consumers.

Recommendation: Mandate the elimination of rebates and force manufacturers to set a Suggested Retail Price. All other prices such as, what distributors pay, what major accounts pay, and what governments pay, should be derived from this index.

Recommendation: Eliminate the impediments to a national insurance market. Let consumers purchase policies on an open national market. Mandate that these policies be transportable from state to state and job to job. Recommend that employers change from specific policy bundle offerings in these arbitrary groups with smaller actuaries into simply offering specific benefit payment amounts to the employee. Mandate that the actuarial be across the full breath of an insurer's policy group. Eliminate high risk pools for all policy holders of a specific policy offering in the same pool.

Recommendation: Enact sweeping and significant tort reform. Following are the recommendations of the U.S. D.H.H.S:

- ✓ Improve the ability of all patients, who are injured by negligence, to get quicker, unlimited compensation for their "economic losses," including the loss of the ability to provide valuable unpaid services like care for children or a parent.

- ✓ Ensure that recoveries for non-economic damages could not exceed a reasonable amount ($250,000).

- ✓ Reserve punitive damages for cases that justify them -- where there is clear and convincing proof that the defendant acted with malicious intent or deliberately failed to avoid unnecessary injury to the patient -- and avoid unreasonable awards (anything in excess of the greater of two times economic damages or $250,000).

- ✓ Provide for payment of a judgment over time rather than in one lump sum and thus ensure that the money is there for the injured patient when needed.

- ✓ Ensure that old cases cannot be brought years after an event when medical standards may have changed or witnesses' memories have faded, by providing that a case may not be brought more than three years following the date or injury, or one year after the claimant discovers or, with reasonable diligence, should have discovered the injury.

- ✓ Informing the jury if a plaintiff also has another source of payment for the injury, such as health insurance.

- ✓ Provide that defendants pay any judgment in proportion to their fault, not on the basis of how deep their pockets are.

Recommendation: In addition to the national exchange marketplace, states should provide a simple framework for participants (consumers), facilitators (enrollment workers, volunteers and others helping consumers find services), providers (people who provide the goods and services) and sponsors (people who pay for goods and services) to communicate with one another and then form Virtual Care Teams. This system should be provided by the state, for use by all, for free. Utilizations would be incentivized by tying reimbursement rates and program dollars to use of the system. If they use this system, the state's costs are lowered; therefore, the paid rates become increased.

Recommendation: Mandate coordination of care and benefits across all available sources.

Recommendation: Preserve the laws that prohibit denial of coverage based on disease state. Preserve subsidies for the purchase of coverage for the economically disadvantaged. Require all policies to be in large national pools to spread the risk. Ban the use of high risk pools that consolidate the risk and create higher premiums to those who are sick and who are at the most risk; spread the risk across the widest population. Continue the elimination of annual and lifetime caps on coverage. Eliminate state-by-state-based Medicaid and fold this service into the Medicare system—that would provide a single safety net for the entire eligible population (saving both the Federal Government and the individual states, cities and counties huge amounts of money), with eligibility based on three primary criteria, age (70 years old), economic status (under $50,000/year for an individual) and/or disability (specific disease states). Enact legislation to stimulate the states to provide a free basic single point of administration for the registration of programs, match offerings to those in need, and the simple coordination of care and benefits for the connection of those facilitating, providing, and paying for services, in order to reduce waste fraud and abuse.

Other Steps

- ✓ Appoint a congressional commission to begin a national values assessment program that would review the values we have as a nation and then compare those values we held prior to 1960 to the values we have held since that time. Using this assessment, initiate a national dialogue on values. From this national dialogue, develop a statement of national values and a plan for education to reintroduce and reinforce these values to our people, particularly our children.

- ✓ Develop a campaign to stimulate individual and corporate philanthropy.

- ✓ Review tort law and identify provisions that are overly burdensome, and/or subject to abusive and wasteful litigation, to volunteers and philanthropic individuals and organizations. Revise the identified code to eliminate over burdensome liability to the individual volunteer assistance, corporate volunteerism, philanthropy, and community-based services in order to remove barriers so that there can be a spirit of neighbor helping neighbor.

- ✓ Review the tax code to identify sections that may reduce or restrict volunteerism or philanthropic activities by individuals, groups and corporations. Revise the existing tax code to stimulate individual, group and corporate philanthropy. In making these revisions, also provide incentives for hard-to-document contributions, like volunteer hours and in-kind donations. In addition, stimulate philanthropic activities incorporated into the core business model of companies and corporations in the newly revised tax code plan.

✓ Appoint a national commission, composed of providers and representatives of every phase and point of care in the healthcare industry, and re-describe the supply chain of healthcare for all. This commission should include; physicians, pharmacists, nurses, therapists, researchers, educators, device manufacturers, venture capitalists, consumers/patients, businesses, both large and small, and philanthropists—in effect, every potential point in the supply chain.

XI. Epilogue

Dare to Dream and You Will Achieve Great Things

We grow great by dreams. All big men are dreamers. They see things in the soft haze of a spring day or in the red fire of a long winter's evening. Some of us let these great dreams die, but others nourish and protect them; nurse them through bad days till they bring them to the sunshine and light which comes always to those who sincerely hope that their dreams will come true.

–WOODROW WILSON

If one advances confidently in the direction of his dreams, and endeavors to live the life which he has imagined, he will meet with a success unexpected in common hours.

–HENRY DAVID THOREAU

All men dream: but not equally, those who dream by night in the dusty recesses of their minds wake in the day to find that it was vanity: but the dreamers of the day are dangerous men, for they may act their dream with open eyes, to make it possible. This I did.

–T. E. LAWRENCE

You see things; and you say, "Why?" But, I dream things that never were; and I say, "Why not?"

–George Bernard Shaw

Imagine . . .

The long road seems endless as you and your wife make the torturous drive from Dulles Airport in Virginia to St. Mary's County. At 4:30 this morning, you'd left your apartment in San Francisco for the last time. The five-hour flight was uneventful, but traveling with your new wife next to you was a wonderfully fresh experience. The middle seat was free, so the two of you were able to spend the flight snuggling. Only a week since your wedding, you truly are on a great new adventure together. Not just the adventure of life with which all marriages begin, you both are moving all the way across the country to start your new life together in a new place.

It all seems to be happening so fast. Just three years ago, you had met Elizabeth Manning at Santa Clara University during your senior year. You simply could not believe, she agreed to go out with you, after you told her that stupid opening line when she introduced herself. You still remember saying, "Wow, your name is Elizabeth Manning? My great, great, great, great grandmother's name was Elizabeth Manning!" You also still recall, how utterly lame you felt when she said, "You think I look like someone's grandmother?" And, you also remember actually then looking at her tall slender very attractive frame and thinking first, "Hell no, she doesn't," and then "Man, what an idiot I am!!!"

But then, Beth laughed at your flustered awkwardness, and since that first moment, it had just gotten better and better. She was interested in who you were as person. She wanted to know everything about you, your family, your doctorate in paleontology, and how you could ever know about such a distant ancestor as the original Elizabeth Manning. At first, it seemed as if you were in an interview that never ended.

The first year with Beth was the best of your life, and the second was even better. You remember the first day that you took off your shirt and let her see the zippered scar down the middle of your chest. You worried that she might dump you, judge you to be defective, because of your history of open heart surgery as a kid. But, she was right there with you, never wavering and always supportive. And, now as you are making this long two-and-a-half-hour drive to your new job and new home, you still can't believe she is now Mrs. Aleck Ford Loker.

When you told her, you'd landed an interview for an assistant professor position at St. Mary's College, you wondered how she would react. But, her interest in history and the fact that your family history is tied to this place so tightly have left you both feeling as if it is fate drawing you here. Beth found a job with the St. Mary's City Historical Society and despite the long drive from the airport, you both really feel like you are coming home.

Your heart problem has haunted you most of your life. Even though you haven't had any symptoms for years, there is always the worry—what if? And, then there was the perennial concern over whether you'd be able to get affordable health insurance when changing jobs. That part is so much easier, now that the law has changed, and you can take your health insurance with you.

When you turned twenty-five, and got your first job, you logged onto the National Health Marketplace (NHM) and signed for your basic health insurance from Blue Cross of Pennsylvania, even though you lived in California at the time. The NHM listed base policies from insurers across the country were at the same price, with the same coverage. You were able to pick any policy you wanted, and chose according to the pricing and features of Pennsylvania Blue Cross's enhanced services options. Your first employer offered you a tax-free benefit bonus of $500 per month to help pay the premiums. You weren't obligated to buy insurance at all, but federal law made it a very attractive option. That $500 monthly bonus would be taxed at 80 percent unless you spent it on an NHM-approved health plan. It made no sense to do anything else with that money.

Beth's policy was with Anthem of California, but when you reached the annual open enrollment she was able to change to your plan, and since all the base policies were the same coverage, her new policy was exactly the same price. Now that you are married, you also receive the marriage discount, and you can afford the maternity option at the same price as you paid for the two individual base plans.

Everyone enrolled in the NHM base plans are members of one giant coast-to-coast insurance pool. The risk for all basic coverage is absolutely shared equally. Now that you are making better money in your new job, you will be able to purchase some additional optional enhancements and since it is all nationally available you can shop on the NHM for just the combination of services and price you want. With your medical history and the easily affordable options now available, it makes no sense for you not to have insurance. While a few years ago figuring out and purchasing insurance was just overwhelming, now it is very simple. Since all base plans from every insurance company are the same, everywhere in the U.S., and the plans all require just one, simple, standard, online enrollment form, everyone has insurance. You can simply select which company you want based on the attractiveness of their options, their reputation and their service offerings. No one you know goes without insurance nowadays.

This is so much better than the old system. With your heart worries, you have always wanted a bit more hand-holding from the doctor, and in this structure, you can purchase just the level of service you want. When you got your first policy, a couple of years ago, like most young people right out of college, you bought the basic policy. The provided services were all at the minimum level, but you had the necessary protection if something unexpected happened. After all, you have a few friends who have had serious accidents. The thought of crashing on your bike or, while skiing, and being left a quadriplegic—well, who in their right mind would take this risk anymore?

Even the basic plan protects you and your new wife from what could be financial ruin. The additional options just bring added choice. Best of all, St. Marys' is offering you $600 per month as a benefit bonus, in addition to your higher salary. Now, you are in a position to get just the combination, of additional services, you and Beth want and need. You know Beth is a very private person, and she will prefer the comfort of the "extended consultation time" option. You also want the extended testing and prevention options. Each company has so many optional choices, and you can add them as you go, with only a few exceptions. When you have both the mandated basic coverage *for everybody and the ability to choose those optional services you prefer based on what you are willing and able to afford from every insurance vendor in the country, you can't blame anyone but yourself in the long run if you don't like what you get.*

When you have little, the base policy sees that you are taken care of, perhaps with few frills, but you don't have to worry. If you want the frills, you can go out and earn and buy them. How did people deal with these issues years ago, when the employer provided you whatever they wanted to? You remember your dad telling you that if you lost coverage and had to purchase insurance, you would have been in a high-risk pool. The premiums, despite the government subsidy, were still higher than you could have afforded. However, in the end, the years of work by the National Healthcare Supply Chain Task Force (NHCSCTF) finally paid off. Now you, and everyone else, can get both what you need and, optionally, what you want.

As you enter St. Mary's County for the first time, you both have this eerie sense that you have been here before many times. You remember your dad's stories about "the county" and as you drive down the old "Three Notch Road" towards St. Mary's City, you recognize many of the landmarks he used to speak about. Beth is so excited that you are going to be staying at Bard's Fields Bed and Breakfast in St. Michael's. Ever the history student, she went online to look up everything available about the original Thomas Loker and his wife, Elizabeth Manning. The state historical society has recognized Bard's Fields as one of the oldest private residences in Maryland.

As you pull into the long, oyster-shell driveway and first see the farm at the back of the property and hear the tires crunch on the shells, you feel as if you have a bit of vertigo. It seems for a second that you are displaced in time. For an instant, you imagine that you see mules pulling plows in the field, driven by the "original teamsters," workers chopping the weeds out of the rows of tobacco, and a tall woman in a dark, long, broadcloth dress, with a blue bonnet, tending to a garden on the side of the house.

The B&B proprietors are happy to see you and eagerly take you on a tour of the home. They know your family history and add to the already exhaustive knowledge that your wife has accumulated from your dad and the internet. As you both retire for the evening, you feel as if you are at home.

After breakfast, the next morning you arrive for your first day of work at St. Mary's College. Your new office is in Kent Hall, the same building where your dad worked years ago. After settling in, you go to the bookstore. There you gaze upward at the ceiling rafters that your dad and Bobby Abell installed so many years ago. You realize that your ancestors were all here, on this very ground, and you know this is your destiny. This is where you and Beth were meant to come to raise your family. When your dad left to find his fortune, he was the last male Loker in the county. Over the past fifty years, while there are many cousins, there have been no Loker surnames left. Yours is the first to reappear. You don't know it yet, but you will be the start of a new generation of St. Mary's County Lokers . . .

"Aleck, it's time to go!" Beth is shaking you awake. "Aleck . . . Aleck, get your ass out of bed! We need to go, or this baby is going to be born right here in the bedroom!"

Quickly, you are up and moving. "OK, baby, let's get in the car and get going," you say.

"Don't tell me mister!" Beth replies. "I was ready before you got out of the damn bed!"

At nine pounds and six ounces, your first child enters the world at St. Mary's Hospital, roaring like a lion for all to hear. She is named Teresa Elizabeth Loker, after your mother and your wife.

Her birth is picture perfect. You and Beth were able to choose the doctor, the anesthesiologist and the pediatrician that you wanted because all doctors in the county accept any of the basic NHM plans and almost all would take the extra coverage from your optional enhancements. In the end, you and Beth were able to choose options providing your choice of midwife delivery teams and extended consultations with a pediatric nutritionist. Surprisingly Beth decided against the private room since she didn't want to put your hard-earned dollars into "such a frivolous want," as she put it in her succinct and direct manner. Most importantly, you got just the delivery team you wanted. Further, they were able to coordinate the care your family receives because you were able to link them together in your Virtual Care Team available through the NHM. Not only can they easily communicate with you and Beth, but they can also communicate with one another just as easily.

At the last minute as you grew more anxious about the delivery, both you and Beth decided you wanted a doctor to be present at the birth, even though the plan called for a nurse-midwife as most people have nowadays. Since Beth really wanted that extra personal attention, she was able to use the online tools to research each of the providers in the area. She also interviewed most of them online and in the end settled on Dr. Jarboe as the one she felt most comfortable with. And, since he has been a pediatrician for a long time, you both knew he could deliver—pun intended!

Your optional enhancements, however, did not cover Dr. Jarboe's fees, so you paid his invoice price through hospital billing. The cost was the same, either way; you had no worry that the fee was fair, because you could check online and compare his fees, education, and efficacy against any other doctor in the area. It was the same with all the people in the room. The pricing was easily available, and it was exactly the same whether, or not, it was paid to the hospital or the doctor. You could be sure the price you paid was within 10 percent of what the insurance company would pay to the doctor, or the hospital—now that there was fair and transparent pricing due to the new healthcare supply chain system.

The supply chain system allowed each provider to set its own price for services, and required publication of those prices on the NHM. As a result, now the published pricing had become a fair and accurate representation of what everyone in the supply chain was paid. Also, since they rationalized the scope of services offered by all the professionals in the supply chain, it became legal for lower-paid nurses and pharmacists to provide more of the simple and routine healthcare services that don't require a doctor's attention. It also opened up much more access for care, because some of these providers, like pharmacists, are always available and do not require appointments.

A few years ago, it was hard to get a simple check-up. It could take weeks to get an appointment. For some, getting an appointment was almost impossible because many doctors were unwilling to accept the available reimbursements from insurers. Your congenital heart condition meant that even when you could get an appointment, you had to drive two to three hours to Washington, DC, or Baltimore. In those days, specialists were all part of a hospital or large group. They simply could not get paid enough from reimbursement, so they would not practice in rural areas where people traditionally were earning less money. Also, they could not afford the liability insurance individually.

If specialty docs did not have a hospital or some other big entity backing them, they could not afford to practice. Now the doctors are free to see the patients who need the higher level of care they are trained for. Tort reforms have lowered insurance costs, so, now doctors can seek smaller practice options. And, most importantly, they all can earn both the basic plan coverage flat service rates and they get a market rate for the optional coverage services. Now, there is more, easy access care for the small, simple issues from the other licensed providers. Also, there is greater availability of doctors—for the more complicated and serious issues—since they are not tied up with the small stuff.

Last year when you cut your hand on the old steel fence in the backyard, you were able to get the wound cleaned, disinfected and stitched up by a nurse practitioner at the local pharmacy. You left the pharmacy with a "theranostic kit" in your bandaged hand. All this was provided quickly, inexpensively and without any appointment and all under your basic coverage plan, for $45. Of course, you could have gone to a doctor, but you would have had to pay for the extra charges—as high as $450—yourself. Or, you could have purchased an enhanced option in your insurance plan to help cover the extra cost of seeing a doctor for this kind of service. According to the theranostic kit instructions, you took the antibiotic pills for three days, then you took the automated test, which came up negative for infection, and then you finished the remaining pills as instructed. This is so much cheaper than going to the emergency room and then following up with a doctor, the way they used to do these things. Of course, if it the test had reported infection, you would have gone back to the pharmacist, who would have given you an alternate kit.

And, while Beth was pregnant with your new daughter, during the entire pregnancy, she only saw the doctor a couple times to review some tests. The rest of the time she went to the local community clinic and saw a nurse who performed all the routine exams, injections and blood tests. You were never worried because you knew the nurse at the clinic was in direct contact with the doctor and all the other members of your team through your Virtual Care Group. You could see all their reports and communications and you knew they were all well informed and fully coordinated on any issues that arose. They could not have been better coordinated if they had all worked in the same office.

The AMA had squealed when this new system began, but, in the end, most doctors got on board. They realized, soon enough, that their time would be worth so much more once they stopped basing their business on the low-cost routine tests. Once they began seeing sicker, and higher-risk patients, their reimbursements per patient grew much higher. Before the change, many doctors were quitting practice or struggling to make money because they could not predict their income and expenses from one month to the next. Today, they have predictable businesses, and they actually can set their price accordingly to what people are willing to pay for their services. They are no longer held hostage to the biggest discount that the cheapest doctor will take. Service is better and more people are getting care.

As you leave the hospital to take your new daughter home, you and Beth are filled with the anticipation of what this new life will bring for your daughter, Teresa, and where your lives together will go. Everything at the hospital went smoothly, and, unlike your ancestors, fear and worry about how you would pay for the birth are not there. You know, they are covered, because of the simplicity of the system, and the choices you have made. And, you know that the funds are there in the system for you and your family, because everyone else has the same access and the same requirement to make good, and fair, choices. You and Beth arrive at your home with your new daughter fully prepared to enter the parenting phase of your lives.

Years pass. It is a Saturday, and you're having lunch with Beth and the children. Teresa, now 9, has darted away from the table to return to her art project in the rec room. Little Aleck, 5, is still propped in his chair, pawing at his sandwich. Baby Rebecca is cuddled in Beth's arms.

The phones rings and, before you know it, you answer the way your father taught you 35 years ago: "Hello, Loker residence—Aleck speaking." Old habits die hard, you tell yourself, as you listen to the voice on the other end of the line. It is Jimmy Pratt, the current resident of Bard's Fields, the Loker family's ancestral home.

"I wanted you to know that my job's taking me outside the county, and I'm looking to sell the house," Jimmy says. "My dad always told me that once he was gone, if none of us wanted the house, we should give you a call before putting it on the market. He always felt that you and your family belonged here and that your kids should grow up here. He liked the idea of returning the property to the family that first found it."

You are speechless. Your mind reels with memories of Bard's Fields. For a moment, you can't feel your legs. You cup one hand over the telephone. "Hey Beth, I got something we need to talk about!!!"

XII. Works Cited

Adams, Samuel Hopkins. *The Great American Fraud.* New York: P. F. Colliers & Son, 1905.

Adams, Stephen B. *Mr. Kaiser Goes to Washington.* North Carolina: The University of North Carolina Press, 1997.

Association, New York Health Plan, interview by New York State Department of Insurance and New York State Department of Health. *Testimony of the New York Health Plan Association* (October 7, 2007).

Atlas, Scott. "10 Surprising Facts about American Health Care." *National Center for Policy Analysis.* March 24, 2009. http://www.ncpa.org/pub/ba649 (accessed January 16, 2011).

Bristow, M.D., Algernon Thomas. "The Economics of Medicine." *New York State Journal of Medicine, Vol IX,* 1909: 481-483.

Brown, E. Richard. *Rockefeller Medicine Men: Medicine and Capitalism in America* . Berkely, California: University of California Press, 1979.

CA Legislative Analyst's Office. *The 2010-11 Budget: California's Fiscal Outlook.* Sacramento, CA: California Legislative Analyst's Office, 2009.

Dossey, Larry. "Creating Disease: Bog Pharma and Disease Mongering." *Frank Lipman MD.* Dr. Frank Lipman MD. 09

2009. http://www.drfranklipman.com (accessed 10 18, 2010).

Feld M.D.,FACP,MACE, Stanley . *What Is Real Price Transparency?* May 24, 2007. http://stanleyfeldmdmace.typepad.com/repairing_the_healthcare_/2007/05/what_is_real_pr.html (accessed February 17, 2011).

Halvorson, George C. *Health Care Will Not Reform Itself.* New York: CRC Press, 2009.

Helms, Robert B. *Health.* March 01, 1999. http://www.aei.org/article/health/the-origins-of-medicare/ (accessed December 16, 2010).

—. "Health." *American Enterprise Institute.* March 1, 1999. http://www.aei.org/article/health/the-origins-of-medicare/ (accessed December 18, 2010).

James P. Cole Jr., DO, FACS, Vijay Nair, MD, FRCS, and Jeffrey Rosen, MD, FACS. *Medical Advances as a Result of War.* Paper, Downers Grove, Il: Advocate Good Samaritan Hospital, 2008.

Kelly, Robert. *Where can $700 billion in waste be cut annually from the U.S. healthcare system? - A Whitepaper.* New York: Thompson Reuters, 2009.

Lagnado, Luciette. "One Critical Appendectomy Later, Young Woman Has a $19,000 Debt." *The Wall Street Journal,* March 17, 2003: 1.

Landsberg, Brian K. ""Pure Food and Drug Act (1906)." Major Acts of Congress ." *eNotes.com.* 2004. http://www.enotes.com/pure-food-drug-act-1906-reference/pure-food-drug-act-1906 (accessed February 29, 2012).

Lister, Joseph. *On the Antiseptic Principle of the Practice of Surgery 1867.* New York: P.F. Collier and Son, 1909.

Lubitz, M.P.H., James, James Beebe, B.A., and Colin Baker, M.P.P. "Longevity and Medicare Expenditures." *the New England Journal of Medicine*, 1995: 999-1003.

Miller, Phillip, Louis Goodman, PhD, and Tim Norbeck. *Physician Foundation Survey - In Their Own Words.* New York: Morgan James Publishing, 2008.

Patricia Scott Deetz, James Deetz. "POPULATION OF PLYMOUTH TOWN, COLONY & COUNTY, 1620-1690." *The Plymouth Colony Archive Project.* University of Illinois. 12 14, 2007. http://www.histarch.uiuc.edu/plymouth/townpop.html (accessed 12 13, 2010).

Porter, Michael E., and Elizabeth Olmsted Teisberg. *Redefining Health Care.* Boston: Harvard Business School Publishing, 2006.

Rettig, Richard A., and Adam Yarmolinsky. *Federal Regulation of Methodone Treatment.* Report to Committee on Federal Regulation of Methodone Treatment, Washington, D.C.: Institute of Medicine (U.S.), 1995.

Shattuck, Lemuel. *Report of the Sanitary Commission of Massachussetts of 1850.* Boston, Massachussetts: State of Massachussetts, 1860.

Staff, stateline.org. *Stateline Top Story.* March 07, 2005. http://www.stateline.org/live/ViewPage.action?siteNodeld=136&languageld=1&contentld=16625 (accessed January 23, 2011).

Thompson, M.D., Gilman. "The Over-trained Nurse." *New York Medical Journal, Vol 83, No. 17*, 1906: 845-49.

US Freedom Foundation. *U.S. HEalthcare Services Retail Price Guide.* Markham, Va.: U. S. Freedom Foundation Health Care Pricing Research Project, 2003.

Various. "Inebriety." *The Quarterly Journal of The American Association for the Study and Cure of Inebriates*, 1892-1903.

Wikipedia. "Plymouth Colony." *www.wikipedia.com.* December 8, 2010. http://www.wikipedia.com (accessed 12 13, 2010).

XIII. List of Tables, Charts, and Figures

XIV. Index

A

B

C

D

E

F

G

H

I

J

K

L

M

Y

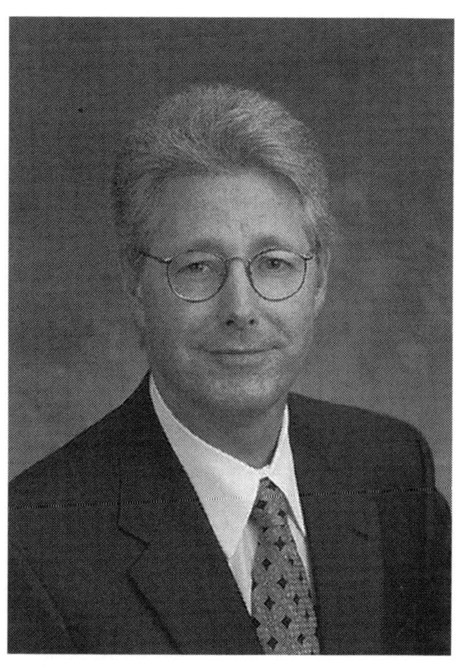

About the Author

Thomas Loker served as Chief Operating Officer for seven years with a company that manages public-funded healthcare benefits for low-income and underserved populations. He has had a long career serving in the fields of science, technology, and healthcare-related industries. He is an active board member in both for-profit and not-for-profit companies. Tom has written numerous articles in the areas of healthcare, technology, politics and the economy, published by California Political Review, Lead-Zine, and others. He has been a quoted expert in numerous stories by NBC-universal, Workforce Management Magazine, Managed Care Advisor, Managed Care Magazine, Menlo Park Patch Newspaper, Physicians Money Digest, BioPharma Insight, and others as well as on radio and television. He maintains his passion for St. Mary's County, its people, and culture by writing short essays published on his blog. When he is not writing or working in business, Tom is also an accomplished photographer.

Prior to this work, Tom published "Delusional Ravings of a Lunatic Mind"—a collection of essays from his popular blog available at

Amazon, Barnes and Nobles, and other bookstores—and with his son Aleck, "Calistoga Ranch – A Photo Collection"—a photo essay of pictures from the Napa Valley area of California focused on Calistoga Ranch, available at Blurb. Com. You can find Tom online at:

www.loker.com
tloker.wordpress.com

Made in the USA
Middletown, DE
28 December 2022